KU-608-906

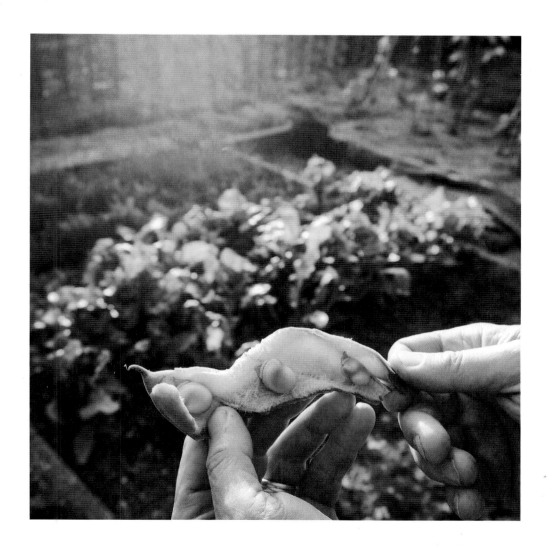

HUGH FEARNLEY-WHITTINGSTALL

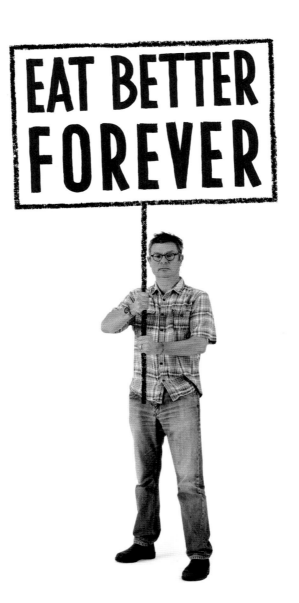

EAT BETTER FOREVER

7 WAYS TO TRANSFORM YOUR DIET

PHOTOGRAPHY BY SIMON WHEELER

BLOOMSBURY PUBLISHING

LONDON · OXFORD · NEW YORK · NEW DELHI · SYDNEY

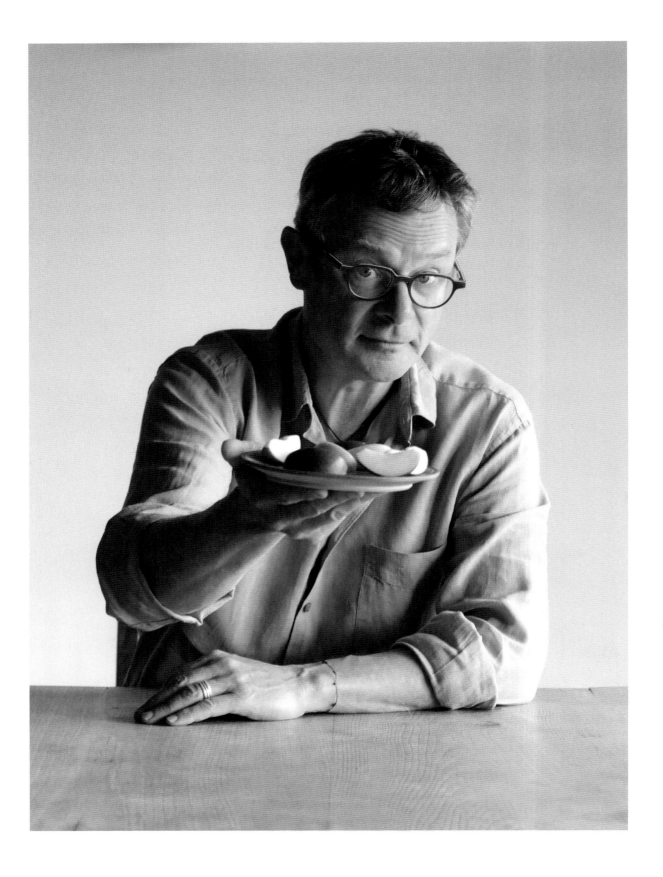

The food we eat is the most important factor influencing our health and well-being. Yet despite (or perhaps because of) a decades-long debate about diet, many of us still feel confused, unhappy, guilty and anxious about what we eat. I want to help change that. And this book is my most focused attempt so far.

More than ever, in the light of the Covid-19 pandemic, it's vital that everybody knows how much making good food choices can do to help us stay well. It's not just the healthy functioning of our digestive systems that's at stake. It's the complex web of activities in every cell of our body – what is collectively referred to as our immune system. So, when we eat well, we don't just function well day to day, we also fight back when viruses and bacteria come to call. We are far better at fending off challenges to our body and, when we do get ill, at recovering quickly.

I believe that a helpful book about healthy eating must not be a negative thing, with long lists of banned foods and dietary restrictions. It needs to lead with a positive understanding of what the good foods are, and it needs to make it easier for us to choose, eat and enjoy much more of them. That's my plan here.

I'm also going to talk about when and how we eat. That's going to help us understand why we eat certain foods that we know we would be better off not eating; and it will help us replace them with the good stuff. We're going to combine clearer understanding with achievable actions – and delicious recipes – so we can eat better, not just for a while, but forever.

Before we get to where we're going, let's look at where we are. Although we are living longer (on average 82 years in the UK), many of us spend our last 20 years or so in poor health, often with conditions which could be prevented through different lifestyles – primarily by eating better. 67% of men and 62% of women are above a healthy weight; a third of us are obese. Around 50% of adults are 'trying to lose weight', usually unsuccessfully. And the age at which our health starts to be negatively affected by our weight gets younger by the year. So it seems that our daily bread – and our extended life span – brings us neither health nor happiness. We *have* to change that.

I believe that the sheer volume of information about diet that now speeds its way backwards and forwards across the globe is actually part of the problem. The constant in-flow of data, advice and opinion that we are exposed to is often contradictory, unrealistic and unhelpful. A great deal of it, in fact, is flam, fashion and faddism. But that doesn't mean we should give up, or dismiss it all. On the contrary, I think it's vital to realise that in amongst the cacophony there is some very sound advice.

The last few years in particular have seen some genuinely useful advances in evidence-based science around healthy eating. This is actually a very good time to mine the seemingly bottomless pit of modern dietary advice for some golden nuggets of true wisdom. Or, in other words, to size up the latest good science and summarise it clearly. That's been my mission for the last two years, and this book is the result.

I want to stress that this is a collaborative effort. I have strong views about healthy eating, based on some pretty in-depth reading and research, but also on my experiences as a chef, writer, cook and broadcaster in the food industry for over 30 years. But I also know the value of discussing those views with people for whom understanding diet and human health is a full-time job. I've talked to many experts in this field, including Dr Giles Yeo, Professor Tim Spector and Professor Mark Mattson, and you'll find them quoted in the text. I've also asked one of the food scientists I most admire, dietitian Dr Michelle Harvie, of the Prevent Breast Cancer Research Unit in Manchester, to read (several drafts!) of this text, and comment and challenge me along the way. Her support has hugely increased my confidence that this book really can help you change.

One problem I see looming large (and my collaborators happen to agree with me) is that the world of diet publishing and the 'wellness' sector continue to orbit around 'single-fix' ideas. Most books offer up one big commitment you can make, one diet plan

you can sign up to, one headline-grabbing concept you can market the crap out of...
Some of those books may help some people, some of the time. But I think we can, and
must, do better than that. And we will start doing better as soon as we stop pretending
that the combined complexities of what we eat, and what our bodies do with it, can be
reduced to a single mantra or one neat idea, be it Paleo, Fasting, High-fibre, Zero-sugar
or whatever. They surely can't because the variables are endlessly... well, variable. We
need to take that into account. I've written this book quite deliberately in order to buck
this 'one big idea' trend.

I've been paying attention to new – and not so new – ideas about healthy eating ever
since, as an undergraduate, I took steps to reduce my student beer (and biscuit) belly.
I've always had a taste for the 'good things' of life – including beer and wine, burgers
and kebabs, fish and chips, and chocolate, cakes and puds. But I have also tried to steer
my appetite towards things I know are good for me. I used to struggle, for instance,
to enjoy certain vegetables, including tomatoes, beetroot, spinach, mushrooms and
sweetcorn. But as a young adult teaching myself to cook, and then a chef learning on
the job, I deliberately set out to find 'better specimens' of these vegetables, and ways
to cook them that I could first tolerate, then enjoy.

Learning to grow food myself massively enhanced this process, and now I have a love
for pretty much every fruit and vegetable under the sun. This journey has taken time,
but it's convinced me that with the right help and guidance we can all make important
changes to the way we eat. We can learn to eat better. And that is so much more
enduring, and important for our health and happiness, than 'going on a diet'.

I've always enjoyed 'good food', but the meaning of that phase has evolved for me.
It still means pleasure-bringing and therefore good for the soul, yes, but also good for
my health, my family's health and the health of my environment. I have never stopped
trying to learn more about what good eating really means, and as a consequence my
eating and drinking habits have evolved over the decades. It's been a meandering
kind of road, but I am now at a place where I'm confident that I'm making reasonable
decisions about what to eat... most of the time! I still make some less good decisions –
a second helping of ice cream, a packet of crisps on the train – but these days I am
much more aware of them. I don't beat myself up about my poorer choices, because
I know I'm making them less often than I used to.

I have developed an approach to eating and living that is working well for me. I'm lighter,
healthier, fitter and less anxious than I have been for years. I sleep better and I cope
with stress better too. So, I want to share that approach with you. But I am emphatically
not about to tell you that if you simply do what I've done, you'll become a new person
and all your problems will be solved. It's crazy to suggest one size fits all when it comes

to health, or even that one 'size' is enough. Tackling several different things, in whichever ways are achievable for you, has got to be the way forward. And it also helps avoid the shameful spectre of 'failure' that haunts every One Big Idea approach. If you entrust all your healthy eating eggs to one ideological basket, so to speak, you've only got to drop it once to feel like you've totally messed up. If you're spinning a few different plates, on the other hand, it's not such a big deal if you take your eye off one of them sometimes.

So, you won't find one single doctrine that sums up my approach. Rather I have a cluster of useful and entirely complementary pathways – seven of them, as it happens.

This manageable bundle of helpful facts about food and health, and the range of sensible, reasonable actions that follow from them, will have different importance for different people. That's the beauty of them: they can be organised into a set of personal priorities that you can keep coming back to and progressing, bit by bit. To me, that reflects real life. It's achievable. And it doesn't leave a scary amount hanging on a single endpoint: 'success', 'smashing your target' or somehow transforming into a 'new you'.

Each of my 7 chapters is built around a simple imperative, be it 'Reduce Refined Carbs' or 'Go with Your Gut': all things you can easily take on board that will make a genuine difference to your health. I've looked at the latest evidence and thinking on each idea and offered up my personal interpretation of them, and even a few of my personal struggles. We all have issues, at times, with food and drink. I've tried to make talking about them acceptable, interesting, even amusing (without ever forgetting this is a serious business). The idea is to help you know more, think more and understand more about food and the good and bad it can do us. And, in order to help you make some useful choices and health-supporting plans, there's a simple summary of 'action points' at the end of each chapter.

To complement all this talking, I have, of course, included a raft of healthy recipes – simple ideas (often *very* simple) for brilliant breakfasts, healthy lunchboxes, satisfying suppers and lovely treats. If you've read any of my more recent books, you'll recognise some common themes: lots of veg and fruit, plenty of whole grains, nuts and seeds, as few processed foods as possible, a smattering of fish, and not much meat. I have avoided obscure or expensive ingredients, and if you find something you consider a bit 'unusual' (spelt, flaxseed, farro) it's because I think it should be less so...

I've kept these recipes as straightforward as I can, but I have dared to assume that you are prepared to do at least a little bit of cooking. I have to be frank and say that if you aren't, then eating healthily is not impossible but certainly harder – and probably more expensive too. If you're kitchen-shy, please don't be put off by this. You have nothing to lose by giving a recipe a go. You may very well surprise yourself...

This is not a weight-loss manual – though it can certainly help you lose weight (without counting calories) in a way that is healthy and, crucially, sustainable. If that's your goal, then my 7 Ways to Lose Weight on pages 188–197 will explain how you can use the book for that. I am writing for anyone who wants to eat healthily, regardless of their current weight. Our Body Mass Index (BMI) is a significant health-marker – but we must look beyond the scales when we think about our health.

Most of the book is about eating and drinking. But it would be foolish to take these out of the context of all the non-food-related decisions we make daily that can affect our health for good or ill – decisions about the way we manage activity, sleep and stress, for example. So, on pages 198–208, you'll find a summary of the other things you can do that will enhance and magnify the benefits of eating better.

Another thing we have to do, unfortunately, is take the modern food environment as we find it – i.e. in a far from ideal state. We must learn to navigate and largely avoid the endless exhortations to eat and drink industrially processed foods that are not good for us. I want to change the environment in which these foods are so ubiquitous, so normalised – and I'm using other platforms, including television, to try to do so.

Government and industry must be held to account when it comes to processed ingredients, junk food advertising, too much sugar and salt in foods. There are, at last, some signs of positive action but we can't afford to wait for them before we make changes ourselves.

For now, it's up to us to make the right choices; and that, in a nutshell, is what this book will help you to do. There are far too many factors affecting our health in a negative way; but there is also a raft of things we can do to redress the balance: steps you can start taking now that, consolidated into new habits, become an effective force.

Even when the food industry is pitted against us, we are not powerless. To make healthy choices, we need science – but we don't need rocket science. Existing and emerging knowledge, common sense and, I think, a little righteous anger, are already pointing us in the right direction.

I've got a pretty good handle now on the things we need to do to be healthy. There's nothing impenetrable about them; they just had to be gleaned and sorted from among the misinformation, the marketing and the mumbo-jumbo. These seven simple insights are the backbone of this book. Take a few of them on board and you'll be heading in the right direction. Pay attention to all seven of them – accumulatively, over time, as it suits you – and you will soon be eating better and feeling better. And not just for a while, or for as long as it takes to shed a few pounds, but for the rest of your life.

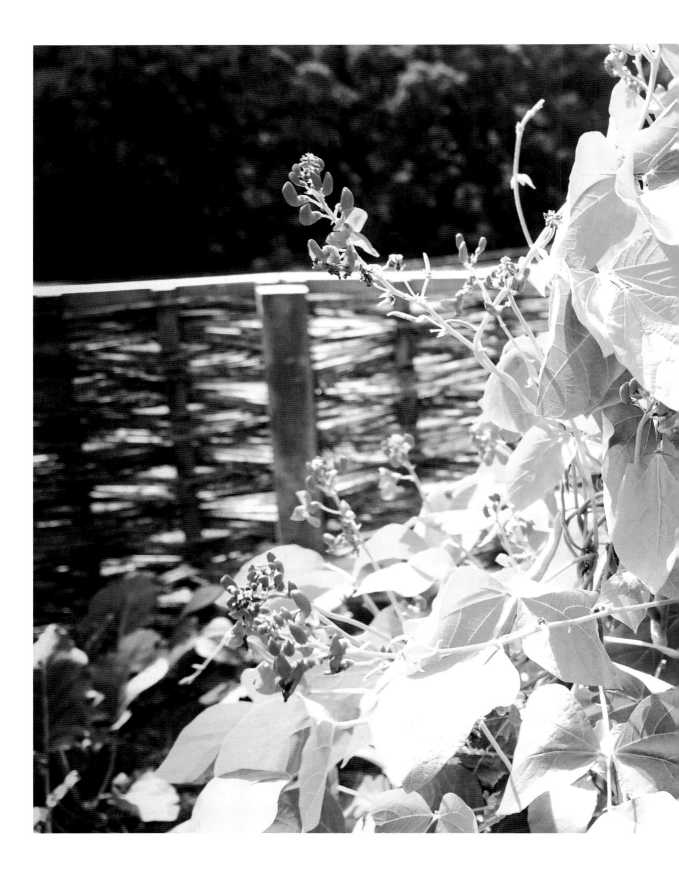

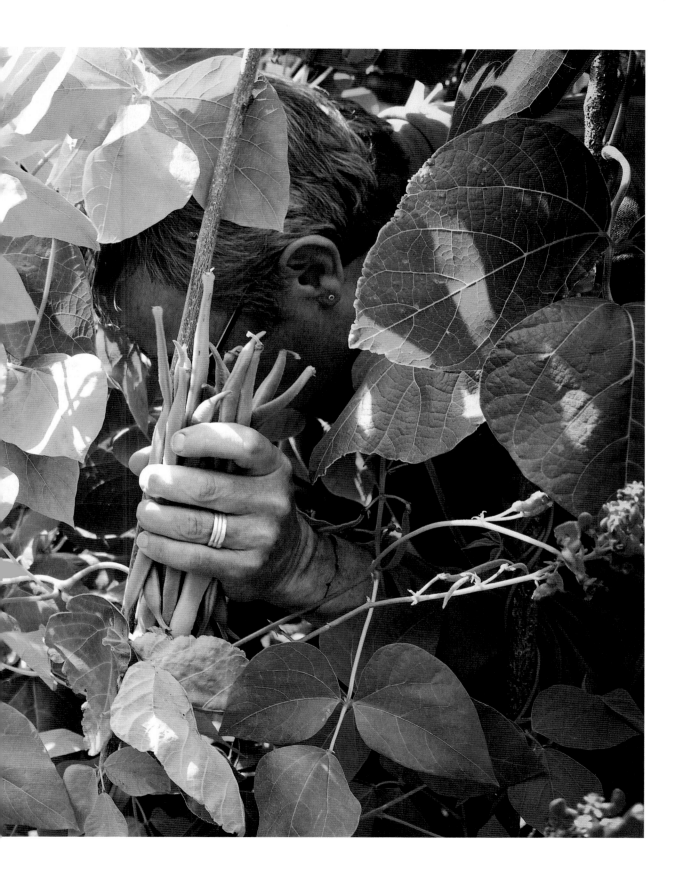

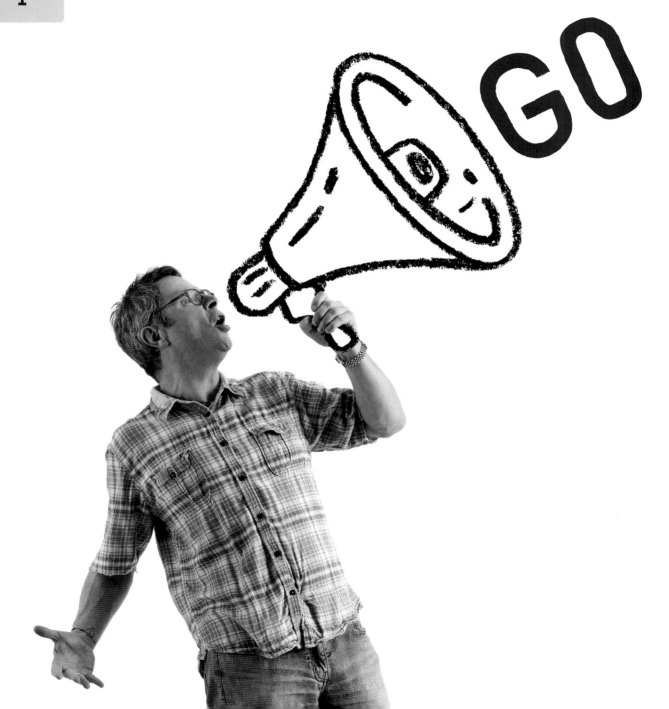

1

WHOLE

I believe I have seven slices of life-changing advice for you in this book. But if you take away one overarching message, please make it this: eat more whole foods. In the often-confusing world of nutrition, this is the one principle that every doctor, scientist and dietitian agrees on. Countless studies back it up. Whole foods protect our hearts and brains and bones. They nurture our gut, help us maintain a healthy weight, and it looks like they can safeguard our mental health too. That's why this chapter is the first in the book. When it comes to a great diet – a nutrient-packed, energy-boosting, body-nurturing, disease-preventing, obesity-busting diet – everything comes back to whole-ness.

SO, WHAT EXACTLY ARE 'WHOLE' FOODS?

The answer is very straightforward, and also much broader than you might think. Whole foods are simply those that have been processed as little as possible, and so remain close to their natural state. They are, if you like, the *original* versions of foods – the original and the best! – of which highly processed convenience foods, created out of refined ingredients, are an unhealthy modern distortion.

For some, I am well aware, the idea of whole foods is loaded with a sense of foreboding, an aura of austerity and self-sacrifice. There is a fear that the 'whole food' bracket comprises only lentils and brown rice and their close relations. And while those certainly are excellent whole foods, loaded with goodness and potentially very delicious too, they represent only a tiny fraction of the whole food palette available to us.

In reality, the term 'whole foods' means every edible fruit, vegetable, nut, seed and herb on the planet, as well as eggs, fish, meat and milk. (We'll get to butter, cheese and yoghurt later.) You can buy plenty of whole foods in any supermarket. Roast chicken and three veg is a whole food dinner; strawberries and cream is a whole food pud; a vegetable curry, made in the right way (with healthy fats and not too much salt), can even be a whole food takeaway. I hope the idea of embracing whole foods is starting to sound a little less daunting...?

WHY ARE WHOLE FOODS SO IMPORTANT?

The obvious and instinctive answer is that these foods are pretty much as nature intended them; they are what our bodies have evolved to digest and use. Packed with the good stuff, such as vitamins, minerals, antioxidants and fibre, whole foods give maximum healthy bang for your buck. That's why studies into many different aspects of diet continually reinforce the whole food point.

One review in 2014, for instance, by researchers at Yale University, looked at all of the most popular mainstream diets, including low-carb, vegan and Paleo, in order to see which was most effective at improving overall health. After comparing the health outcomes associated with many different eating regimes, the scientists agreed there was no overall winner. But, by noting certain common elements among these diets, they drew one clear conclusion: 'A diet of *minimally processed foods close to nature*, predominantly plants, is decisively associated with health promotion and disease prevention...' they said. These are my italics. You should make them yours too!

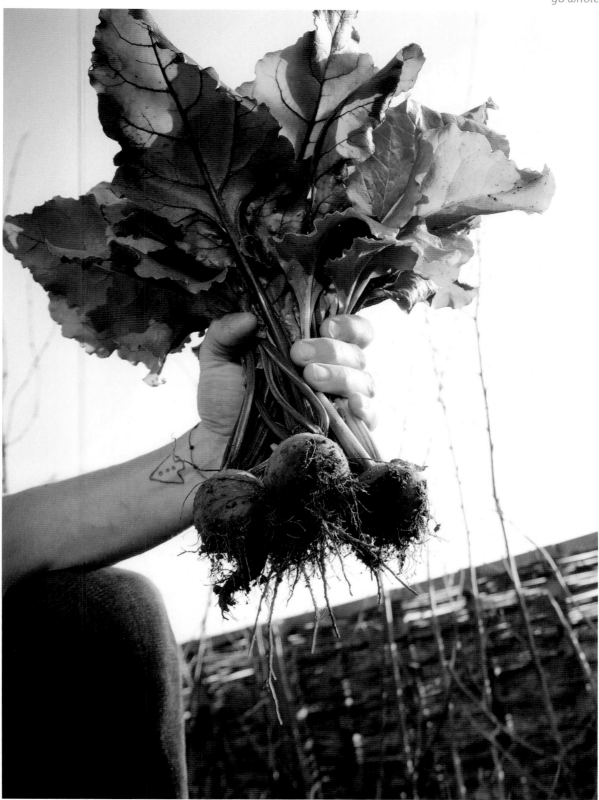

More recently, exciting research from the 2017 SMILES study in Australia showed improvements in depression when people adopted a healthy whole food diet.

The thing I love about the unambiguous principle of 'Going Whole' is that it is so positive. And it offers real hope. For example, a major piece of international research called the Global Burden of Disease Study concluded in 2019 that bad diets now kill more people worldwide than tobacco. The study estimated that *one in five* deaths globally is associated with poor diet. Just pause to digest that for a moment. It's a pretty grim statistic... until we decide to flip it. Because the authors went on to say that the biggest issue, even beyond the terrible stuff we eat, is the great stuff we *don't eat*.

The worst damage to our health is done by the *absence* of healthy foods. Embracing this insight can change everything. It means our first step should be to increase our intake of fantastic whole ingredients, before we worry about anything else.

GOING WHOLE IS ABOUT MORE, NOT LESS

Going Whole is about deliciousness, not denial. It means piling into a smörgåsbord of fresh vegetables, fruits, nuts and seeds, unrefined whole grains and healthy oils. It can absolutely include meat and dairy too, if you like; it just means eating them in moderation and switching to whole (or whol*er*) versions, like unprocessed meats and unsweetened natural yoghurt. (Wholeness is not absolute, but relative, as we'll see.)

Of course, Going Whole also means eating less of some things: less of the foods that aren't whole, the junk foods and refined ingredients that are making so many of us ill and overweight. I'll go into more detail on that later. The key point here is that focusing on the positive – on eating more of what's good – means you won't have so much room, in your shopping basket, kitchen, fridge or stomach, for foods that are nutrient-sparse and that may be actively harmful. In short, if you start building your meals out of whole ingredients, you will automatically start eating better. You won't be able to help it.

Going Whole doesn't have to be instant, and it doesn't have to be total. My diet is healthier than it's ever been but I still snaffle the odd bag of crisps, and the occasional chocolate bar. The difference is that now, when I do, I'm more conscious that they are not contributing to my physical health. I acknowledge the short hit of pleasure they give, which is appreciated as just that, while reminding myself they do nothing good for my body. And so, I'm determined that they should be the exception and not the rule. In the end this is about balance, and about *shifting* the balance. For far too many, junk is now routine, and whole foods just an occasional encounter. It's time to flip that around.

WHOLE AND WHOLER

Many ingredients come into our kitchens entirely whole and unprocessed – vegetables and fruits are the most obvious. But I'm not proposing a diet consisting entirely of *totally* unprocessed fare. There are plenty of ingredients that have undergone a bit of processing that we can definitely include in the healthy whole foods bracket.

The 'processing' of such foods usually has history on its side, and is relatively simple. You could say it's mechanical, rather than industrial or chemical: the grinding of whole wheat into wholemeal flour; the crushing of seeds into 'cold-pressed' oils; the mixing of fresh milk with live yoghurt to produce... more live yoghurt.

By contrast, it's the highly refined, 'ultra-processed' modern foods that we need to be wary of. Most of these owe their existence to sophisticated industrial techniques, and are often modified and preserved by a plethora of industrially produced additives.

When you're deciding whether or not to put something in your shopping basket, consider the following:

Ask yourself: what has been done to the raw ingredient in order to produce this? If it's a whole food like a potato, an egg or a fresh chicken, the answer is going to be 'not much at all'. If, on the other hand, you're looking at a packaged muffin or a box of batter-coated chicken nuggets, the answer is 'quite a lot' – i.e. it's not very 'whole'. Generally, the less foods have been altered, rearranged or combined with other foods – the better.

The number of ingredients listed on the back of the pack is a useful pointer. The more ingredients there are, then very likely the more processed that food is. Completely whole foods like fresh fruit and veg have no ingredients lists at all!

Ingredients that sound industrial, chemical or baffling – such as hydrogenated palm oil, 'lactic acid esters of mono- and diglycerides of fatty acids' or 'copper complexes of chlorophyll' – are clear indicators that the food is highly processed.

Wholegrain breads and pastas can be a really good source of fibre and healthy carbs. Of course, even these 'brown' versions are processed to some extent, but some are far more processed than others. Look for those that contain fewer ingredients, and, in particular, fewer additives – things like palm oil, preservatives, emulsifiers, colours and flavourings.

WHOLE V PROCESSED

The following table shows the difference between some everyday whole foods and the processed products that are distorted versions of them. To boost your whole food tally, base your shopping, cooking and eating on the sort of foods listed in the green column rather than the blue one. For some, that might mean quite a major shake-up. But I'll also bet there are foods from the green column in almost every kitchen in the land. If you can lay your hands on an egg, an apple or a carton of milk, you're in whole food territory already.

Whole food	Processed version	What's the difference?
Chicken	Chicken nuggets	Only about 50% chicken; refined flours, salt and flavourings added
Fish	Fish fingers	Only around 60% fish; refined flours and salt added
Potatoes	Hash browns	About 90% potato; salt, flavourings and stabiliser added
Onions	Battered onion rings	Only about 45% onion; refined flours and salt added
Tomatoes	Tomato ketchup	About 70% tomato; sugar and salt added
Apples	Apple sauce	About 70% apple; sugar, fructose syrup, modified starch and preservative added
Oranges	Orange squash	Only about 20% orange; sweeteners, flavourings and preservatives added

If you start with whole foods, you will often have to do some 'processing' yourself, of course. That's what cooking is. But home cooking is not usually the kind of processing that takes away good stuff and adds bad stuff – as with the refined and processed foods I have highlighted. It's the simple preparation, combination and assembly of good, whole ingredients.

So, whole grains need cooking, fish needs baking, tomatoes need slicing. But eating whole foods does not have to be a labour-intensive business. It's true that I cannot offer you a healthy lunchbox recipe that's as easy as unwrapping a Big Mac. But I can offer you one that's ready in 10 minutes, tastes amazing and will do you a whole world of good.

CAN'T WE JUST POP PILLS?

Maybe you're thinking the idea that we all need to go 'back to basics' and eat whole foods is a bit retrograde. Can't we just buy supplements to add back the good bits that are missing from junk food? Can't we get our vitamins and minerals, maybe even the increasingly elusive fibre, from pills and 'fortified' foods?

The short answer is no. It's true that some supplements may be useful for specific problems and deficiencies. If your doctor tells you that you need to take a specific supplement, then you should take it. But the idea that a battery of pills can replace good food is completely bogus. There's little evidence to support the effectiveness of many vitamin supplements, and some have even been shown to be harmful. Taking high-dose supplements of vitamins A and E can increase the risk of cancer, for instance.

When you eat a whole food you are invariably getting more than one good thing. There is vitamin C in oranges, but also fibre, folate and antioxidants. Walnuts give us omega-3 but also vitamin E, fibre and phytonutrients (see page 32) with anti-inflammatory properties.

In addition, we know that the interrelation between different nutrients in a food is very significant – one nutrient will often assist the absorption or metabolisation of another. Nuts, for example, which contain lots of unsaturated fats, also contain lots of antioxidants, which keep those fats stable and stop them oxidising. The iron found in some fruits and vegetables comes packaged up with natural vitamin C, which aids its absorption. This complex interrelationship is called 'food synergy' and it's something we can't hope to replicate in a pill, or even a shelf full of pills. It's one more powerful argument for a diet based on whole foods.

SOME SIMPLE WHOLE FOOD SWAPS

Instead of
a sugary breakfast cereal...

Have a portion of jumbo oats or medium-coarse oatmeal – cooked as porridge or soaked overnight with orange juice (see page 227).

Instead of a white bread sandwich with cheese and pickle...

Try a wholegrain flatbread with hummus and sliced pepper or grated carrot.

Instead of
a bag of crisps...

Try unsalted raw nuts. Or take a completely different route with a couple of 'hard-boiled' eggs.

Instead of
a chocolate biscuit...

Eat some whole almonds or raw cashew nuts with a couple of squares of dark chocolate (minimum 70% cocoa solids).

Instead of
a shop-bought smoothie...

Just have a portion of whole fresh fruit.

Instead of grabbing a sugar-sweetened cereal bar...

Carry a little pot of nuts, seeds and raisins or dried apricots.

Instead of
heating up pasta sauce from a jar...

Toss cherry (or other) tomatoes in a tray with a little oil, garlic and herbs and roast in a hot oven for 20 minutes or so, until they burst and release their juices. Stir into wholemeal pasta.

Instead of
a curry ready-meal...

Roast a trayful of chunky chopped veg (e.g. sweet potato, cauliflower and onions) with bashed garlic cloves, curry powder and a dash of oil in a hot oven. Finish with flaked almonds and serve with brown rice and natural yoghurt.

THE 'WHOLE' FAMILY

It is important to remember that a good diet – a diet of whole, healthy, unprocessed foods – is no less vital for a young person than an older one. There's a perception that we only really need to start worrying about our health when we hit 50, our waistlines expand and our cholesterol heads north, and that youngsters can 'get away with' eating any old crap they fancy. It's just not true.

There are a few differences in precise requirements: children need a bit less fibre, for instance; and some foods, such as whole or chopped nuts, are inappropriate for the very young. But the basic message is simple – our children need healthy food just as much as we do. They need it now, and to help them build healthy habits for life.

Good health is built day by day, from the moment we are born. Children who don't get plenty of fresh veg, fruit and other whole foods are missing out on essential nutrients during their most crucial stage of development. Diets high in sugar, fat and salt can impact a child's immune system and lead to obesity and the ill health that comes with it. The better the food you feed your kids while they are growing up, and the more you can help them maintain a sensible weight, the greater their chances of a healthy adulthood, right into old age.

That's not to suggest any of us of more advancing years have missed the whole food boat. Far from it. These changes will help everyone to have a healthy, balanced immune system, and as Covid-19 has grimly insisted, that benefit can be literally life-saving. The Go Whole project needs to be family-wide and age-deep.

Helping kids to love the good stuff

You don't have to tell me that it's generally harder to get kids to eat chickpeas or cabbage than coco pops or chicken dippers. We find it hard not to tussle with them as they reject anything green, or anything crunchy or anything leafy, refuse sauces or 'wet' food, or don't like different foods 'touching each other' on their plates! Convincing youngsters to limit their consumption of refined, processed foods – and eat more fruit, veg, whole grains, pulses and all the other good foods I've talked about – is not easy. Not at all. But there are ways and means, dare I say 'tricks' even, that can help us succeed.

Play to their strengths: if your kids only like raw carrots and peas, say, don't despair, that's two great whole foods they *do* like. So, let them have their fill as often as possible, even as you offer up new foods for them to try alongside.

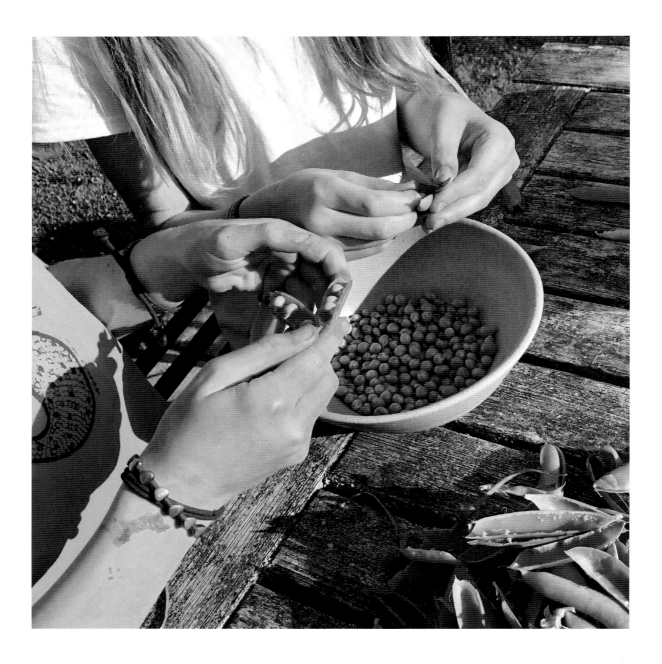

Here are a few observations and suggestions that might come in useful:

Be a good role model. A parent who baulks at broccoli or says 'yuk' to sprouts is not helping their child. Focus on the fruit and veg you do love, and let them see you loving it! The more, healthy whole foods you tuck into, enthusiastically, in front of your children, the more normal and desirable those foods will seem.

Let them play with their food. This can build children's confidence around new foods and encourage them to accept healthy ingredients. One study has shown that 3–4-year-olds who were encouraged to play with fresh fruit and vegetables – picking them up with their hands, squashing or bending them, making pictures with them on a plate, with no pressure to actually eat them – were more willing subsequently to taste not only those fruit and veg, but also others that hadn't been part of their play.

Take the pressure off. Encourage kids to try healthy foods but don't force or bribe them. The old, 'you can have ice cream once you've finished that cauliflower' ploy is hugely counterproductive, creating conflict and reinforcing the idea that veg is a trial to be undergone. Take the pressure off yourself too – if one particular mealtime hasn't gone the way you wanted it to, shrug it off and move on.

Understand the biology. It's perfectly natural for small children to be cautious, even fearful, around new or unfamiliar foods. In our distant past, this trait would have been highly desirable – an inbuilt instinct that protected newly mobile young humans from ingesting poisonous or dangerous foods 'in the wild'.

Get them shopping, prepping, cooking and growing with you. This is a key way to break down that fear and unfamiliarity. The more ownership and agency a child feels over the food they are eating, the more receptive they are likely to be to it.

Let them serve themselves. Enabling children to build their own meals gives them a feeling of control, importance and what psychologists call 'self-efficacy'. It boosts children's confidence in themselves, and in the food they are eating. Telling your child that they can help themselves from a big dish in the centre of the table can inspire them to try something new.

Be patient. Don't rush any of the above. Better eating is a long-term project – for you, for your children, for the whole family. Taking it seriously, but slowly, reduces anxiety all round.

FUNDAMENTAL, FILLING FIBRE

One consequence of the decision to eat more whole foods is that you – and your family – will also eat more fibre, without even trying. This is great news, and it's worth understanding why.

Fibre is incredibly important for our bodies. In our white-bread Western world, we eat far too little fibre and that is having profound effects on our health. Low fibre intake is associated with a greater risk of killer diseases such as heart disease, type 2 diabetes, stroke, and breast and bowel cancers. We also know that a high-fibre diet helps reduce the long-term weight gain that is in itself a powerful factor in ill health.

The beneficial effect of upping the fibre in your diet can be rapid. One study undertaken in 2014 put a group of people from rural South Africa and a group of African Americans on a two-week food swap. The South Africans started eating a high-animal-protein, low-fibre diet of burgers, meatballs, hash browns and mac 'n' cheese, while the Americans switched to a diet of fruit, veg, maize, fish and pulses. This gave them 55g of fibre a day (three times the amount of their usual Western diet). After just 14 days, the high-fibre African diet led to dramatic changes in the bowel, reducing inflammation, changing the gut bacteria (see page 77) and lowering levels of toxic substances associated with cancer.

What exactly is fibre?

Fibre is not one single homogeneous substance, but is made up of various kinds of plant material, including cellulose, lignin, pectin and chitin, and molecules known as beta-glucans and polysaccharides. What all of these have in common is that they form part of the 'tough stuff' in plants. Most often they are found in a plant's cell walls – i.e. they literally hold the plant together. These fibrous elements are all types of carbohydrate but their defining characteristic is that they are not broken down in the human digestive system in the same way as other carbs.

Why is fibre good for us?

It's precisely the fact that we can't easily digest fibre that makes it so important. It is the manner in which it passes through us, and what it does on the way, that brings the benefits. For a start, fibre slows down the first stages of digestion – it literally makes our stomachs empty more slowly. Not only does that mean we feel fuller for longer, but it slows the release of glucose into the blood and helps avoid undesirable spikes in blood sugar. That's hugely helpful in reducing food cravings.

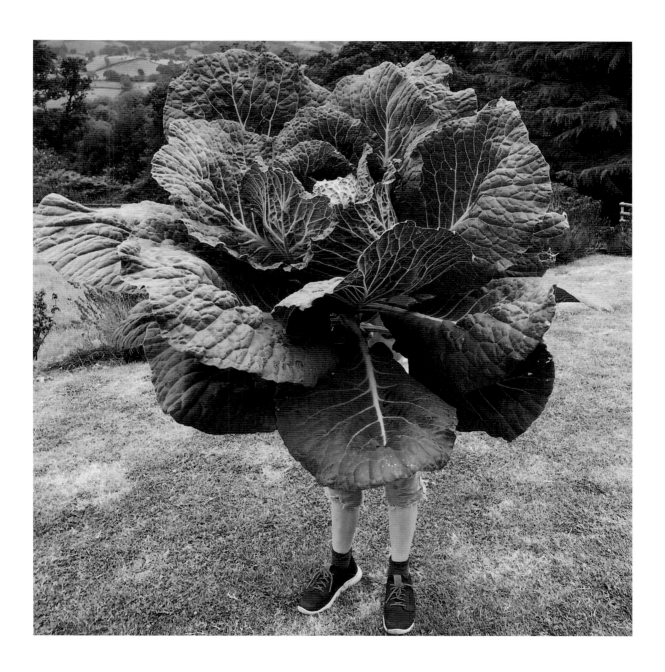

After passing through the small intestine undigested, fibre reaches the large intestine, where most of our good bacteria live. I'll talk more about these beneficial bugs in Chapter 3: suffice to say, cutting-edge science is now revealing them to be incredibly important for our health. They affect many things, including immunity, but also appetite, metabolism and mood. Fibre fosters and feeds these friendly bacteria, allowing them to flourish and do their thing.

Fibre keeps you regular too, as everybody knows. And it's worth stopping to think about why that matters. Constipation is not just deeply unpleasant, it can be utterly debilitating – and it's costing taxpayers a fortune. One report revealed that in 2017–18, this horribly common condition cost the NHS in England an eye-watering £162 million, with on average nearly 200 people a day admitted to hospitals because of constipation alone. Even if it doesn't hospitalise you, constipation increases the risk of problems like piles and urinary tract infections.

Constipation also means, of course, that waste is being held inside for longer, during which time some waste products can be reabsorbed by the body and others may start to break down and produce toxins.

Research is ongoing as to whether constipation is a direct risk factor for cancer (some studies suggest it is, some that it isn't), but it's clear that the longer food takes to pass through the bowel, the greater our contact with potentially harmful substances. It's simply not good for us to hold on to our waste for too long.

Where do we get fibre?

There are two types of fibre: soluble and insoluble. We need them both. And that's easily achieved if you eat a good range of fruit, veg, whole grains, pulses, seeds and nuts. Many of these contain both types, and this is one of the most compelling reasons to get regular helpings of all of them into your diet.

There are some rather fun and unexpected sources of fibre too: a mug of coffee gives you around 1g of soluble fibre, while dark chocolate has approximately 1g of fibre per 10g square. Another healthy, high-fibre snack is popcorn – though it's less healthy if it's covered in butter, sugar or salt! None of these should be your prime sources of fibre, but it all adds up.

Insoluble fibre is plentiful in whole wheat, in the tougher parts of fruit and veg, such as the skins and stalks, and in nuts and seeds. It's bulky and doesn't change much as it passes through us, except to absorb and hold on to water. It helps to keep your colon nice and healthy, moving everything along.

Soluble fibre partially dissolves in the digestive tract to form a sort of gel. Oats and barley are rich sources, and soluble fibre is also found in pulses, fruits and vegetables. It makes us feel full and is brilliant for our bacteria. But it also actually binds itself to cholesterol, helping to remove it from the body.

Foods that are low in fibre are – you guessed it – refined grains (especially 'white' flours), sugars and fats, and the products based on them such as white bread, cakes, biscuits, sugary drinks and snacks. Animal foods such as meat, fish, dairy and eggs don't contain fibre but are still useful for other nutrients.

How much fibre do we need?

In 2015, the government changed their advice on how much fibre we should be eating, upping the recommended amount for an adult from 23g to 30g a day. Their report explained that a pretty exhaustive review of data showed 'intakes of 30g per day and above are associated with the greatest health benefits in reducing the incidence of cardiovascular diseases, type 2 diabetes and colorectal (bowel) cancer.'

Now, when you compare it to the 100g of fibre from tough wild plants that our Stone Age ancestors probably ate every day – or even the 55g contained in the modern rural South African diet mentioned earlier – 30g sounds pretty modest. But in the context of the average Western diet, 30g is a lot of fibre. It's certainly way more than most of us are getting – around three times as much, on average. So, is it a sensible or achievable amount for us to aim for?

I think so – not least because it will encourage us to cut right back on refined ingredients and 'ultra-processed' foods, reduce animal products, and eat lots of plant foods, all of which are smart steps anyway.

In truth, to get the levels we need, we should be thinking about fibre at pretty much every meal, even snacks. You cannot bag yourself 30g by simply having an apple after your cornflakes or a portion of baked beans with your fry-up (a medium apple has 4–5g fibre, half a can of beans 7–8g). But an apple and a stick of celery, a portion of carrots, and two slices of wholegrain toast will get you halfway there. And if your breakfast is oat granola with fresh fruit and seeds, your lunch is a big salad including chickpeas or lentils, your dinner is a veggie curry with brown rice and you snack on fresh fruit and whole nuts, you will have completely nailed it.

What's more, along with the roughage, you'll also be getting a rich array of vitamins, minerals, healthy carbs, fruit and veg. A daily diet like that may require a step-change for many of us, but it's completely doable – and well worth doing!

That daily fibre figure doesn't have to be exactly 30g, of course. It's a nice round number, and an ideal amount, but in practice, few of us are going to sit down and start calculating the grams of fibre we eat at each meal – and nor should we. Fibre-counting is probably ultimately as unhelpful and soul-destroying as calorie-counting.

But since it's now so blindingly obvious that fibre is one of the keystones of good health, we need to be thinking about increasing it *every time we eat*. So mentally swap the figure of 30g for the phrase 'a lot', fill your shopping basket with unrefined whole foods and you'll be very much on the right track.

Easy does it: FODMAP foods and the wind of change

One of the important functions of fibre is to absorb and hold water as it passes through the gut – this is one of the ways it helps to keep us regular. But it does mean it's important to increase your water intake at the same time as you increase your fibre intake, to keep everything working well.

And yes, fibrous foods can make you fart. Again, this is a sign of how they work – they are fermented by those teams of good bacteria in our colon. Jerusalem artichokes, for example, are legendary for their flatulatory effects precisely because they are powerful 'prebiotics', feeding the good bacteria in our guts: gas is the by-product.

Some people are more affected by this process than others. If you suddenly ramp up the fibre in your diet, you and your nearest and dearest might really feel these effects, so it's not a bad idea to work up gradually.

Even then, some people do have a problem with high-fibre diets, particularly with what are known as 'FODMAP' foods. FODMAP stands for 'fermentable oligosaccharides, disaccharides, monosaccharides and polyols'. It's a description of a range of natural sugars found in some foods.

Once in the large intestine, FODMAP foods start to ferment. That happens in everyone, but for some people it can cause discomfort, gas, bloating and other IBS symptoms.

FODMAP-rich foods include onions and garlic, pulses, cabbage, broccoli and cauliflower, stone fruits, apples and pears – as well as wheat and milk. If you find any of these have an adverse effect on you, there are ways to deal with the problem. Speak to a doctor or dietitian about a low-FODMAP diet – which can help to identify trigger foods. You can still find plentiful other sources of fibre.

WHAT ABOUT CALORIES?

Calorie-counting works for some people, over the short term, when they are trying to lose weight. But as a general approach to healthy eating, I reckon it sucks. It's hard to enjoy food if you see it only as a set of energy units: the higher the count the 'worse' the food is – so you'll have to eat less of something else, or pound it out on a treadmill.

Such soul-sapping thoughts aside, calorie-counting is a *terrible* way to judge the goodness of foods. In fact, it can direct you away from the whole foods that will benefit your body most. Extra virgin olive oil is crazy with calories. And is it good for you? Extremely. A giant, toffee-flavoured rice cake on the other hand might be 50 calories. You could eat a whole pack for breakfast, lunch and supper and still be in calorie credit. But with their refined grains, sugar, colours, flavours and emulsifiers, they sure as hell aren't whole – and there's barely a gram in them that's going to do you good.

So, before you start fretting about calories, just ask, 'Is this a whole food?'. If the answer is yes, then it's got the fibre and nutrients nature gave it and it's very likely to be good for you – as long as you consume it in sensible amounts.

Now consider this: the average Briton in mid-Victorian times ate 4,000–5,000 calories a day – far more than the average of 2,500–3,000 we consume today. Yet, these recent forebears did not suffer an obesity epidemic. They had health issues, certainly, but weight-related diseases were not prevalent. They were more physically active than us, which accounts for a lot of the extra calories. But there's more to it than that.

Dr Giles Yeo, at Cambridge University's Department of Clinical Biochemistry, gave me this insight: 'We eat fewer calories now, but they are different calories,' he says. 'The processed and refined foods we eat these days mean there are far more "available calories" on the average plate. If you eat 100 calories' worth of highly refined table sugar, your body will absorb 95–97% of those calories. If you eat 100 calories of whole sweetcorn, or peas, you don't absorb the same percentage. Some of the calorific energy in the veg remains bound up in the fibre that helps move it through your system.' In short, high-fibre whole foods make fewer calories available as they pass through us.

That's a massive deal. Dr Michelle Harvie has calculated that if an individual increased their fibre intake from 12g a day (the woeful national average) to the recommended 30g, they would effectively reduce their daily calorie uptake by around 125 calories. That's pushing a thousand calories a week – a couple of small meals' worth.

You don't need to remember these numbers – you're not counting calories! But it's good to know that when you switch to whole foods, you're no longer asking your body to store so many calories that it may not need.

YOUR WHOLE FOOD LARDER

It's hugely helpful if your whole food mindset is reflected in the contents of your larder and fridge. So welcome in some new staples, alongside the tinned tomatoes and pasta. Dried and tinned pulses, and nuts, seeds and whole grains should be the dominant force on your dry store shelves. And if opening your fridge doesn't present you with swathes of green and splashes of whole-fruity colour, then it's time for a new kind of shopping list that puts the fresh and the whole ahead of the altered and the made.

Vegetables and fruit

The biggest, richest cornucopia of whole foods is furnished by the plant kingdom, with veg and fruit at the top of the tree. They are the finest of whole foods and loading your plate with them on a daily basis is the simplest way to overhaul your diet for good.

Gifts for our over-worked, under-nurtured, stressed-out modern bodies, whole fruits and vegetables offer plentiful fibre – along with valuable vitamins and minerals. In addition, plants contain natural chemical compounds called phytonutrients. These benefit the plant in some way, helping to protect it from infection or sunlight, for example. The good news is that when we eat those plants, their phytonutrients are also beneficial to us. In fact, they are one of the reasons that fruits and vegetables are so crucial for our health.

There are thousands of different phytonutrients – carotenoids in carrots, lycopene in tomatoes, phenolic acid in tea and coffee. Science has yet to work out precisely what they all do for us, but we know they are *protective*, preventing and repairing damage in our cells and tissues. A fruit- and veg-rich diet can reduce the risk of things like heart disease and stroke, it's linked to a lower risk of cancer, and it improves bone health too.

The key to getting more fruit and veg into your diet is variety. It's an important principle in healthy eating in general – so important that the next chapter is devoted to it – but variety is particularly applicable to fruit and veg because they offer it quite naturally, with so many families in so many forms. A spinach leaf is just *so* different from an apple, as a beetroot is from a raspberry; and the differences in shape, colour, taste and texture represent differences in the many, many good things they contain.

Capitalise on this glorious range and scope by getting as many different fruits and vegetables as possible into your daily diet – into every meal in some way if you possibly can. Five a day is great but six, seven, eight or ten is better! The evidence is that the more whole fresh fruits and vegetables you eat (and tinned, frozen and dried fruit and veg all have a part to play too), the greater the benefits.

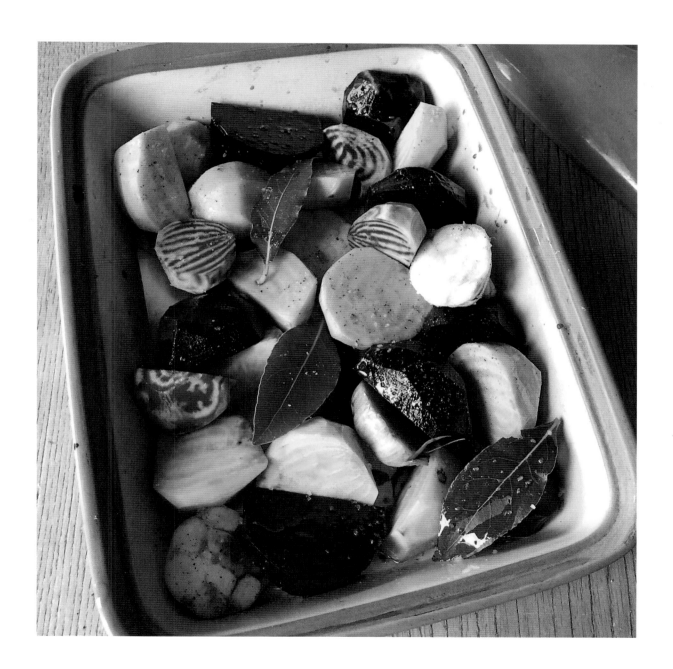

Expanding your family's veg horizons

If you know that vegetables are under-represented in your kitchen, here's something that can really help: a family-oriented vegetable cook-off. The basic idea is to grab a bunch of different vegetables – ideally five at a time – and cook them very simply, or not at all, then get everyone to try them and give them a score, using a different colour. You don't have to follow the list of veg here, and you don't have to do all your tasting at the same time, but try to get the whole family together for each session.

Veg	Vegetable Score		
	Raw	Steamed or boiled	Roasted
Beetroot			
Broccoli			
Cabbage			
Carrots			
Cauliflower			
Celeriac			
Courgettes			
Fennel			
Green beans			
Kale			
Leafy greens			
Parsnips			
Peas			
Sprouts			

1 = I'm not a fan   **2** = I don't love this but I can eat it   **3** = I quite like this
4 = This is delicious!
Raw = thinly sliced, grated or chopped, with a trickle of good oil, a squeeze of lemon, pepper and a tiny pinch of salt. **Steamed or boiled** = until just tender, with a touch of good oil or butter, pepper and a little salt. **Roasted** = in chunks with a trickle of good oil, pepper and a pinch of salt at 190°C/Fan 170°C/Gas 5 until tender and starting to brown.

You might be surprised at the vegetables you like, or how a different way of preparing a once-rejected variety makes it more tempting for someone in the family. A touch of butter or oil can help, and a tiny scrap of grated garlic in warmed butter or oil – on greens and beans, especially – can be catnip for some people too. It's certainly helped my kids eat more veg. You only need a little though: a walnut-sized knob of butter or a tablespoonful of olive oil is ample for a 4-person helping of veg or salad.

Anything that scores 2 or above from everyone is veg gold! If it turns out, for example, that half the family can tolerate roast beetroot, while one member quite likes it and another thinks it's great, then the door is open: now you can tweak, layer and dress. Serve roast beetroot wedges with crunchy seeds, with tender leaves, with juicy cherry tomatoes, with a little crumbling of cheese or a spoonful of creamy yoghurt. Make a tangy dressing with olive oil and cider vinegar or lemon juice, throw on some fresh herbs – chives, parsley, basil – and add a little salt and pepper. Now we're talking!

You don't have to come up with your own recipe of course – Google 'roast beetroot salad recipe' or 'best beetroot recipes' and await the deluge. And if beetroot *hasn't* yet floated the family boat, there are dozens of other veg (and fruits, nuts, grains and seeds) on your radar now, just waiting to get into your kitchen, and reveal their charms.

A note on potatoes

Spuds are often demonised because they are a source of starchy carbs. It's true that they can send your blood sugar up fairly quickly. And, for some, daily spuds are almost as much of a religion as daily bread – at which point they can become similarly problematic (see page 109). But skin-on potatoes are a natural whole food and a good source of fibre and nutrients, including vitamin C. It's all about balance and moderation. So, mix up your carbs to avoid eating spuds every day.

Most of us love a spud that's been crisply fried or roasted with a generous dash of oil or dripping, but we don't need telling that's not a healthy choice. It's marginally healthier if you leave the skins on, but even then it's best to make those chips and roasties an occasional outing, to avoid processed potato products like waffles and hash browns, and to rein it in on the buttery mash too. By all means include boiled new potatoes or jacket spuds in your diet reasonably regularly, keeping portions moderate: 200g per serving is plenty for the average woman, around 300g for a man. No need to weigh, though – a potato roughly the size of your fist is about right (see pages 170–1). You can up that a bit if you are very active. And, of course, it's always a good idea to partner spuds with plenty of other, more colourful veg.

Pulses

Pulses include kidney beans, butter beans, haricot beans, lentils, chickpeas, split peas, peas, soya beans and broad beans. Plain, traditional tofu, which is made from soya beans, can be counted as a pulse too. All of these are increasingly recognised as wonderfully beneficial foods. For example, there's a fascinating body of work centred around what are called the 'Blue Zones' – places where people live exceptionally long and healthy lives (see bluezones.com). Researchers studying five of these communities, in quite different parts of the world, have identified several factors they have in common that seem to explain their robust good health. One key thing that people in Blue Zones all share is a diet that is emphatically plant-based – and includes lots of pulses.

Pulses are a great source of protein, fibre, vitamins, minerals and unrefined, slow-burning carbs. They reduce cholesterol and – this is really important – they fill you up. One study in 2016 showed that adding just one serving of pulses a day to the diet led to a small amount of weight loss without any deliberate cutting down of other foods – this is almost certainly because of the 'satiety factor'. Of course, it's also hugely helpful that pulses are, for the most part, as cheap as chips – but a very much wiser choice!

So, whether dried, tinned or frozen, pulses are a whole food essential. Dull? They can be, if served in glaring isolation. But whiz them into a garlicky hummus with some roasted roots (see page 277), add them to a zingy curry (as on page 330), or toss them with some shredded leaves and a punchy dressing (see page 254), and pulses are as vibrant as they are virtuous.

Whole grains

The Western diet includes a lot of grains, particularly wheat, but they are nearly always highly refined (into white flours) before we eat them. This is not good. Refining, in one fell swoop, turns a great raw ingredient (the whole grain) into a potentially unhealthy one that can cause a number of problems (which we'll come to in Chapter 4).

Unrefined whole grains, on the other hand, have been linked to an amazing range of health gains. This is largely down to the fibre they contain, the benefits of which we have just discussed. But they also come with a substantial package of other nutrients, including vitamins (especially B vitamins), minerals, polyphenols, antioxidants and even protein. Whole grain intake is associated with a reduced risk of heart disease, stroke, cancer (particularly bowel cancer), respiratory diseases, infectious diseases and type 2 diabetes. It may even reduce the likelihood of developing depression.

Whole grains include brown, red, black or wild rice, oats, whole wheat grains or 'berries', bulgar wheat, whole spelt and pot barley, and a trendy new grain (actually very ancient)

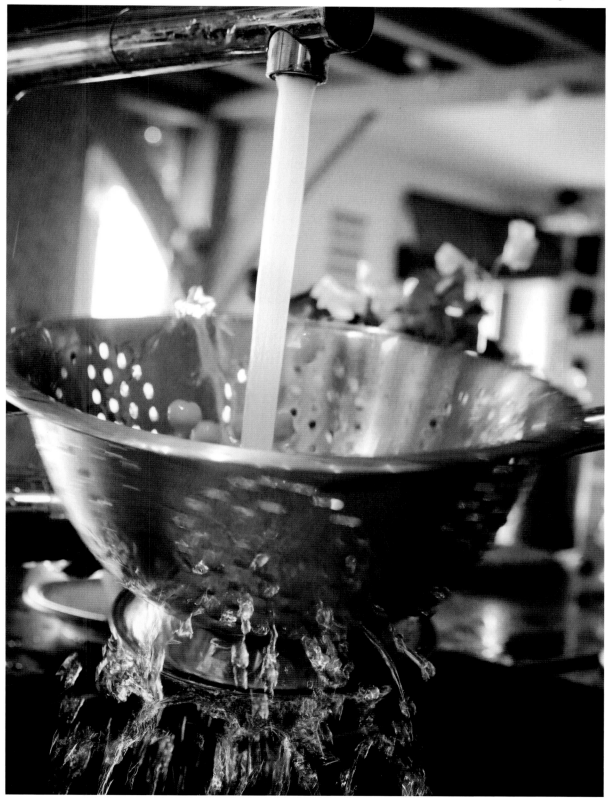

called emmer or farro. Sometimes grains like spelt and barley are described as 'pearled'. In this state they are not technically whole grains since some of their bran is polished away, but they are still much higher in fibre than, say, white rice. Whole buckwheat and quinoa are sometimes called 'pseudo-grains' because they are actually seeds, but you can cook and serve them like grains and they are very nutritious.

Whole grains, including wheat, rye, spelt and buckwheat, are used to make wholegrain bread, noodles and pasta, too. These are more nutritious than standard white versions and they usually have much more fibre, though not all are equal in their fibre-providing potential. A good rule of thumb is to apply the 10:1 test. Look on the 'nutritional data' panel on packaged wholegrain products: if there is at least 1g of fibre listed for every 10g carbohydrate, you're onto a good thing.

Whole grains – and foods based on them – take longer to digest and be absorbed, which is good for your blood sugar, and, as with those pulses, for your satiety. For example, brown rice is more filling than white, so a smaller portion will do you. If you are used to loading your plate with white rice, try brown instead and you may find you'll be happy with half of your usual portion. Swapping 'brown' for 'white' with other 'made' carbs such as white bread and pasta also makes sense, and again, portion-wise, less will feel like more.

We don't need to go overboard on whole grains: making them part of your diet is a great idea but they only need be a moderate part. Dr Michelle Harvie, an expert in healthy weight loss, feels that the conventional advice to base every meal around starchy carbohydrate is misguided. 'Wholegrain carbohydrates are an important part of a healthy diet,' she says, 'and I certainly don't advocate low-carb diets. But we really don't need starchy carbs like bread and rice at every meal. There's a danger they can take the place of the fresh veg that ought to make up about 50% of our diet, as well as the healthy fats and proteins which are really satisfying and help to stop us overeating.'

I whole- (excuse the pun) heartedly second this. It seems to be almost a religion in Britain that we must have a big dose of carbs – bread, pasta, spuds or rice – at every meal. But reducing or altogether replacing the carbs on my plate is increasingly a choice I'm happy to make – particularly when the replacement is a good helping of pulses. These give me protein and carbs and fibre too, and from a taste and texture point of view they can play a similar creamy, starchy role to our favourite carbs.

So, if I've got plenty of beans in my chilli, I'm often happy to have it with a big green salad rather than a pile of rice, or a baked potato. High-fibre carbs such as spelt and barley, good wholegrain breads, skin-on spuds and wholemeal pasta will never be strangers to my plate – I like eating them and I love that they do me good. I just don't feel obliged to dish them up daily.

Nuts and seeds

Nuts and seeds are fantastic whole foods: high in fibre and protein, rich in antioxidants and flavonoids, and usually containing quite concentrated amounts of key nutrients such as selenium (Brazil nuts), magnesium (almonds, cashews and peanuts), omega-3 fatty acids (walnuts and linseeds) and B vitamins (pistachios). And the *different* nutrients that each of these nuts offers bolsters the compelling case for variety that I'll be making in the next chapter...

Studies have linked various types of nuts and seeds to a range of health benefits, from weight loss and lower cholesterol to reduced inflammation and even protection against cancer and stroke. Eat a broad range and view them as little health-bombs to sprinkle, mix and munch, boosting the goodness of anything you add them to. You're going to be encountering plenty of them in the recipe section, so get some in and enjoy!

Nuts and seeds sometimes get a bad rap, because they are quite high in fat. But that fat is of a natural, healthy kind. Moderation is the key: nut butters without added sugar or salt, for example, can be a great whole food ingredient, but it's easy to overeat them. So, swap in a few whole nuts and seeds when you can – try my seedy toast on page 232.

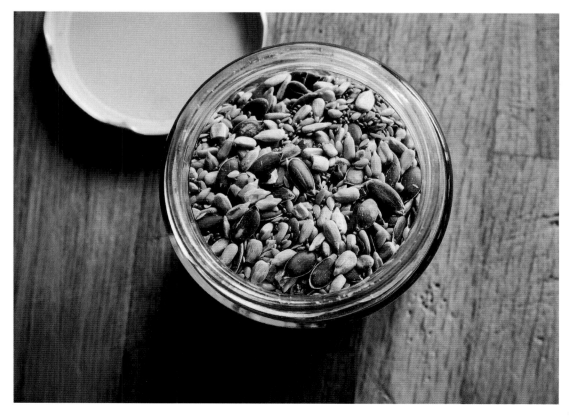

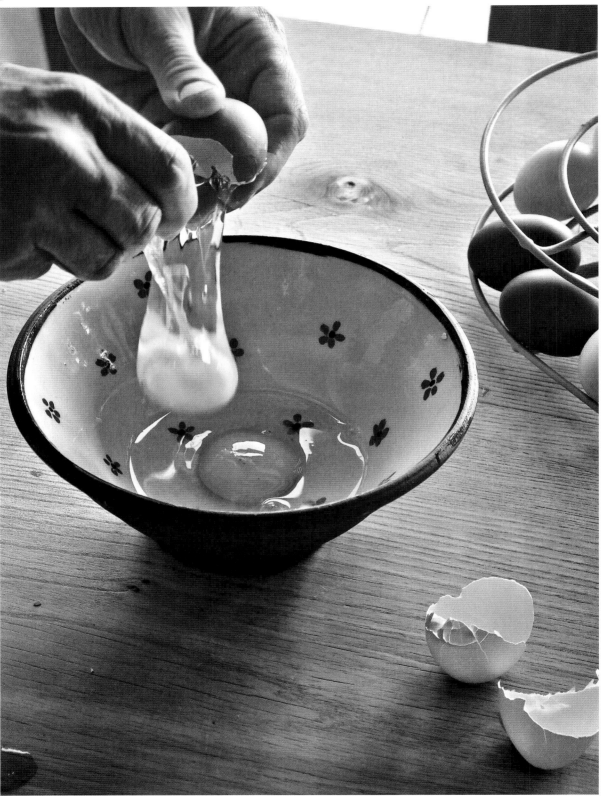

Eggs

Eggs come to us perfectly formed with nothing added and nothing taken away. High in complete protein and various essential minerals and vitamins (including vitamin D), they are inexpensive, filling and very versatile. The idea that they will raise your cholesterol has been debunked. It's true that egg yolks are rich in cholesterol but, for most people, cholesterol in the diet does not raise levels of bad cholesterol in the blood.

Organic or free-range systems offer a more natural and stimulating existence to egg-laying birds, which is a vital consideration, to my mind. But there's another bonus: eggs from grass-fed hens also have significantly higher levels of vitamin E and essential omega-3 fats, with one grass-fed egg contributing about 10% of our daily omega-3 requirement (eggs from caged hens offer only half that).

Dairy

Not everyone chooses to eat dairy products. Not everyone *can* eat them – in fact around 65% of the world's population is lactose intolerant. And although dairy offers us protein, calcium and various vitamins, it isn't essential to human nutrition. So, if butter, cheese, milk or yoghurt are off your menu, for any reason, you don't need to worry. However, minimally processed dairy products can definitely be considered healthy whole foods.

I still enjoy dairy but I eat less than I used to. For starters, high dairy consumption drives poor welfare in the massively pressurised dairy industry. And while I like dairy, I don't think it's *necessary*. Eating less dairy is one way to reduce your intake of saturated fats (which, for most of us, is probably not a bad idea, see page 120) and I have cut back on butter and cheese (I used to eat a lot). Ice cream is also a rarer treat than it once was!

I prefer full-fat dairy products to reduced-fat or skimmed versions. They are more satisfying and more delicious (two important qualities I want from my food). At around 4% fat, whole milk is hardly a high-fat food anyway. If you prefer low-fat dairy products, be aware that some are highly processed and padded out with sugar, thickeners and stabilisers. Others, like skimmed milk or low-fat plain yoghurt, have simply had their fat removed – so if you want to reduce your intake of calories they can certainly help with that. Whether full- or low-fat, go for the least processed dairy: plain milk and yoghurt are very different propositions for your body than a chocolate milk drink or sugary yoghurt in a squeezy plastic pouch!

As I'll be exploring in some depth in Chapter 3, live-cultured dairy products such as yoghurt and kefir, and also some unpasteurised cheeses, can be an excellent way to boost your all-important gut bacteria. I eat one or other most days, often with fresh fruit, fruit compote (page 224), or my overnight oats (page 227).

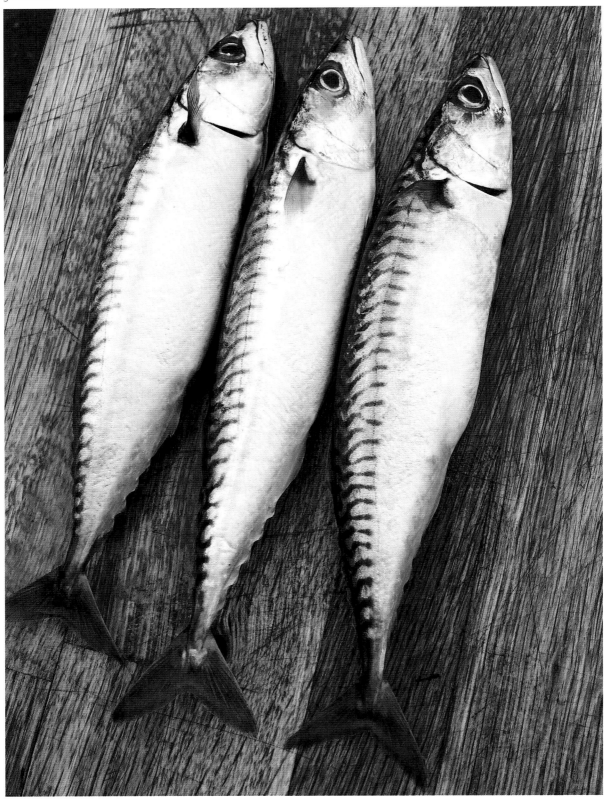

Fish

If you're not vegetarian or vegan, then fish is a fantastic whole food to include in your diet. There's good evidence that people who regularly eat fish – particularly oily fish – have less heart disease and stroke. This is largely attributed to the omega-3 oils that fish contains (all fish have it, but it's more concentrated in oily fish). It could also be partly down to other nutrients, as well as the simple fact of fish nudging out less healthy proteins (like red and processed meat) from our diets.

You shouldn't panic if you *don't* eat fish – you can get omega-3 from plant sources including linseeds/flax seeds, walnuts, chia seeds, rapeseed oil and walnut oil. It's not known if plant sources of omega-3 have exactly the same effect as including fish in your diet, but to get the equivalent amount of plant-based omega-3 as you would from eating two portions of oily fish a week you need one of these each day: 1 tsp flaxseed oil, 1 tbsp rapeseed oil, 1 tbsp flax seeds, 1 tbsp hemp seeds, 12g walnuts or 2 tsp chia seeds. My overnight oats (page 227) and seedy toast (page 232) can oblige.

At least one portion of oily fish a week – such as mackerel or sardines – is a great choice. (Pregnant women shouldn't have more than two portions.) Enjoy white fish and shellfish in addition to that. Mussels are a great choice as they are mostly sustainably produced, and bursting with good things, including those omega-3s.

Choose sustainably caught wild fish, or organic farmed fish. Generally, mackerel, sardines and herring/kippers are good sustainable oily-fish choices. Farmed salmon and trout are much more problematic – they are fed largely on fishmeal made from wild fish, and the sourcing of that is often unsustainable. Organic fish-farming addresses that issue by using feed sourced mainly from the offcuts and trimmings of fish already caught for human consumption. It's not a perfect solution, but it's way better than feeding farmed fish on wild fish harvested solely for that purpose.

If you're struggling to maintain an activist's zeal in sourcing sustainable fish, then there are guides to help you. Look for fish with the blue MSC eco-label 'tick', or consult the Marine Conservation Society's online Good Fish Guide before you go shopping for fish: mcsuk.org/goodfishguide/search.

Meat

Meat used to be seen as essential to a 'normal', healthy diet, with vegetarian and vegan regimes viewed as lacking something, and potentially unhealthy. But the pendulum is now swinging very much in the other direction. So much so that it's moving towards a consensus that meat-free diets, if based on a balanced array of good whole foods, represent some of the optimum ways of eating for well-being.

The landmark EAT-Lancet study in 2019, authored by 37 experts from 16 countries, concluded that a benchmark healthy diet should include only a low to moderate amount of poultry and little or no red meat or processed meat. Consumption of red meat, the authors explained, particularly cured meats like ham and salami that contain nitrate-based preservatives and a lot of salt, have been associated in different studies with an increased risk of stroke, type 2 diabetes, heart disease and some cancers.

This is not the same as saying 'red meat will give you heart disease and cancer', but it is a useful warning. It is also a fact that lower consumption of meat often goes hand in hand with higher consumption of vegetables, fruits and whole grains, and with other healthy choices. And, as you will have gathered, that's where we are heading!

Environmentally speaking, the impact of the meat-heavy diet that dominates our planet is disastrous. Not only is livestock farming massively resource-hungry, swallowing up great quantities of crops, power, fuel and water, but meat production is a key factor in climate change. The farming of animals – particularly in intensive systems – releases huge volumes of greenhouse gases. Recently, researchers at Oxford University concluded that a global switch to plant-based diets could 'save up to 8 million lives by 2050, reduce greenhouse gas emissions by two-thirds, and lead to healthcare-related savings and avoided climate damages of US $1.5 trillion'. In other words, eating a lot less meat is one of the best possible ways to save our bacon.

'White' meat, such as chicken and other poultry, is seen as the healthy option, simply because it isn't red meat. And it's true that it isn't associated with specific health risks in the same way. But that doesn't mean we need to eat piles of it; even white meat should only make up a small part of our diet. We already eat more protein than we need and the environmental and welfare issues relating to poultry farming are grave.

If you choose not to eat meat at all, and you apply a little forethought and planning to your diet, you can eat exceptionally healthily. However, unprocessed meat from well-raised animals is a nutritious whole food, and a diet that includes a modest amount of well-chosen flesh can be a healthy one.

If you're going to eat red meat, then keeping your consumption to a maximum of 70g a day, or 500g a week, is sensible. The simplest way to do this is to just keep several days a week meat-free. This is what we've done at home, since I first made the conscious decision to recalibrate my cooking around an expanded repertoire of plant-based food – about 10 years ago now. These days we have more days without meat than with. Meat now has indelible treat status – and processed meats like bacon and salami are really an occasional indulgence. One of my hopes for this book is that it will encourage and empower many others to forge a similar plant-laden, meat-light path.

As ever, I take a 'nose-to-tail' interest in the livestock that gives us meat. Fresh offal like liver and kidney is highly nutritious, and a good ethical choice if it comes from organic or free-range animals, because it means a fuller use of the carcass. So, if you eat meat, include some offal from time to time. Try not to rely on liver alone as too much of this can lead to excessive levels of vitamin A. I particularly like lamb's hearts.

Now let me be more explicit about animal welfare: I urge you to choose organic meat, and dairy. It represents a better life for the animals we kill for meat (that means more space and a more natural, outdoor environment, as well as natural food suited to the species). For me that's an ethical must. But there's a health factor too: organic livestock rearing often directly correlates with higher levels of healthy omega-3 fatty acids – from feeding on grass rather than concentrated industrial animal feeds. The nutritional bonus may not be huge but, for me, it's one more reason to choose organic. Here's another: antibiotic use in organic farming is tightly controlled, whereas the rampant use of antibiotics in conventionally farmed animals, in addition to all antibiotic use worldwide, is now threatening human health via the spectre of antibiotic resistance.

Organic meat is more expensive because it reflects the cost of humane as opposed to inhumane farming. But if the price tag puts a natural check on our meat consumption (editing it down from two or three times daily to perhaps three or four times weekly) then I think that's all to the good.

I reckon I'm making a reasonable fist of practising what I preach – but I could do better. Most of the meat I eat is reared very locally – some of it right here at home. It's all either free-range or organic. I feel increasing satisfaction from a run of meat-free days, and I plan to go further, and notch up whole weeks of meat-free eating. I think that's where we all need to be heading – for our own health, and for the health of our planet.

Replacing meat

Of course, there are some processed veg products – like Quorn (based on a type of fungus) and TVP (textured vegetable protein, made from soya flour) – that have been largely designed to fill 'the meat space' for vegetarians and vegans. I'm not completely convinced by them. They definitely aren't whole foods and they don't feature in my cooking – I prefer to use whole pulses, and occasionally tofu. But I know some people find them really handy when switching to a more plant-based diet. Be aware, though, that the more processed forms – veggie nuggets, pies, vegan 'bacon' and sausages, ready-meals etc. – can be full of refined ingredients and are no healthier than their meaty equivalents. Vegan junk food is an emerging market that needs to be approached with caution!

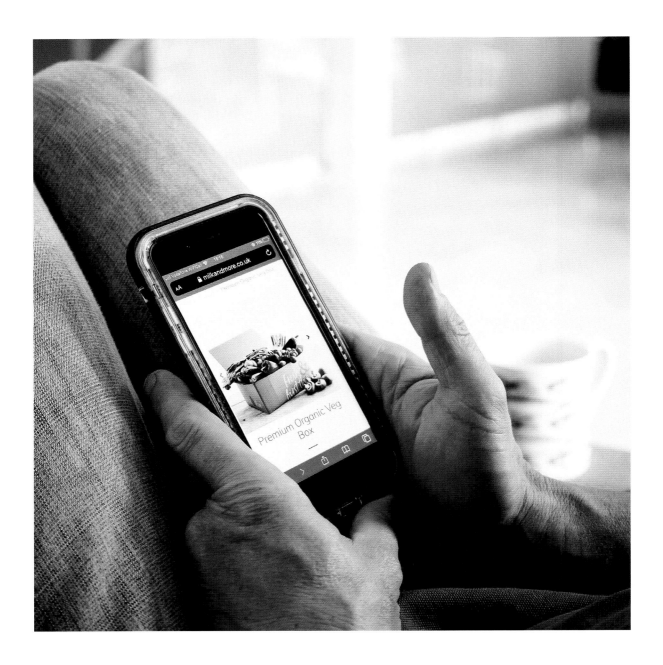

SHOP SMART

Shopping, of course, is where Going Whole actually starts. Bring the good stuff into your home, and it's right there where you need it. Keep the unhealthy stuff out of the larder and fridge, and it's a whole lot easier to keep it out of your mouth!

Shopping healthily in the environment of the average supermarket isn't easy, of course. After all, retailers make a lot of money from peddling processed fare. Thinking ahead is the best way to stay on track – and also a sure-fire route to wasting less and shopping more economically. It takes a few minutes, maybe, but you'll be repaid tenfold.

So, look at what's already in your fridge and cupboards, plan your meals for the next few days (at least roughly) and only get what you need. This might sound absolutely bleeding obvious but many of us don't shop like this anymore. We are so busy that we swing by the nearest retailer on our way home and just grab what looks tempting. And of course, that may well be glossily packaged ready-meals, fresh-baked pastries and heavily promoted BOGOF deals on family-sized pizza.

In an ideal world I'd urge you to shop small and to shop local, visiting greengrocers, independent fishmongers and butchers, bakers and farmers' markets, and perhaps to order a regular organic veg box delivery. I do all these things and, in combination, I think they offer the most sustainable way to shop. They give you access to more homegrown goods, more seasonal produce, more information and advice, less packaging and less plastic. They also bring you closer to the story of where your food is coming from – and that's a great way to feel better about what you are eating.

But I know that shopping like this is not realistic for many people, certainly not all the time. And if you are among the million people who live in one of Britain's food 'deserts', with little or no access to shops selling fresh fruit and veg, it is not an option at all.

However, whether you buy food in supermarkets, corner shops, markets, wholesalers or online, a determination to resist the processed in favour of the whole – or at least wholer – is something you can always take with you.

Tackling Britain's shocking food deserts, and the poor public transport, inadequate funding and social inequality that have created them, should be a priority for our government at national and local level. Until that happens, the onus remains on individuals to make the smartest choices possible, to look for everyday items like brown bread, tinned beans and frozen sweetcorn, maybe fresh apples or bananas – most of which should be available even in small corner shops. Even takeaways usually offer some kind of salad or coleslaw – my local chippy sells great mushy peas!

Time, effort and money

Will changing your diet to include more whole foods and fewer processed foods cost you more in terms of time, faff and money? To the first two points, I'd say yes, a bit. Whole foods often require a certain amount of prep. Their opposites – 'convenience foods' – have earned their name for a reason. But they could just as accurately be titled 'processed foods' or 'poor foods'. And that's the healthy way to think of them.

Whole foods are not *in*convenience foods. They're just normal foods. They are not always instant, but they can be pretty snappy – an easy lunchtime omelette with cherry tomatoes and sliced spring onions doesn't take much longer than making a sandwich, for instance. Time doesn't equal effort either: a groaning dish of spicy roasted veg might demand an hour in the oven but it doesn't require much prep time. You can also cook in bulk and spread the overall effort of preparing food over a few meals. There's a growing army of food writers, chefs, bloggers and teachers – myself among them – falling over themselves to offer easy, quick, low-effort recipes for healthy foods. So, finding something simple to do with your favourite whole food ingredients won't be a challenge.

But I don't want to make unrealistic promises. To eat really healthily, we have to be prepared to put in at least a little time in the kitchen. The total non-cook is at a big disadvantage, being dependent on ready-meals, takeaways, and other factory-made foods that lead you down the aisle of the less whole, and the more processed. There is no judgement here, this is not about laziness. Not cooking isn't always a choice. Often people don't cook because they don't have access to shops selling fresh ingredients, or the equipment needed to store food or cook with it. Sometimes people are just too exhausted or consumed with day-to-day stress to have the time or energy to cook.

I'm convinced that the fact so many of us are struggling with even the basics of cooking is a huge part of the health and obesity crisis we are facing. It's a difficult problem to deal with here – in a book which is inevitably loaded in favour of those with the will and the wherewithal to do at least some basic cooking. I've been addressing this wider issue on TV, and through working with the Food Foundation and the Soil Association on initiatives including Veg Power (vegpower.org.uk) and Food For Life (foodforlife.co.uk). We need better food education, including the basic skills of cooking, for all, and it has to become easier for people to get hold of the right raw ingredients. I will continue to press for the political engagement that I believe is essential if we are to become, once again, a nation of competent cooks.

The monetary cost of Going Whole is a trickier issue to pin down, although it is certainly related to whether or not you are willing and/or able to spend a little time in the kitchen cooking (or sometimes simply assembling) those healthy plates of food. You don't have to be a mathematician to see that a loaf of sliced white and a couple of tins of budget beans costs a lot less than, say, the ingredients for my nutty beany beetroot curry on page 330. But a lot of the whole foods that I advocate are cheap: onions, cabbages and carrots, apples and bananas, oats and brown rice, beans and lentils, eggs, frozen peas, a glass of good old tap water on the side. At the same time, I accept that fresh herbs, spices, nuts and seeds, good oil, meat and fish certainly push your shopping bill up. But then I would argue that these are the things we tend to need in smaller quantities.

And, of course, unhealthy treats can be costly too. It's well worth sitting down and totting up how much you spend each week on all of your food and drink. Then look at how much of that goes on takeaways, pre-packed puddings, crisps or chocolate – and you should probably put booze on that list too! (see Chapter 6). Reducing spending on any of those things frees up money that could be redirected towards healthy whole foods.

The overall cost of a healthier diet is the sum of the new whole foods you'll be buying *minus* what you would have spent on ready-meals, unhealthy snacks, takeaways and other foods you are no longer buying; i.e. the cost of the *change* to an overall healthy diet as opposed to the weighing up of individual healthy *ingredients*. It may well be that a new healthy whole food diet won't actually cost you a whole lot more.

If you don't (excuse the pun) buy this, if your experience is that you need less money to eat badly than you do to eat well, then the question has to be: is a good diet worth it? Well, my answer is a resounding *YES*. Sometimes it feels painful to even have to make the economic case for better eating. And that's because I feel I am, in part, fighting a cultural battle – one waged on the other side by advertisers on behalf of multinational food brands and huge food retailers, for decades now. They have been trying to persuade us that food – the very sustenance that builds our bodies and brains, and has the power to keep us well, or make us ill – is the best area of the household budget to target for savings. I think the opposite. I think it's the *worst*.

I realise I'm striding into a minefield here, especially as I am not managing a tight food budget myself. I understand that can be very irritating to those who are counting the pennies every time they do the family food shop. But I'll risk that. Because it seems to me that, if you can possibly manage it, it has to be worth tweaking your household spend to include more whole foods, boost your family's fibre count, and lose some of the additives and processed foods that may well be doing you and your family harm.

I believe that, over time, this will help you not only to stay well, but also to build a resilience and positivity based on the knowledge that, when it comes to food, you are doing the very best you can. And that's something that, whatever life puts in your path, could ultimately prove priceless.

ACTION POINT RECAP

1 Whole is the goal – for everyone, every day

Go whole in your thinking first, and your shopping, cooking and eating will follow. Understand that choosing whole foods over processed foods, whenever you can, is the simplest and most powerful way to make your diet healthier. It's a principle that applies to the whole family, young and old, and it needs to be a long-term project, a lasting change, not a temporary regime or quick-fix intervention. Make it your daily goal to choose ingredients that have had as little done to them as possible.

2 Shop whole, shop smart

Plan healthy meals, write whole food shopping lists for them, and try to stick to them. If you want to be spontaneous when you are shopping and try new things – try new whole foods!

Be mentally prepared when you shop; ignore those towering walls of snacks, biscuits and chocolates in displays sited so you have to bump into them. They are there to make money out of you, with zero regard for your health or well-being.

Remember the simplest way to sort the whole (or wholer) from the processed: read the back of the packet. The fewer ingredients listed, and the simpler they sound, then generally the less processed that food will be. Better still, choose foods that don't have packets at all, apart from their own skin. And don't shop hungry!

3 Fill half your plate with plants

Get unprocessed plant-based foods, especially fresh fruit and veg, to dominate your diet at every main meal. Reduce the space you give on a plate or in a pan to starchy carbs, meat and dairy products and make way for beautiful salads, crunchy slaws, creamy dips, hummus, roasted veg, stir-fried veg, steamed veg, sauced veg and raw veg (recipes coming up!). Think half-a-plate-of-plants and your daily veg count will go through the roof!

4 Make meat a treat

Eat less and better meat. The more meat you eat, the less space you have on your plate and in your belly for fibre-rich plant foods. That's a case for not only eating meat less often, but scaling down the meat portion when you do eat it, leaving more room for the really good stuff... My rule of thumb is to have more days without meat than with. If you're currently a daily carnivore, then start with deleting meat a couple of days a week and go from there.

5 Raise your pulse rate

Eat more beans, lentils, chickpeas and other pulses. They are brilliantly useful in going whole, helping you to eat less refined carbs, and less meat too. Remember that these plant foods occupy a brilliant position on the spectrum of healthy foods, being both protein-rich veg *and* healthy, high-fibre carbs rolled into one. Tinned is fine, and very easy. So, swap them in to favourite meals, adding generously to both meaty and veggie stews and sauces, and even serving alongside roasts.

If you think plain pulses are 'boring', then toss them in spices or light, punchy dressings (garlic is magic with pulses, as are fresh herbs). And try serving chickpeas and tinned beans with your favourite pasta sauces, instead of the pasta – or combined with a small portion of wholewheat pasta.

6 Swap white for brown... and use the 10:1 rule

Increase your whole grain intake and the level of fantastic, health-giving fibre in your diet by swapping white bread, rice, noodles and pasta for 'brown', or wholemeal, versions. Check labels for fibre and remember the incredibly handy 10:1 rule – look for at least 1g of fibre listed for every 10g carbohydrate.

7 Think quality, not calories

Know that 'low-calorie' does not mean 'good for you', and remember there is very little nutritional virtue in highly processed low-calorie foods such as diet drinks and reduced-calorie confectionery and snacks, or even low-calorie ready-meals. Remind yourself: the promise that they are healthy is completely empty. The goodness in whole foods, by contrast, may come with a few calories attached but, providing we are not overeating, that shouldn't trouble us.

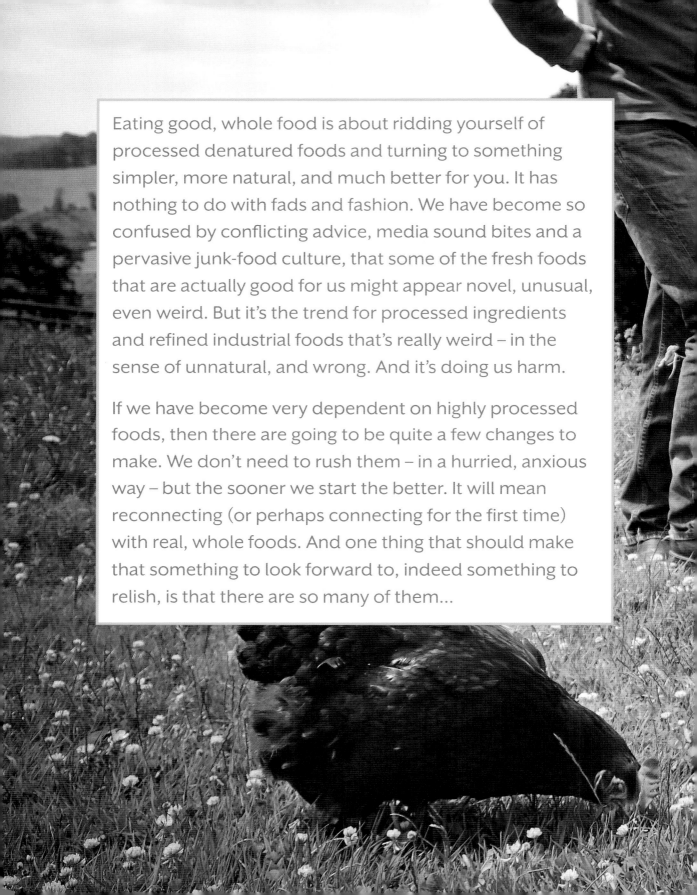

Eating good, whole food is about ridding yourself of processed denatured foods and turning to something simpler, more natural, and much better for you. It has nothing to do with fads and fashion. We have become so confused by conflicting advice, media sound bites and a pervasive junk-food culture, that some of the fresh foods that are actually good for us might appear novel, unusual, even weird. But it's the trend for processed ingredients and refined industrial foods that's really weird – in the sense of unnatural, and wrong. And it's doing us harm.

If we have become very dependent on highly processed foods, then there are going to be quite a few changes to make. We don't need to rush them – in a hurried, anxious way – but the sooner we start the better. It will mean reconnecting (or perhaps connecting for the first time) with real, whole foods. And one thing that should make that something to look forward to, indeed something to relish, is that there are so many of them...

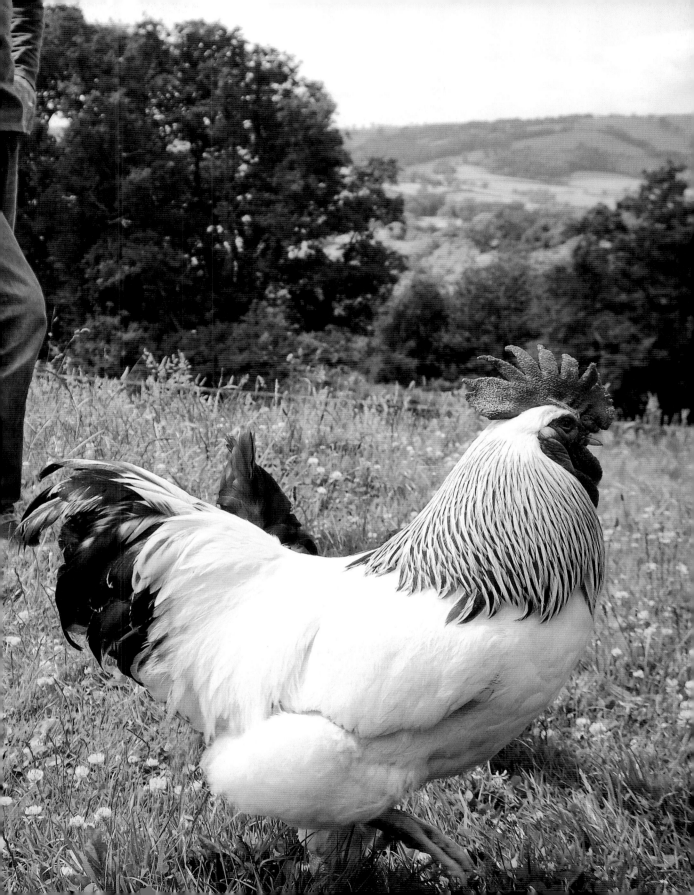

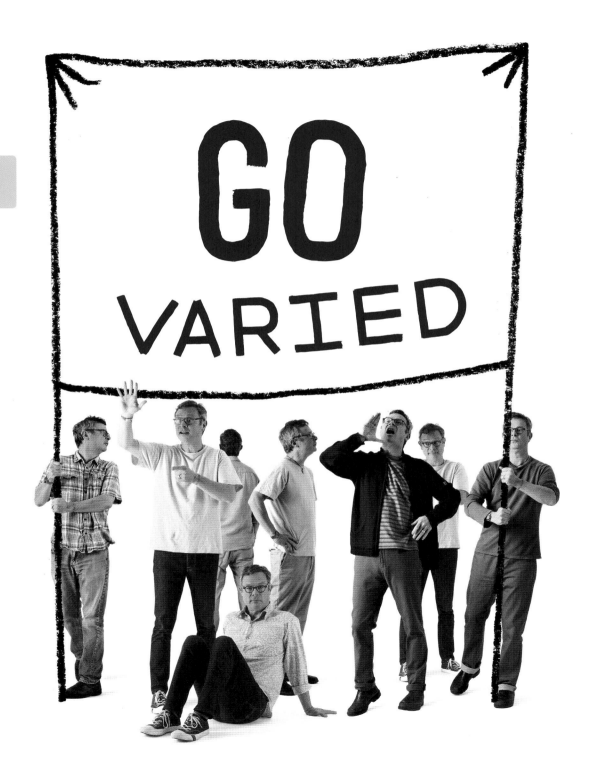

2

No way of eating can be called healthy if it isn't varied. And, just like going whole, going varied is a pure positive. By definition, it's about more, not less. It's an antidote to boredom, and the key to replacing old, bad habits with new, good ones.

By contrast, lack of variety is a downer in so many ways. Industrial monoculture is at the heart of our food problems. Fill vast fields with identical crops, and whole ecosystems will suffer: soil is depleted, birds, insects and animals die out, diseases thrive – unless you whack them with poisonous chemicals.

The same is true of our own personal ecosystems: our bodies. If we feed them with a narrow and unvaried diet, we are at greater risk of disease and medical dependence. No single food can protect against cancer or diabetes, cure high blood pressure, end obesity or guarantee good gut health. But in combination, lots of different, nutrient-packed whole foods just might.

DIVERSITY: THE KEY TO GOOD HEALTH

To go back to biological basics, varied diets are what we are supposed to eat; they are what our bodies need. It's easy to question this – after all, there were no richly stocked supermarkets in the Paleolithic era. Is a highly varied diet actually natural for human beings? It turns out the answer is yes.

A quote from science writer Ann Gibbons, published on Nationalgeographic.com, is telling. As part of a feature on the evolution of human diets, Gibbons interviewed biological anthropologist Professor Clark Spencer Larsen. 'When he describes the dawn of agriculture, it's a grim picture,' writes Gibbons. 'As the earliest farmers became dependent on crops, their diets became far less nutritionally diverse than hunter-gatherers' diets. Eating the same domesticated grain every day gave early farmers cavities and periodontal disease rarely found in hunter-gatherers... When farmers began domesticating animals, those cattle, sheep and goats became sources of milk and meat, but also of parasites and new infectious diseases. Farmers suffered from iron deficiency and developmental delays, and they shrank in stature.'

Larsen isn't the only scientist to see the narrowing of the human diet as an unfortunate modern trend. In a paper from 2018, Washington University researchers Jacob Eaton and Lora Iannotti wrote, 'A survey of hominin diets over time shows that humans have thrived on a broad range of foods. Earlier diets were highly diverse and nutrient dense, in contrast to modern food systems in which monotonous diets of staple cereals and ultra-processed foods play a more prominent role.'

This is something of a revelation. We often think of settled agriculture – the cultivation of grain crops and raising of livestock – as the dawn of civilisation. This isn't necessarily wrong – the food security from agriculture allowed communities to settle and populations to grow. But we shouldn't confuse food security and population growth with healthy eating and quality of life.

And this holds true today: we may think our modern diets are varied, but for far too many of us they are anything but. There are more than 10,000 edible plant species on the planet but fewer than 200 of them are now used for food, and an astonishing 60% of the calories human beings get from plants come from just three crops: wheat, rice and maize.

Processed foods in particular, which are now so ubiquitous in our lives, draw hugely on an extremely small group of ingredients: sugar, refined white wheat flour, refined vegetable oils, maize (as corn syrup and maize flour) and white rice. This is the stuff which, when it comes to dominate our diet, can do us so much harm.

What's more, even the modern fruit and veg we eat is very different to the wild plant foods our ancestors gathered, which would have shown more diversity even within individual species. The wild blackberries we pick in the autumn, for example, are actually the fruit of hundreds of different micro-species, often growing together cheek by jowl. Brambles are not the only species to show such diversity. In our wild past, food might have varied from bush to bush, from tree to tree.

This is very different to the fruit and veg in modern retailers, where each type is typically represented by just one or two highly bred and standardised commercial varieties. This doesn't mean, of course, that modern fruit and veg isn't good for you, but it's one more argument against only eating one or two types of it. In short, modern processing and global food availability have taken much of the natural variety out of our diet. We need to put it back in.

Hitting all the right spots

Eating many different types of whole food, including different varieties of veg, fruit, pulse, nut, seed and grain, means you're far more likely to get the full complement of nutrients you need. Fibre, for example, can be both soluble and insoluble; we need both, ideally from lots of different fibre-rich foods. Technically, you could get the recommended 30g fibre a day by tipping 5 tablespoonfuls of wheat bran on your breakfast in the morning, but that would be an exceptionally bad way to do it because pure bran is rich in phytic acid which can reduce the absorption of some minerals, including calcium, iron and zinc.

The concept of food synergy (see page 21) is also central in a varied diet – the synergy in question being between the vitamins, minerals and other nutrients in whole foods that often enhance and amplify each other. So, the vitamin C in fruit and veg increases the absorption of iron from pulses and leafy greens, for example, while our bodies take up the fat-soluble antioxidant lycopene from tomatoes best if they are eaten with natural fats like olive oil or avocado. There is a phrase I like, whose origin I now can't place: 'A constellation of protective nutrients'. That's what we're after.

There's a growing consensus, too, that a varied diet is essential to good gut health, which in turn is essential to... pretty much everything, as I'll discuss in the next chapter. Science is just beginning to understand the complex miracle that is our gut microbiome, but one clear conclusion so far is that a healthy biome is a varied one, and that the simplest way to create that inner diversity is to feed and nurture our friendly gut bacteria with lots of different whole foods.

THE MORE THE MERRIER

Research points to the fact that, when it comes to fruit and veg consumption, more is better. Five portions a day is great, but ten is terrific – because there appears to be a direct relation between the amount of veg and fruit eaten daily and a reduction in risk of stroke, heart disease and cancer. (Make sure those healthy plant foods are *replacing* some of the less healthy foods in your diet, not just being added on top of them!)

Consciously varied eating will help us achieve a high plant count and that constellation of protective nutrients that comes with it. We're always going to struggle to achieve the kind of intake of veg and fruit that will keep us well if we don't mix it up and eat lots of different types. It's easy to realise that a sumptuous shopping basket bursting with fresh produce is highly nutritious and appetising. By contrast, investing all your healthy eating hopes in just a few favoured foods – bunch after bunch of bananas, for example, or kilos of frozen peas – isn't going to do it. To put it another way, if we met our vitamin A requirement just by eating carrots, we'd all turn orange. That's got to tell you something.

Variety then, is our ticket out of both nutritional imbalance and dietary tedium. But there's more to it than that. To quote the World Health Organization: 'The benefits of eating a wide variety of foods are also emotional.' Variety means a range of flavours, colours, textures and styles. It makes food interesting; and if it's interesting, we're much more likely to want to eat it. Variety is the thing that should help us banish for ever the outmoded idea that healthy food is boring – all limp lettuce and bran flakes. Could there be anything more depressing than the notorious grapefruit or cabbage soup diets that both had their moment back in the last century? Grapefruit and cabbage are fantastic foods to eat, of course – but for *every* meal, day after day? Who could stick to that regime? Who would want to?

Variety, diversity and plurality are great on the micro-level then, in terms of individual ingredients, but they have a much broader meaning when it comes to healthy eating too. There's a reason why this book is based on 7 Ways to eat well, not just one. It's become clear to me that when it comes to eating better, the savvy approach is to change more than one thing. Ideally much more. We set ourselves up for failure if we become tunnel-visioned or limited in any way, putting too much pressure on ourselves, and pretty much ensuring that we miss out some important stuff to boot.

There are many ways to eat better and it's vital that not one of them should be taken in isolation. Moreover, they all enhance and anchor each other. Eat more whole foods and you will also be eating more fibre and being good to your gut. Stop snacking on junk and you'll be increasing your mindfulness around hunger and eating. Skip the fizzy drinks and you've created space for water and fresh fruit in their stead.

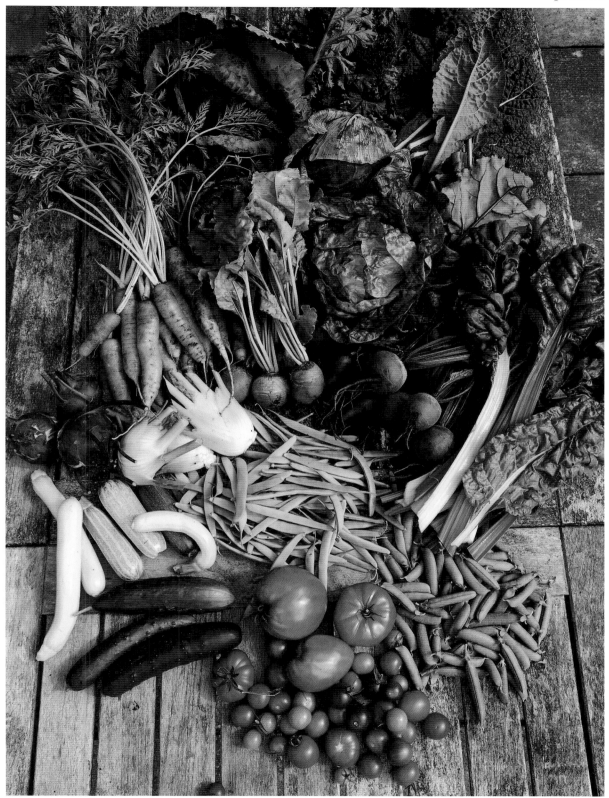

Weaving many different healthy strands into your diet not only amplifies the effect of each, it gives you a safety net too. Just switching to wholegrain bread isn't enough to overhaul your diet, nor is giving up chocolate biscuits, eating an apple a day, or incorporating more whole grains and pulses into your cooking. They are all great ideas, though, and if you do all four you'll really be getting somewhere.

This diversity also provides some insurance against the inevitability of the occasional less-good choice. So, if you do succumb to the choccie biccies once in a while, but you've still got the brown bread, beans, and apple boxes all ticked, then you are in good shape. (Swap the biccies for my oaty nutty chocolate 'tiffin' on page 390 and you're well away!)

Let's be honest, very few people – certainly not me – will be able to eat really well, really healthily, all the time. We all sometimes choose foods that aren't good for us, or have too much wine, or just simply overeat. Some of us do it a lot, some a little. I think you've got to aim high, but it's good to know that if you tackle several different areas of your diet at once then the things that aren't so great, whatever they may be – the takeaway, the birthday cake, the giant caramel latte – are at least put in a very different context. The odds are still in your favour.

Most of the things that have gone wrong in our diets are about a total lack of balance – the unprecedented dominance of refined and processed foods, the ubiquity of poor-quality bread, of sugar, of alcohol. Even the loss of distinction between times when it's appropriate to eat and times when it isn't – the fact that the green light to graze is always on. In this challenging environment, keeping variety as a central principle in your diet – and your lifestyle – is the best way to give yourself a fighting chance. A varied, holistic approach to eating and living well is more productive, more flexible, more enriching – and far more likely to succeed.

In terms of boosting our immune systems and keeping us well, variety × wholeness is genuinely a multiplication, not merely an addition. In a world that has experienced Covid-19, where we know that problems like heart disease and diabetes can make us more vulnerable than ever, choosing foods that help keep such problems at bay is more than smart, it's vital.

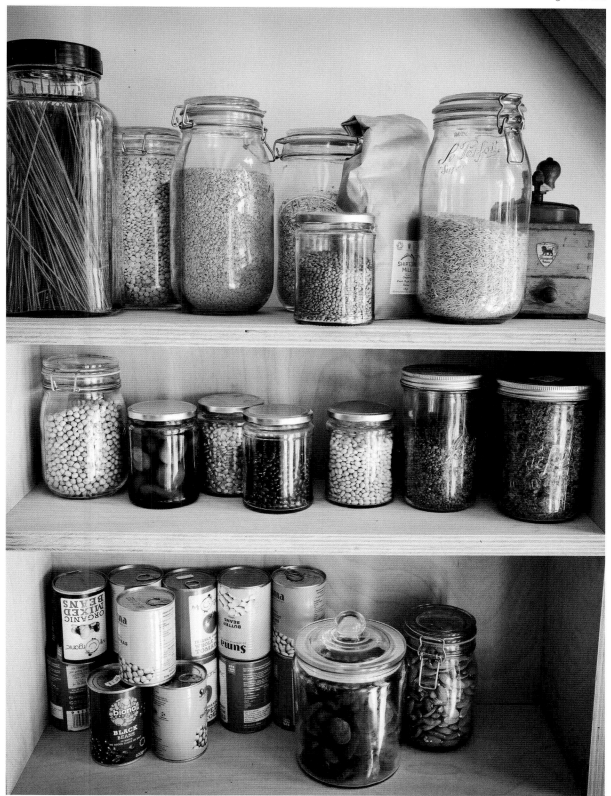

TIME FOR A VARIETY AUDIT...

It's a really good idea to take a long, hard look at how varied your diet is (or isn't) at the moment. So, I'm going to ask you to carry out a simple survey of what you are eating over a three-day period. Ideally, that will include one weekend day – so you could pick a Thursday, Friday and Saturday, or a Sunday, Monday and Tuesday (but if another three-day stretch happens to work better, that's okay).

Feed that info into a tally chart like the one overleaf, breaking down your food into the listed categories. Don't be concerned about the quantity in each serving now (there are ideas on portion control coming up in Chapter 7), just note the frequency.

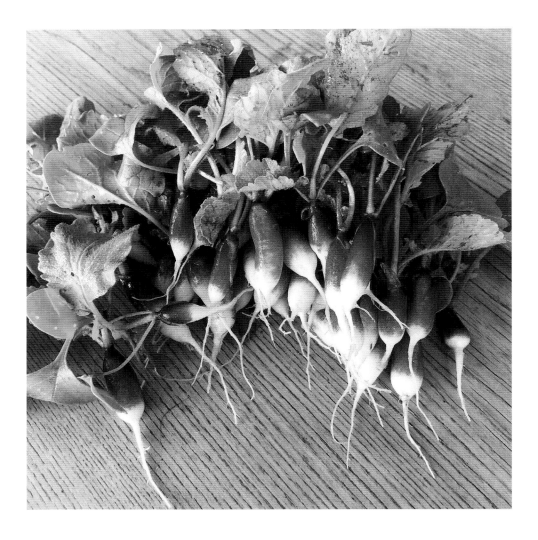

So, for peanut butter on white toast, give one tick for white bread and one tick for nut butters. For bangers and mash, put a tick for processed meat, one tick for potatoes and one tick for any other vegetable you had too.

This isn't a strictly scientific exercise, but it's a good way to focus your mind on the diversity, or otherwise, of what you eat. Try to account for every single thing you eat over the three-day period. One great way to do this is to take a picture of all your meals and snacks (including the biscuits you have with your tea!). Then you can do the tally at the end of each day, or even all in one go at the end of the 3 days.

I've left drinks out of this for now. That's not because I don't think they are important, quite the opposite. What you drink is *so* important for your health that I've got a whole chapter on that coming up.

As an at-a-glance indicator of a richly varied diet, you're looking for those tally marks to be spread out across the boxes – lots of different marks in lots of different boxes. But I don't need a crystal ball to predict that many people will find a veritable thicket of ticks accumulating in the lower part of the third column, where I've placed the less healthy choices – the refined foods that many of us eat too much of. If you end up with lots of tallies in 'white bread and bread products' and a generous clustering in 'cakes, pastries, puddings, biscuits' or 'crisps and other packaged snacks', and rather fewer ticks than is ideal in 'pulses', 'leafy greens', 'tree fruits' and 'whole nuts', don't panic. It's also likely to be the case for many others.

The whole point of doing this is to help you see where you are, and visualise where you would like to be. It is, of course, entirely within your power to change the spread of the tallies, by expanding the variety of your food shopping, and the diversity of the choices you make every time you cook, eat and snack. And you can start right away.

Then you can use this chart not only to plot where you are now, but to measure your progress over the weeks ahead. Redo the tally for a three-day period every couple of weeks, or even every week if you are really going for it. I've been road-testing this audit among friends and family, and the results have been really positive: 'This was quick and easy to do,' said one, 'and it highlighted a few things I hadn't thought about – for example, I eat a good amount of veg but not a great variety.'

If you make good progress over the coming weeks, you can congratulate yourself as the heavy cluster of ticks in that final third column category thins out, and spreads its way back up the chart. Note the new foods you have tried, and enjoyed, and bring them back for a regular outing. I predict (again, no crystal ball needed) that you will find this commitment to diversifying your diet is its own reward, bringing more pleasure and interest to your cooking and eating, and helping you to feel better fast.

FOOD VARIETY AUDIT

DAY 1 DAY 2 DAY 3

Veg

- [ ] [ ] [ ] Brassicas: broccoli, Brussels sprouts, cabbage, cauliflower, kale, pak choi etc.
- [ ] [ ] [ ] Leafy greens: chard, spinach, spring greens etc.
- [ ] [ ] [ ] Salad leaves: lettuce, rocket, watercress
- [ ] [ ] [ ] Other salad veg: celery, chicory, cucumber, radishes
- [ ] [ ] [ ] Peas and beans (fresh or frozen)
- [ ] [ ] [ ] Alliums: onions, leeks, spring onions
- [ ] [ ] [ ] Mushrooms
- [ ] [ ] [ ] Root veg (except potatoes): carrots, beetroot, celeriac, parsnips, swede etc.
- [ ] [ ] [ ] Pumpkins and squashes
- [ ] [ ] [ ] Tomatoes (tinned or fresh), tomato sauces (not ketchup!)
- [ ] [ ] [ ] Peppers
- [ ] [ ] [ ] Avocado
- [ ] [ ] [ ] Aubergines and courgettes
- [ ] [ ] [ ] Potatoes

Fruit

- [ ] [ ] [ ] Tree fruit (fresh): apples, pears, plums, cherries, nectarines, figs
- [ ] [ ] [ ] Berries (fresh or frozen): blueberries, raspberries, strawberries etc.
- [ ] [ ] [ ] Citrus fruit: oranges, grapefruit etc.

DAY 1 DAY 2 DAY 3

- [ ] [ ] [ ] Grapes
- [ ] [ ] [ ] Bananas
- [ ] [ ] [ ] Dried fruit

Nuts and seeds

- [ ] [ ] [ ] Whole nuts
- [ ] [ ] [ ] Whole seeds
- [ ] [ ] [ ] Nut butters

Whole grains, cereals and pulses

- [ ] [ ] [ ] Oats/porridge/granola
- [ ] [ ] [ ] Wholegrain/brown bread (including sandwiches, rolls, wraps, pizza etc.)
- [ ] [ ] [ ] Oatcakes, rye crackers
- [ ] [ ] [ ] Brown, red, black or wild (i.e. wholegrain) rice
- [ ] [ ] [ ] Whole barley, spelt, bulgar wheat
- [ ] [ ] [ ] Whole quinoa, whole buckwheat
- [ ] [ ] [ ] Wholegrain/brown pasta
- [ ] [ ] [ ] Pulses (tinned or dried): beans, chickpeas, lentils

Eggs, dairy and alternatives

- [ ] [ ] [ ] Eggs
- [ ] [ ] [ ] Cheese
- [ ] [ ] [ ] Yoghurt or kefir
- [ ] [ ] [ ] Cow's milk (except in tea and coffee)

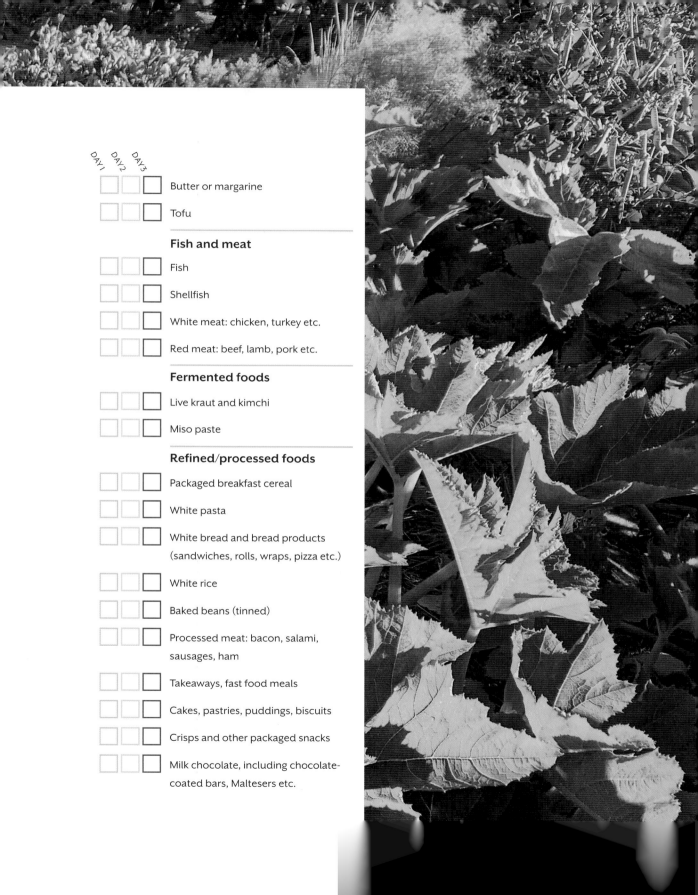

DAY 1 DAY 2 DAY 3

☐ ☐ ☐ Butter or margarine

☐ ☐ ☐ Tofu

Fish and meat

☐ ☐ ☐ Fish

☐ ☐ ☐ Shellfish

☐ ☐ ☐ White meat: chicken, turkey etc.

☐ ☐ ☐ Red meat: beef, lamb, pork etc.

Fermented foods

☐ ☐ ☐ Live kraut and kimchi

☐ ☐ ☐ Miso paste

Refined/processed foods

☐ ☐ ☐ Packaged breakfast cereal

☐ ☐ ☐ White pasta

☐ ☐ ☐ White bread and bread products
(sandwiches, rolls, wraps, pizza etc.)

☐ ☐ ☐ White rice

☐ ☐ ☐ Baked beans (tinned)

☐ ☐ ☐ Processed meat: bacon, salami,
sausages, ham

☐ ☐ ☐ Takeaways, fast food meals

☐ ☐ ☐ Cakes, pastries, puddings, biscuits

☐ ☐ ☐ Crisps and other packaged snacks

☐ ☐ ☐ Milk chocolate, including chocolate-
coated bars, Maltesers etc.

To maintain momentum, you might well find it helpful to establish something like a New Foods' Day, picking one (or two) day(s) a week to trial new recipes that are bursting with fresh, vibrant whole food ingredients. It doesn't matter which night(s) of the week it is – but it is definitely helpful to name the day(s) so you can make it a dependable weekly occurrence. Ideally, the recipes should be plant-based, or at least plant-led, and take in ingredients and food groups that you know from your Variety Audit you could do with more of.

Of course, I would love you to choose recipes from this book, plenty of which lend themselves well to more plant-led family suppers. But there are countless other healthy options online, in the papers, and in the crop of tempting new plant-heavy cookbooks that have appeared in the last couple of years.

If you're looking for an easy way in, try several variations on the effortless technique of veg-roasting. It's a great way to boost the flavour of everything from onions and leeks to cabbages, caulis and sprouts, taking in tomatoes, peppers, courgettes, aubergines and even beans and peas. There's barely a veg you can't oil, season and whack in the oven for really great results. To help you on your way, there's plenty of foolproof veg-roasting winners in the Vital Veg Mains recipe chapter that starts on page 326.

It's important not to put too much pressure on yourself or your family. If a new recipe gets a thumbs down from the troops, or is just too much hassle, you never have to cook it again. But if it wins approval, please do cook it again. The recipes that go down best can be woven into your regular repertoire. And keep trying *at least* one new one every week!

And while you're mixing it up midweek with new recipes, there are other ways to help build variety naturally into your diet...

EAT WITH THE SEASONS

Seasonal eating may seem on the face of it to be narrowing your options, but for me it is completely synonymous with the commitment to variety.

There is no paradox here. It's not as if eating every food in the supermarket once a week is a real or sensible option for achieving diversity. Seasonality on the other hand gives you the perfect rationale to explore a rich variety of foods, particularly vegetables and fruits, when they are at their best (and most local).

To shop and cook seasonally (and, as far as possible, locally) offers up *natural* diversity, taken at a sensible pace. On the plant front, this means leafy greens, salads, fresh peas

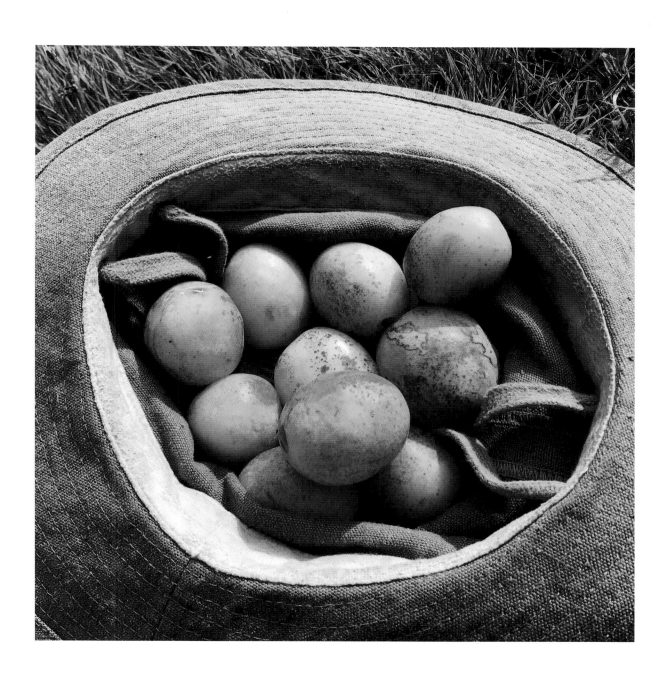

and green beans tend to dominate the summer months, along with native berry favourites such as strawberries and raspberries. As the days begin to shorten, apples, plums and pears join brassicas and roots, and courgettes and aubergines.

It is a rhythm that can take you all around the plant kingdom, right through the year. So instead of having imported green beans every Sunday with your roast dinner, month in month out, or a banana every day in your lunchbox, you'll encounter the full glorious gamut of plant foods that our temperate climate and fertile soils have to offer.

This can be true not just in terms of individual ingredients, but *within* those ingredients. A sweet, waxy little new potato in May is a very different ingredient to a big, earthy maincrop Maris Piper in December. The same goes for carrots, beetroots and other roots, not to mention peas and beans, which can be tiny, sweet and tender or big and starchy and eminently blitz-able or mash-able.

There are always more than enough fruits and vegetables in season to ring the changes on an almost daily basis, should you choose to. But I really don't think you should worry about some vegetables recurring frequently, even almost daily, when they are in season. After all, you won't be eating that vegetable in isolation. And the seasons of all the other vegetables, fruits and herbs you might want to eat it with will be different, ebbing and flowing at varying times. Variable plate-fellows and diverse recipes and cooking techniques will more than see you through.

As gardener-cooks know, even a glut of a vegetable shouldn't lead to repetition or monotony. Having a glut of something, far from stifling creativity, often breeds it. Pickles and ferments add gut-friendly diversity to your diet (see pages 282–7) and veg-laden soups, pasta sauces and curries can be stashed in the freezer, to be called on when an effortless supper is needed. The decision to stretch the seasons by preserving and freezing in this way is one I believe should be taken and controlled by the home cook, not foisted on us by year-round availability of imported foods in our supermarkets.

Cooking 'glut' ingredients, or even very familiar and available veg like carrots, cabbage and even potatoes, in lots of different ways, isn't just thrifty, it's actually very good for you. And it's an important part of the way in which 'variety' is so healthy in our diets. You can absorb more vitamins from raw carrots, for example, but you'll get additional antioxidant beta-carotene from them when they're cooked.

Likewise, raw apples provide valuable vitamin C and potassium, but if you stew them they release pectin, which can be healing for the gut. All in all, there are excellent reasons to eat lots of different vegetables and fruits, cooked (and *un*cooked) in lots of different ways...

LESS WASTE, MORE VARIETY

It might sound counter-intuitive to say that making sure you use the very last scrap of an ingredient can lead to more varied eating, rather than less. But it's true. My long-running love-affair with leftovers (so often the basis of the finest meals!) has convinced me that meeting the challenge of not wasting a single morsel is a sure-fire way to foster creativity and diversity.

Whether it's a lunchtime fridge-forage or a weekend what-the-hell-am-I-going-to-do-with-this? moment, using stuff up has led me to try more new combinations and test more new techniques than following conventional recipes ever could. I habitually, deliberately, cook too much of stuff. I'd rather cook the whole cauli, or half a bag of lentils, rather than 'just enough for supper', knowing that the leftovers will be lunchbox gold, or a handy addition to a sustaining soup or salad.

I've made brownies that use up spent coffee grounds (which, along with the wholemeal cake flour I now regularly use in my baking, increases the fibre). I used to discard the vegetables I put in my stocks, but now I save them to make a tasty hash, or combine them with just enough of the stock to blitz into a soup. These I'm more than likely to top with further random leftovers – toasted nuts and seeds, a poached egg, some of those consciously leftover lentils, the last scraps from a roasted chicken...

This kind of thrift can help foster new techniques and approaches that add further to your commitment to plant-led diversifying of your diet. For example, the thick ribs and stalks of cabbages, kale and cauliflower can easily be grated for adding to slaws. But they can also be sliced and quick-pickled in cider vinegar, or even lacto-fermented in the kind of live kraut whose praises I'm going to be singing in the next chapter (see also the recipes on pages 282–4).

This zero-waste point does bring up the issue of being prepared to cook, as I have discussed on page 48. It's hard to be resourceful and thrifty and creative if you are reluctant to set foot in the kitchen. But I promise you that any effort you put in to redirect trimmings and leftovers into your upcoming cooking will be repaid many times over in terms of personal satisfaction – and delicious, variety-rich meals, that will help keep your heart healthy, as well as warm its cockles.

ACTION POINT RECAP

1 Eat lots of different things...

View every meal as a fantastic opportunity to enjoy a *variety* of delicious whole foods. Good, unprocessed ingredients are the key to better eating, and the benefit you get from them will be massively enhanced if you include as many different ones as you can. This is how you guarantee that your body gets everything it needs.

2 ...in lots of different ways

Even trying different ways of preparing a single ingredient – carrots, for instance, or onions – opens up a range of nutritional benefits. And, of course, different cooking methods, different flavours and seasonings, and different recipes all add to the deliciousness and vibrancy of a diet based on whole foods.

3 Embrace the new...

Unless your diet is already richly varied, then increasing the diversity of what you eat means trying new things – probably new vegetables and fruits, new spices and herbs, and perhaps dried or tinned pulses. It's also likely to involve trying new recipes, and different styles of cooking. So, be prepared to step outside your comfort zone. Try not to reject new things until you've tried them a few times, and in a few different ways. You owe it to yourself! You don't have to completely overhaul your diet overnight. But you do have to be ready for change.

4 ...and go with the flow!

Eat with the seasons, eat what's local, eat what's fresh and good today – and waste none of it. These sound principles are the basis of all sustainable cooking, but they are also at the root of healthy, varied cooking. Allow them to gently guide you into trying new things. Then you will feel good *about* yourself, even as you feel good *in* yourself.

Be curious: let yourself be inspired by other cooks, books, and recipes online. Be flexible when you are shopping: start making choices that aren't just the ones prescribed here, by me, but that you own, and you know are good choices! Tweaking recipes according to what you have to hand (lots of different whole foods!) is liberating. Developing the confidence to do so is a huge step forward in bringing greater variety into your cooking.

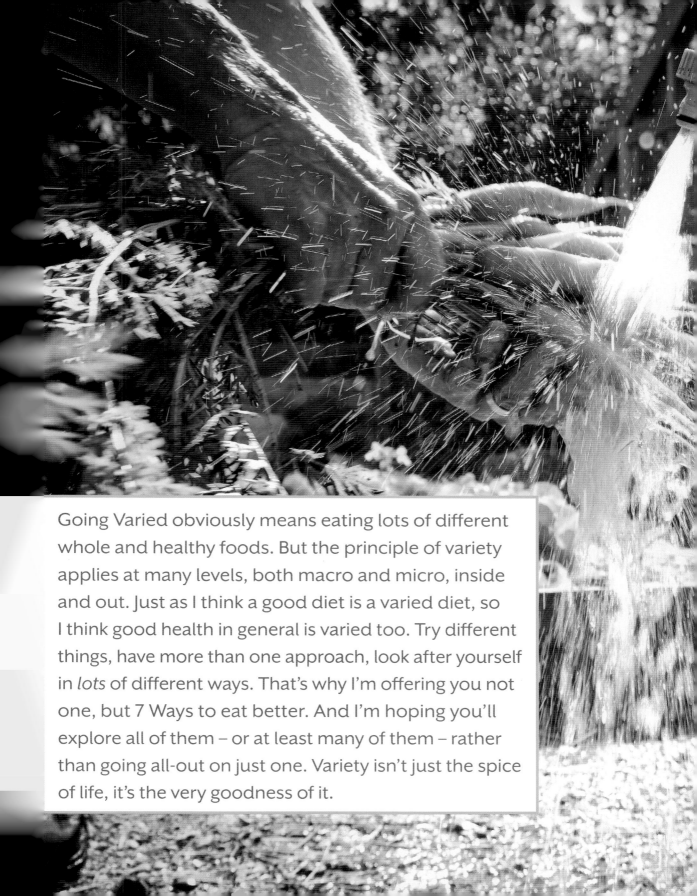

Going Varied obviously means eating lots of different whole and healthy foods. But the principle of variety applies at many levels, both macro and micro, inside and out. Just as I think a good diet is a varied diet, so I think good health in general is varied too. Try different things, have more than one approach, look after yourself in *lots* of different ways. That's why I'm offering you not one, but 7 Ways to eat better. And I'm hoping you'll explore all of them – or at least many of them – rather than going all-out on just one. Variety isn't just the spice of life, it's the very goodness of it.

3

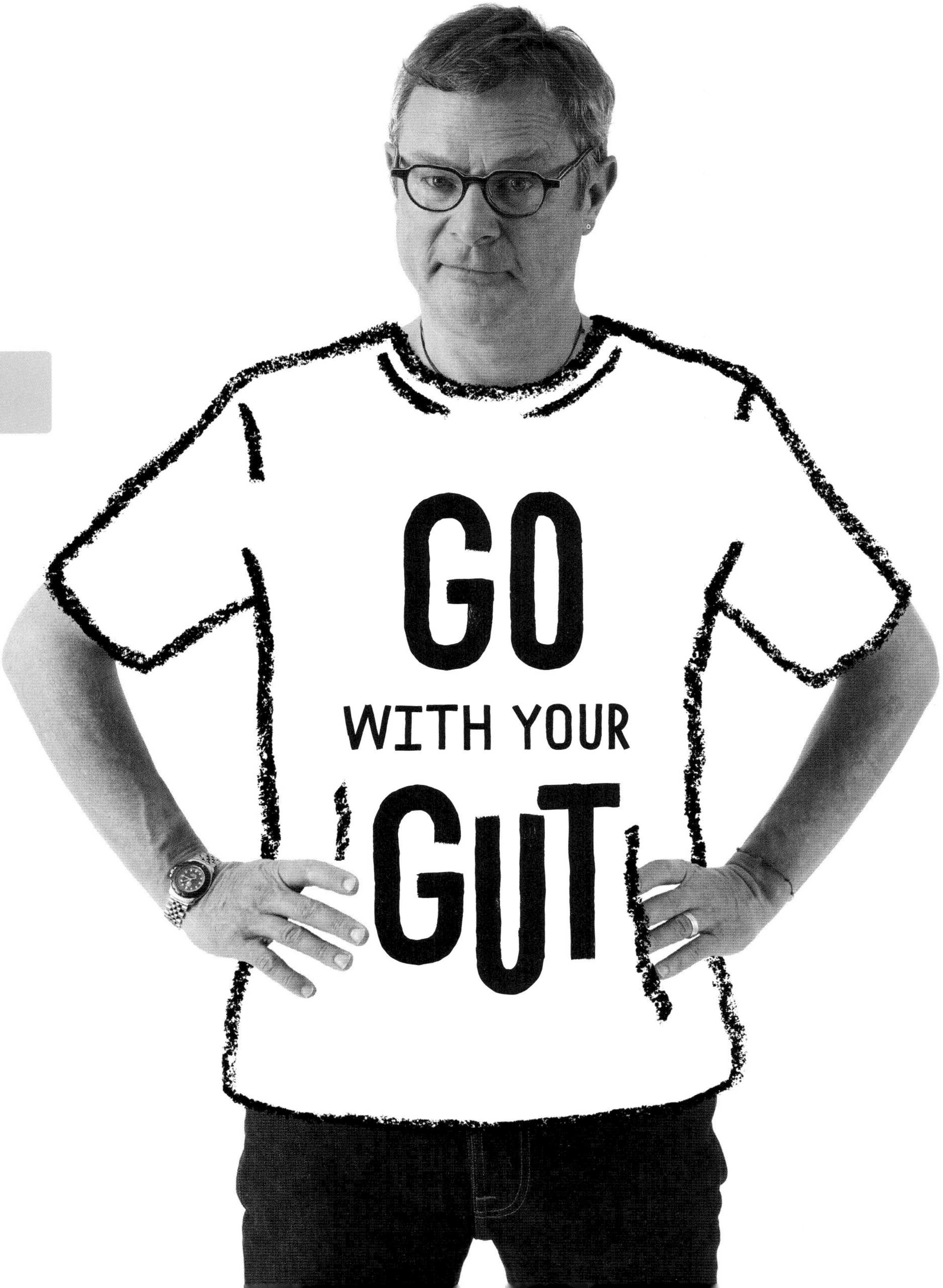

There is a new frontier in our understanding of human health, an area where research is revealing amazing things that we really didn't know before. It looks like it can provide some of the answers to vital questions: 'Why do we get sick?', 'Why do we get depressed?', and even, 'Why do some people gain weight when others don't?'

This new frontier is not 'out there' somewhere. It's very much 'in here' – and right now I'm pointing at my belly. By directing their attention inward, focusing their rigorous investigations into the dark and hitherto mysterious world of our intestines, scientists are casting new light on many aspects of our health and well-being. It's all happening in the seething mass of fermenting food and bacteria that is called our 'gut biome' or 'microbiome'.

IT TAKES GUTS

The last decade or so has seen a revolution in our understanding of the human gut. And while it might have begun in the rarified world of laboratories and medical conferences, that knowledge has rippled outward so that now even the average layperson on the street knows that 'bacteria' is not a dirty word, that there are in fact many 'friendly' bacteria living inside us, and that they do extremely good work. (Or, at least, they do if we let them.)

But what you may not know – what I certainly didn't realise until recently – is just how incredibly influential these bugs seem to be on so many different aspects of our health. The more I discover about this area, the more utterly amazed I am.

The human gut is not merely a tube along which our food is transported, releasing nutrients on the way. It is one of our main lines of defence against illness, the site of huge numbers of information-carrying nerve cells (neurons), and a factory for vital substances, including neurotransmitters and hormones. Our gut bacteria – collectively known as our gut 'microbiome' – play an integral part in all of this. And through their activity, and complex interactivity, they can influence just about every part of our bodies.

It's no exaggeration to say that a healthy gut is as important as a healthy heart or a healthy brain – because a healthy gut is *contributing* to a healthy heart and brain! In fact, alongside our genetic make-up, and our immediate experience and environment, gut health is being confirmed as one of the principle factors that determines our health and, potentially, our longevity.

From the point of view of self-care, that is *huge* news. While we can't change our genetic make-up, or do a great deal to alter our immediate environment, we can do a whole bunch of things to improve our gut health – and thereby our general health – because it is highly responsive to the food we eat.

Gut bacteria: more is more

Scientists believe that our gut bacteria have evolved with us over hundreds of millions of years; we're not talking about any old bugs here, these are highly adapted microbes, specialists at living and working in the human gut.

Individual bacteria are microscopically small: 1,000 of them, placed side by side, would measure approximately one millimetre. And there are trillions (that's 1,000,000,000s, if numbers of noughts help you grasp the scale) of them in our gut.

That vast population comprises hundreds of different bacterial species – some more helpful than others – and, just to add to the complexity, no two people have exactly the same bacterial profile. Our guts are unique – a bit like our fingerprints, except that they are changing all the time. While we all have the same five or six basic family groups of bugs, the balance of individual species within those families can vary enormously.

It's an incredibly complex picture, but there is some clear advice emerging: essentially, the greater the overall diversity of your gut bacteria, the better for your health. Tim Spector, Professor of Genetic Epidemiology at King's College, London, is an expert on the human gut. His book *The Diet Myth* describes many of the revelatory discoveries in microbiology that have taken place recently, and his work points compellingly to our microbes as the missing link in so many areas of health and well-being.

He has a simple message regarding the best way forward for all of us. 'It's quite clear to me that a diverse gut is a healthy gut,' says Tim. 'In adults, the greater the richness and diversity of different microbial species, the better. There is an association between reduced bacterial diversity and disease. A species-rich gut ecosystem is more robust, and better able to defend us against the environmental and biological challenges of daily life. In addition, the greater the number of bacterial species, the greater the number of protective chemicals they produce.' Remember the constellation of protective nutrients – it gets a massive boost from a healthy gut.

Feeding our friends

So, what's going on in there? After we eat, the food we've swallowed spends a few hours passing through the stomach and small intestine. What's left then enters the large intestine (or colon), where the great majority of our gut bacteria live. They feast on whatever they get, fermenting it, breaking it down and continuing to make more nutrients available as they do so. But they don't just extract the good stuff that's already there. They make some new good stuff, too – which I'll come to in a moment.

Different bacteria respond to different foods, so what you choose to eat can really alter the balance of your gut microbes. If you want to positively influence your health by cultivating a diverse gut biome, there is one principle thing you need to know: beneficial bacteria – the ones that make the good stuff, which improves our health and well-being – respond well to high levels of fibre. On the most basic level, looking after your gut is that simple: eat plenty of fibre.

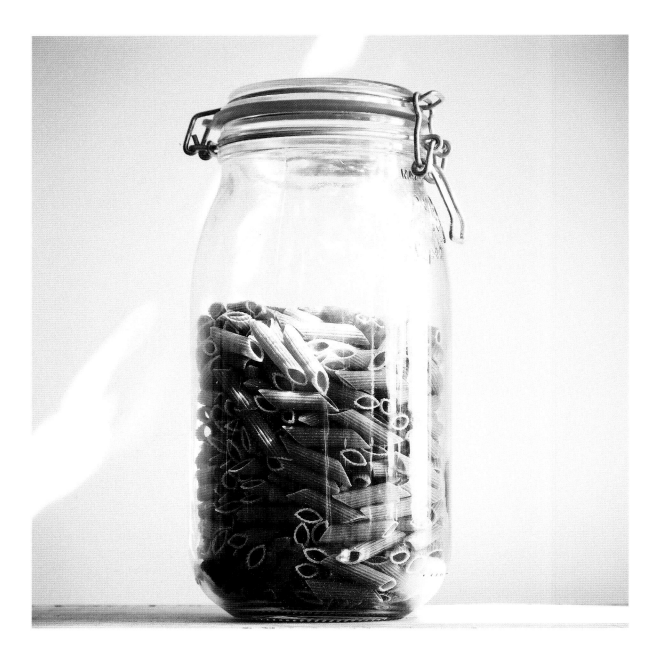

UP THE FIBRE FOR THE SCFAS!

So our friendly bugs are using fibre to make extremely important substances, including 'short chain fatty acids' (SCFAs). It's worth clocking that term – it's one I predict we will be hearing a lot more in the future. SCFAs are central to our health and the more fibre we eat, the more of them our gut microbes can produce. There are several types of SCFA – the most abundant being acetate, propionate and butyrate – and these three perform many different jobs, not just in the gut itself, but throughout our entire system.

Perhaps most crucially, SCFAs nourish the immune cells that line our gut, and prevent damage and inflammation to the gut wall. Their role is still not fully understood, but these combined functions of providing good energy and anti-inflammatory protection for our gut seem to be vital in bolstering our resistance to disease. The flip side is that when our gut isn't well-nurtured, and our biome is less diverse and more compromised, we may become more susceptible to inflammation and serious illness.

There's more: astonishingly, SCFAs can affect not only how much energy we extract from what we eat, but also how we burn or store that energy. They help keep our blood sugar stable, modulate appetite and can even influence the types of food we choose. All of which goes to explain why there seems to be an association between a person's gut-bacteria profile and their weight. Scientists have already discovered that people with obesity tend to have a different bacterial profile to lean people and, crucially, that changes in the diet can alter those profiles.

It's worth pausing to digest (sorry!) the consequences of this. It could imply that a concerted effort to eat more whole foods and more fibre will not merely improve your gut health, but increase your *inclination* in the long term to eat more whole foods and fibre, further improving your gut health and your resistance to serious disease. So, positive changes in your diet that may seem hard to maintain at first could become easier over time, as the virtuous circle of improved gut health kicks in.

Now I may have run with that idea just a little further than the clinical evidence can currently support, but I can relate to it from personal experience. As I have researched and understood the benefits of a healthy gut biome, I have made a conscious effort to eat even more whole and fibre-rich foods than I used to. There are more pulses and whole grains, whole fruits and vegetables and also live and fermented foods (of which more shortly) in my diet than there ever have been before.

And if at first this felt like a bit of an effort, I can honestly say it doesn't any more. These foods are no longer just the things I *think* I should eat more of; they've become the foods I actually *desire*. And it seems I have my gut to thank for this excellent state of affairs.

I sent these exact thoughts to Tim Spector with this simple question: 'Tim, is this a bit far-fetched?' He replied: 'This is a new science, we don't have all the definitive answers, and many of the experiments have not yet been done in humans, but there is no doubt that improving our gut health is pivotal to our well-being. It is quite possible, based on the evidence, that your gut microbes can produce chemicals that can indeed affect your mood and even your food choices. So keep them happy and keep eating your veg and fermented foods!'

GUT FEELINGS

SCFAs are not the only vital substances produced in our gut. Perhaps the most fascinating recent discoveries about our microbiome are the links it appears to have with our feelings. Research is revealing that gut bacteria can affect your mood, via something called the 'gut-brain axis'.

This isn't as weird as it sounds: most of us know that nervousness or anxiety can be felt physically in the gut as 'butterflies'; and you may be one of the many people who find their bowel habits change when they alter their routine or go on holiday. These are examples of the brain having a direct effect on the gut. But we now know that communication happens the other way around too – in fact it turns out there is much more information going gut-to-brain than brain-to-gut.

Substances produced by the gut and in the gut that pass into the bloodstream and affect the brain include 'feel-good' neurotransmitters like dopamine and GABA (gamma aminobutyric acid – low levels of which are linked to anxiety). Serotonin is another one – in fact, a lot of the serotonin in the body is found in the gut, not the brain! Our microbiome can modulate hormones too, including oestrogen.

All of this has enormous and very exciting implications. As with obesity, people who are suffering with depression have been shown to have different bacterial profiles to people who are not, while one analysis of several studies in 2019 concluded that changes to gut bacteria could precede a reduction in anxiety symptoms. Our microbiome could be the mechanism through which our diet influences our mental health. It certainly looks like fostering a diverse and flourishing biome through healthy, varied high-fibre eating can be good for your head as well as every other part of you.

And that adds to the credibility of the idea that improving our gut biomes might further incline us towards healthy, high-fibre eating. This is speculation but, if the recognition of the good it's doing us is emotional, as well as intellectual, isn't that likely to have a much more profound effect on our long-term behaviour?

BOOSTING YOUR BIOME

The field of microbiome research is very new and very complex. Scientists know that gut bacteria influence the rest of our bodies in a profound way, but they are still learning exactly how. We don't yet know the ideal types and numbers of different bacteria required for optimum health. To pinpoint things clearly, some researchers use specially designed probiotic supplements to manipulate the levels of certain bacteria in order to see if they might affect specific problems or confer measurable benefits. Through research like this, we may well get to the point where carefully tailored cocktails of live bacteria can be used to treat a range of illnesses.

We are not there yet – but that's no cause for dismay. And we needn't wait for special supplements and the last scientific word on which bacteria can do what for us, to begin the process of improving our gut health. We can start nurturing and nourishing our gut biomes right here and now, simply by eating well.

One of the most uplifting things to come out of that gut-anxiety study analysis I just mentioned is that the most efficient way to achieve positive changes in the gut is via a healthy diet, rather than through probiotic supplements. It's also clear that our gut bugs can respond rapidly to dietary changes, good or bad (remember the African–American food swap on page 26). So you might start feeling the benefits of upping your fibre before you can say gamma aminobutyric acid!

'The best way to foster bacterial diversity is through a varied whole food diet,' confirms Tim Spector. 'Definitely not a boring diet – you want lots of different veg and fruit, plus whole grains and nuts. And a lot of other delicious things can be really beneficial too: yoghurt, unpasteurised cheeses, dark chocolate, olive oil, garlic and spices, coffee and tea, a little red wine. The worst things for your gut are ultra-processed foods and artificial sweeteners.'

GOING LIVE WITH PROBIOTICS

So Going Whole in Chapter 1, and Going Varied in Chapter 2 have already put us absolutely on track for improving our gut health. What else might we do?

Well, mounting evidence indicates that you can further nurture your gut via two very simple routes: probiotic and prebiotic foods. As with increasing your fibre intake, it's a good idea to increase your intake of these gradually, to give your digestive system a chance to get used to them.

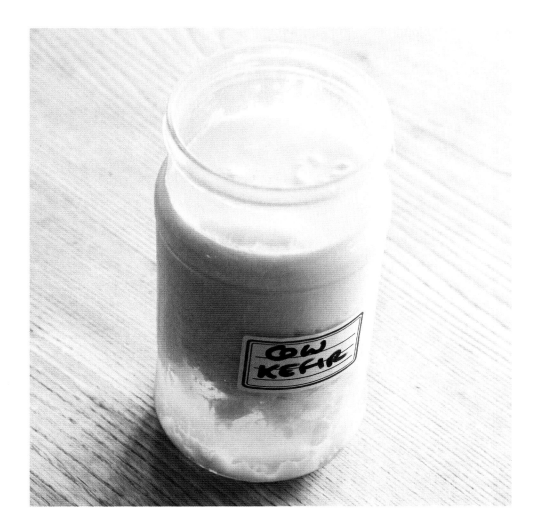

Probiotic foods and drinks are those that already contain live, beneficial bacteria and so can increase the diversity of bacteria in your gut. Usually these are fermented foods, with the bacteria that naturally cause the fermentation being the ones that remain in the product.

For those bacteria to still be active, the food needs to be 'live'. Heat kills bacteria – good and bad – so pasteurised products and cooked foods are no longer 'live'. (In dairy products like yoghurt and cheese made with pasteurised milk, fermentation happens after pasteurisation so they are still live.) Many products have selected bacterial cultures added by the manufacturer too – most notably 'bio' yoghurts. The strains of bacteria chosen for these are known to be relatively resistant to stomach acid and

go with your gut

so a proportion are likely to reach the gut alive. They include bacteria from the lactobacillus and bifidobacteria groups, both of which have been shown to have benefits. Bifidobacteria, for example, can help stimulate the immune system and fight off pathogenic microbes, while they appear to be depleted in people with inflammatory bowel disease, irritable bowel syndrome, obesity, allergies and autism.

Common probiotic foods and drinks

Yoghurt Especially 'bio' yoghurts that have been enriched with additional live cultures such as bifidobacteria and lactobacillus.

Kefir A tangy, yoghurt-like food often taken as a drink, though thicker, spoonable types are available (you can get water-based kefir too).

Kombucha A fermented, slightly fizzy, tea-based drink containing live bacteria (see my recipe on page 244). Do check the sugar content of branded kombuchas as some have more than others. Aim for kombucha with no more than 4.5g sugar or 18 calories per 100ml. And keep your serving to a couple of glasses (or one 330ml bottle) max.

Kraut and kimchi Along with other fermented vegetables (unpasteurised).

Miso and tempeh Both fermented soya bean products (unpasteurised).

Cheese Some traditional cheeses made with raw milk contain useful live bacteria. This includes unpasteurised, mould-ripened or blue cheeses – basically ones where bacterial activity is pretty obvious! Some aged hard cheeses are probiotic too, including traditional unpasteurised Cheddars.

These probiotic foods can be bought in health food shops, and are often available from supermarkets too. I've embraced pretty much all of the above, to varying degrees, and the 'three '3 Ks' – kombucha, kefir and kraut – have become almost constant presences in my kitchen. Sometimes I buy them, and sometimes I make my own, which I find highly satisfying. I'm sure you will too, which is why I have included recipes for them, on pages 244, 246 and 282.

Benefits of fermented foods

It is difficult for science to prove the specific benefits of eating probiotic foods or to explain exactly what they do to us. It's impossible to say, for example, 'yoghurt cures colds' or 'sauerkraut reduces cholesterol'. Both the foods themselves and our bodies' responses to them are complex and highly variable so isolating a single cause and effect relationship is very tricky.

However, exciting findings are accumulating: there is good evidence that probiotic yoghurt can help in conditions such as antibiotic-associated diarrhoea in children, gastroenteritis and allergies. Some research suggests that probiotics can help with IBS. In more than one study, regular yoghurt-eaters have been shown to have a reduced risk of type 2 diabetes. Consumption of the Korean-style fermented cabbage, kimchi, meanwhile, has been linked to a reduction in blood pressure and insulin resistance, which can in turn improve heart health and reduce the risk of type 2 diabetes.

Many researchers also think it's not just the bacteria in fermented foods that bring benefits. The action of those bacteria means the foods themselves are already partially 'pre-digested'. This can make it easier for our bodies to process them, and specifically for our guts to turn them into good things like SCFAs.

Fermented foods may also be more nutritious because bacteria can release 'bioactive' compounds with beneficial properties, as well as removing undesirable elements, such as phytic acid – a substance that can bind to minerals and stop the body absorbing them. Live bacteria make lactic acid, which may have anti-inflammatory effects, as well as B vitamins. 'Lactic fermentation' is what's going on when you make live kraut and kimchi (see my recipes on pages 282–7).

Fermented foods have been consumed for millennia, in most parts of the world. They have long been part of the traditional whole food diets that we in the West have, to our great detriment, been drifting away from. There's a powerful case for bringing them back, and I'm certainly an enthusiastic convert.

I try to eat live, fermented foods on a daily basis, as a way to boost my body's ability to take care of itself. And I'm not flying solo on this at home. Somewhat to my surprise, these ferments have become family staples. I've got my wife pouring kefir onto her breakfast muesli and, after the inevitable 'smells a bit farty' comments on his first encounter with kimchi, my eldest son is now obsessed with the stuff. And everyone loves kombucha – my youngest daughter says my homebrew is 'almost as good as the shop-bought ones'!

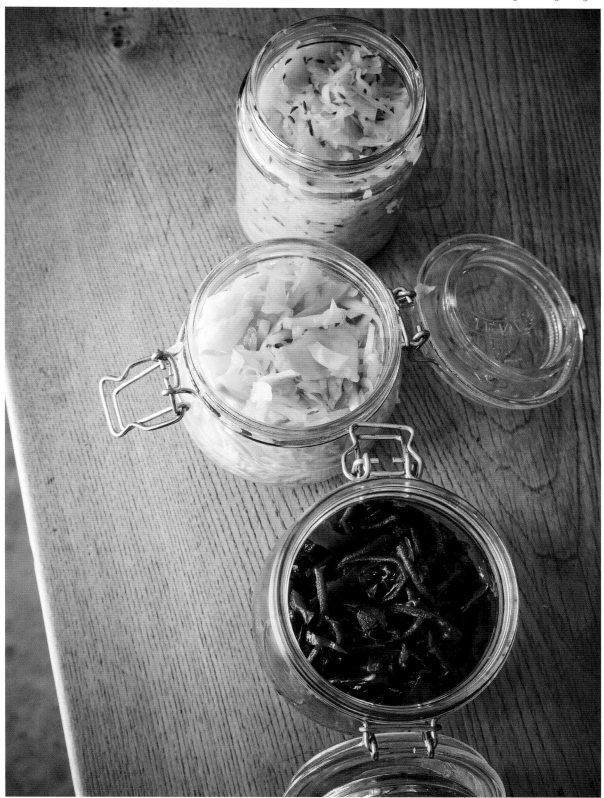

PREBIOTICS AND POLYPHENOLS

A *pre*biotic food doesn't contain any live bacteria, but rather is something that feeds and fertilises particular good bacteria and helps them do their thing. One of the best natural prebiotics is a form of soluble fibre called inulin, as it boosts the numbers of bifidobacteria. Inulin is found in high amounts in Jerusalem artichokes, garlic and dandelion greens, and in useful amounts in leeks and onions, asparagus, whole wheat and rye, and bananas. All these ingredients are good for you in other ways too, so they are brilliant things to include in a varied healthy diet.

Inulin is not the only prebiotic fibre, though. Others include beta-glucan, found in barley and oats; pectin, found in many fruits, but particularly apples, plums and citrus; and oligosaccharides found in pulses. Almonds, pistachios, flax seeds (linseed) and pumpkin seeds are prebiotic too. These foods can all feed your good gut bacteria.

Polyphenols are a particular type of phytonutrient (see page 32); i.e. compounds found in plants that are beneficial to human health. There's good evidence that polyphenols help to boost our good bacteria and quell the bad ones – acting, in effect, as prebiotics.

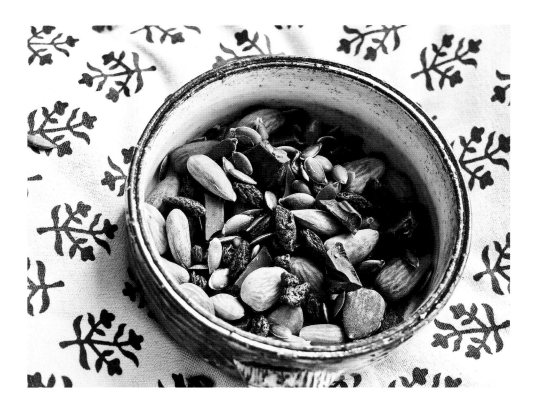

Polyphenols are found in fruit and veg, cereals and seeds but also in tea, coffee, red wine and cocoa. That is not a licence to eat tons of chocolate, but snacking moderately on nuts, seeds and a little dark chocolate can play a part in a healthy, gut-friendly diet.

Probiotic and prebiotic supplements

There's a huge range of products available these days designed to help improve the diversity of your gut bacteria, the most popular of which are probably yoghurt-based probiotic 'shot' drinks (which often contain quite a bit of sugar), and probiotic capsules containing 'billions' of freeze-dried bacteria.

The best way to nurture your gut is with real, whole foods, as these are what our bodies have evolved with. Real foods, including fermented foods that contain a range of live microbes, offer unique, complex and complementary packages of nutrients that our bodies can efficiently digest and use. These cannot be replicated by freeze-dried powdered bacteria in a capsule.

That's not to say supplements are useless, though they certainly can be expensive. Professor Tim Spector believes some probiotic supplements may be useful for some people – particularly if their gut bacteria is really compromised through illness or a course of antibiotics – but given that each person's existing microbiome is as unique as their fingerprint, it's a bit of a lottery as to how a standardised capsule or yoghurt drink will affect it.

I have used capsule probiotics after taking antibiotics (see overleaf). And I have tried one or two of those probiotic drinks, but found them far too sweet for my taste (which is saying something!). I'd rather consume unsweetened (or sweetened by me) natural organic yoghurt and kefir – which I do regularly. And I ring the changes with the brands I choose, as I know that different companies use different starter cultures based on different groups of bacteria. So why not mix it up?

Concentrated *pre*biotic supplements, mostly based on galacto-oligosaccharides or inulin, are also now widely available. I haven't tried these myself. Again, the consensus is that they could be useful for treating specific issues by delivering good amounts of concentrated, isolated prebiotic fibre to the gut, helping to nurture and 'fertilise' a flourishing biome. But bear in mind that too much can have some adverse affects, such as excess gas or trapped wind (see FODMAP foods on page 30) and that they may lack benefit if you don't already have the right microbes to digest them. So racking up real whole foods remains the priority.

THINK ABOUT ANTI-BIOTICS

There are things that are bad for our bacteria, which can be regarded as *anti*-biotics. That includes actual medical antibiotics – the kind we get from the doctor when we're ill, which are sometimes absolutely necessary, even life-saving. Unfortunately, however, anti-biotics will kill off good bacteria along with the bad. So if you are taking or have recently taken a course of antibiotics it is a very good idea to make a concerted effort to rebuild your levels of good bacteria. This may be the time to take a course of capsule probiotic supplements. That's something I have done in the past, and would do again. But it's even more important that you keep up, or even boost, your gut-friendly eating, on all the fronts we've discussed.

'Anti-biotic' is a term we might also use for things other than medicine that can shift the balance of our bugs in an unhealthy direction. These include processed foods and too much alcohol. Artificial sweeteners are another problem – they have been linked, with horrible irony, to an increase in the kind of gut bacteria that are associated with obesity. Stress and lack of exercise are also associated with poor gut health (see pages 200–3).

SHOULD I HAVE MY GUT BACTERIA ANALYSED?

It's now possible to have your own personal gut bacteria tested. There are companies (easily found online) who, for a fee, will analyse a stool sample and provide you with a description of your microbiotic 'fingerprint'.

It's a tempting prospect. Once you know there's this teeming microbiome inside you that is so crucial to health, it's quite natural to want to know how yours is shaping up.

And I have done it myself! The particular company I used sent me some pretty detailed feedback, including scores from 1–10 across various parameters, such as overall biome diversity, probiotics, butyrate (a short chain fatty acid which is considered a key indicator of health), presence of fibre, and B-vitamin synthesis (which depends on the gut biome). These scores are based on population percentiles – i.e. comparison with other people who have had their gut tested – so a score of 1 indicates you are in the lowest 10% for diversity or SCFAs or whatever, and a score of 10 indicates you are in the top 10%. I also got a very long list of the Latin names of bacteria types that were present, and not present. As you can imagine, that didn't mean a lot to me!

The expert view on such tests is that they certainly aren't necessary for improving your gut health, and should be taken cautiously, as they are quite hard to interpret and to follow up on. This is not like having a simple blood test for, say, low iron levels, that can then be dealt with using a common supplement. For a start, composition of the gut can change by the day so you'll only be getting a very brief snapshot. In addition, there is still so much more to find out about our guts. No one yet knows with precision what all those bacteria are doing, exactly what an individual's microbiotic fingerprint means or what should be considered 'normal'.

Some people who have had these tests report feeling at a loss regarding what to do with the data they get, and I can relate to that. My scores were a relatively reassuring bunch of 7s, 8s and 9s. Yet I found myself wondering if I should try and take my already pretty gut-friendly eating to another level, in pursuit of a set of 'perfect 10s'. In the end I decided that was not such a healthy idea! I have no immediate plans for a follow-up test but I probably will check it out again in a few years' time.

Some of these biome-testing companies are starting to link microbiome testing with personalised diet plans and recommended foods, which you can update on your own personal account or phone app. These are then cross-referred to recipes and, in some cases (mostly in the US so far) to online sales of certain foods and supplements. It's a fast-moving field, certainly, but we should be wary of how it's being commercialised.

If you are setting out on a mission to transform your gut health through smarter food choices, then using these tests to confirm your progress can be motivating. I have a friend, Steph, who did take 'before and after' microbiome tests, either side of a pretty radical reboot of her diet. As a very busy professional, she was a 'grab and go' eater, with a fondness for chocolatey treats and salty snacks. Her initial gut biome diversity score was a mere 3.

With a bit of input from me, Steph made a concerted effort to Go Whole and Go Varied, and also to introduce fermented foods to her diet. She retook the test after just 6 weeks and found her scores had changed radically. Her overall gut biome diversity score had risen to a 7! Steph told me she found the whole experience both shocking and helpful. She hasn't given up chocolate and crisps, but she's dialled them right down, just as she's dialled up the whole foods – especially fresh veg.

So taking a couple of tests might prove edifying or inspiring, particularly if your diet isn't good to start with. They are pricey, however (at least £120 a time). By all means splash out if you're curious. But bear in mind they are very much part of a developing field, rather than the last word on gut health. The fact is we already know that a high-fibre, whole food diet with plenty of prebiotic and probiotic foods is a very simple, safe and effective way to nurture your own microbiome and boost your gut health. You don't need take an expensive test to confirm that.

SITTING PRETTY

There's some more new information related to our gut health that I am profoundly moved by, quite literally, and that I would like to share. It's got a bit less to do with what goes into the gut, and a bit more to do with the what comes out. Or, to be more accurate, with the *way* things come out. Now this is a delicate area, but an important one, so please read on.

A few years ago, I discovered the work of a brilliant young German microbiologist named Giulia Enders. She has dedicated herself to studying our guts, what makes them work well and what makes them unwell too. A good deal of what I've said in this chapter is influenced by her research. And if you want to take your understanding of the human gut to another level, then her book *Gut* is not only fascinatingly informative but a genuinely entertaining read!

One thing in the book that really grabbed my attention relates to, shall we say... the engineering of elimination. Or, more bluntly, how we position ourselves for a poo. Most of us in the West sit on a porcelain throne, of course. But in terms of human history, this is a relatively recent and relatively localised practice. For centuries, people would always do their business while squatting – and millions of people worldwide still do.

This matters because the way most of us sit on our shiny white loos leaves our bowel in a position that is actually not very conducive to letting go, with a loop of muscle holding our lower internal sphincter closed and the route from gut to butt somewhat contorted. Squatting, on the other hand, in a position where the knees are higher than the hips, encourages the sphincter to open and creates a more direct passageway from bowel to bum.

There is plenty of evidence that this posture makes pooing quicker and easier, and, given what we know about the physical and financial cost of constipation (see page 28), that's reason alone to give it a try. But Enders suggests it does more, facilitating a more complete elimination of our bowels, and so releasing the pressure in our rectum that can lead to nasty conditions including haemorrhoids (piles) and diverticulitis.

This is in part supported by the fact that incidences of these health conditions are significantly rarer in countries (mainly in the East) where squatting is still far more common than sitting on a loo. I say 'in part', because these also tend to be countries where the national diet is higher in whole foods and fibre, so this could account for some of the effect.

To me, this shift in pooing position seems an obvious commonsense complement to a healthy diet – it's one more way to be good to your gut.

The good news is that if you fancy trying a squat, you needn't abandon your comfy, warm bathroom for a hole in the back garden. You can easily create a comfortable semi-squatting position by putting your feet on a block or step, placed in front of the loo. This will help to elevate your knees, and encourage you to lean forwards slightly.

Indeed, you can now buy specially designed bits of bathroom furniture for this very purpose – known variously as 'Squatty Potties', 'poop steps', 'toilet steps' and the like. And many people have bought them, myself included. Some are expensive, but others cost a tenner or less, and I reckon that's money well spent.

It's worth knowing that you can easily improvise a loo-step, too. Any box or block that is sturdy enough to take the weight off your feet, and about 20–30cm high, will do the job. When I'm travelling and staying in hotels (or even in other people's houses!) I often commandeer a waste paper bin, turned upside down if necessary, to use as an impromptu loo-step. And in the loo next to my office at home (where I'm writing right now) I use a pile of old cookbooks.

So as you can tell, I'm a total convert. I found Giulia's explanation of the benefits of squatting compelling. It's worked for me and it still does – 3 years on. I don't think I will ever go back.

BRINGING IT ALL TOGETHER

I realise that not all of us are completely comfortable contemplating the connections between the food we eat, and how effectively our body is eliminating what remains of that food a day or so later. But these things are so important, and so vitally connected (by that brilliant bit in the middle – our beautiful guts), that I really believe it is worth putting aside such scatalogical squeamishness. So I don't mind admitting (and I hope you don't mind hearing) that I feel a genuine satisfaction, both physical and mental, in sensing and observing that this whole rather miraculous system is working well.

And in the end I think it's not merely gratifying, but genuinely motivating, to know that what's making it work well is the good food choices I am making – particularly the ones I've talked about in this chapter. It encourages me to continue to make them every day, and to think about how I might make even better ones in the future.

These kinds of thoughts will feed very usefully and positively into the mindful approach to eating we're going to explore in Chapter 7. For now, let's resolve to harness them for the simple but compelling reason that when our gut works better, our whole body and brain work better too. And that will help us to feel great, from head to toe.

ACTION POINT RECAP

1 Go Whole and Go Varied – again!

Follow the action points of the first two chapters and keep following them! This is unquestionably the best way to develop and maintain a healthily diverse spectrum of gut bacteria.

2 Go live

Eat more probiotic and prebiotic foods – they are a fantastic way to nurture your gut bacteria. Consider making them the first thing you eat in the day (at least on some days) as this is one way to maximise their effects. Yoghurt or kefir and a banana for breakfast is a great idea. And there's certainly no reason not to have a spoonful of kraut or kimchi with your breakfast eggs and wholegrain toast (see page 238). Fermented foods are also an easy win when putting together a quick lunch or lunchbox (see the recipes on pages 282–7). And when you sit down for a family supper, why not put the kimchis and krauts on the table as tummy-loving condiments?

3 Avoid the antis

Do your gut a further favour by avoiding things that are not good for it – notably highly processed foods, artificial sweeteners, and alcohol. Unfortunately, antibiotic medicines are not beneficial to our gut bacteria either. However, they are sometimes vital and you should take them if your doctor tells you to. It's a good idea to make a special effort to look after your insides when you take them – by eating lots of gut-friendly foods.

4 Ask your gut!

Before you eat anything, ask yourself, 'Is this good for my gut?'. That might sound like an odd thing to do, as you sit down to a meal or start on a snack. But asking that question can encourage you, for example, to leave your fruit (and some vegetables) unpeeled (more fibre), or to choose whole raw nuts instead of roasted salted ones (more polyphenols). And it can nudge you to healthier gut-friendly snacks, like oatcakes and cheese with kraut (instead of chutney!), berries with fresh yoghurt, or dried fruit and nuts with a square or two of dark chocolate. You may even find it helpful, as I do, to visualise these lovely whole foods travelling down inside you and being gratefully received by a host of happy hungry bugs!

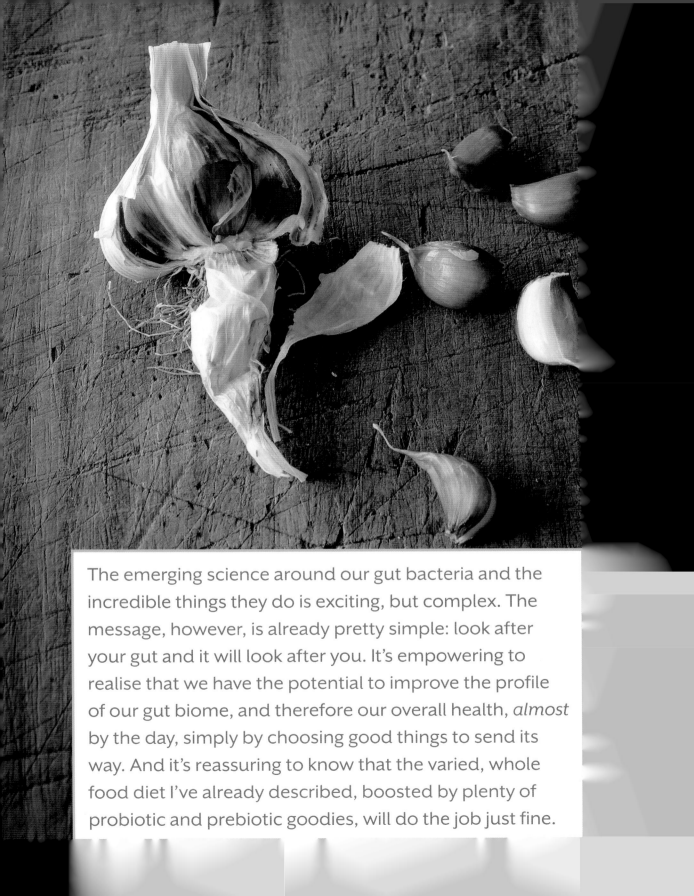

The emerging science around our gut bacteria and the incredible things they do is exciting, but complex. The message, however, is already pretty simple: look after your gut and it will look after you. It's empowering to realise that we have the potential to improve the profile of our gut biome, and therefore our overall health, *almost* by the day, simply by choosing good things to send its way. And it's reassuring to know that the varied, whole food diet I've already described, boosted by plenty of probiotic and prebiotic goodies, will do the job just fine.

4

REDUCE REFINED CARBS

Now we come to the stuff that we need to eat less of. If I could avoid this bit I would. I think we prime ourselves to succeed when we think more about what we *can* do and what we *can eat* than what we should avoid.

Happily, many less-healthy foods will fall away naturally as we dial up fibre-rich whole foods and the sheer variety of what we eat. But there are some baddies we need to focus on and take active steps to dial down.

For me, this isn't just about individual action. It needs addressing by government. If, as a nation, we want to step out of the growing shadow of obesity, and all the related illness it brings, then almost all of us need to eat fewer refined carbohydrates. They are the opposite of whole foods, and have pretty much the opposite effect on our health. Yet they are everywhere, and we are being urged to eat them wherever we turn.

Taking action on obesity is, at long last, on the government agenda. Now we need the action to match the rhetoric.

I am not advocating an out and out low-carb diet. There is nothing wrong with carbohydrate in itself. It is one of the three main building blocks of human nutrition (the other two are protein and fat). Found in many plant foods, carbohydrate is an integral part of the complex, nutritious, well-balanced package offered by whole fruits, vegetables, pulses, nuts, seeds and grains, and a good source of energy.

In fact, fibre is a form of carbohydrate – a natural, complex form of it. And, as I've discussed, fibre is something we desperately need more of in our diets, not less. Low-carb diets that cut out whole grains, starchy vegetables and fruits can make it very hard to get enough fibre.

So, the complex carbohydrate contained in natural, whole plant foods is really not a problem – this is exactly the kind of carbohydrate we need. But the minute you start tinkering with it, the trouble begins.

SO, WHAT EXACTLY ARE 'REFINED CARBS'?

Refined carbs are processed, by stripping out fibre-rich cellulose and bran for example, which takes away not only fibre but most of the nutrients that were originally part of the package too, leaving you with easily absorbed calories – and very little else.

Take sugar, for example. It starts off as part of a plant – either the chunky roots of sugar beet or the thick, bamboo-like stems of sugar cane. Both plants have plenty of fibre and healthy nutrients. But the sugar in them undergoes an extraordinary mechanical and chemical journey before it arrives in our kitchens. The original plant is chopped or crushed and soaked, the resulting fluid is treated with lime and carbon dioxide, filtered and boiled to a syrup, crystallised, centrifuged, 'washed' and dried. The fibrous body of the original plant is a distant memory and even the brown, syrupy molasses component of the sugar, which contains vitamins and minerals, is usually removed too.

Sugar is one of the major refined carbohydrates in our diet. The other is refined grain – particularly white flours derived from wheat, maize and rice. To make these flours, the original whole grain is stripped of its bran and its germ, which together contain around 75% of the grain's nutrients, including fibre, B vitamins, vitamin E, iron, copper, zinc, magnesium and various phytonutrients. Without the bran and germ, you're left with the endosperm, the bulky part of each grain, which is soft, starchy and easy to digest.

In short, refining robs carb-based foods of their nutritional value while making them very easy to eat, in quantity. Think about how soft and woolly-textured white bread can be: it's really not difficult to put away several slices without feeling full.

Most of us buy packets of sugar and white flour to make the occasional cake or batch of cookies, or we perhaps dip into the sugar bowl in order to sweeten our tea. And if that's all we were talking about, we wouldn't have such a problem. But those domestic examples are only the tip of the refined carb iceberg. Sugars and refined grains are *everywhere* now because they are the building blocks of both long-standing staples, like white bread and pasta, and many new, highly processed foods.

WHAT FOODS CONTAIN REFINED CARBS?

In combination, refined sugars, syrups, flours and starches are central to a huge range of modern processed foods, including:

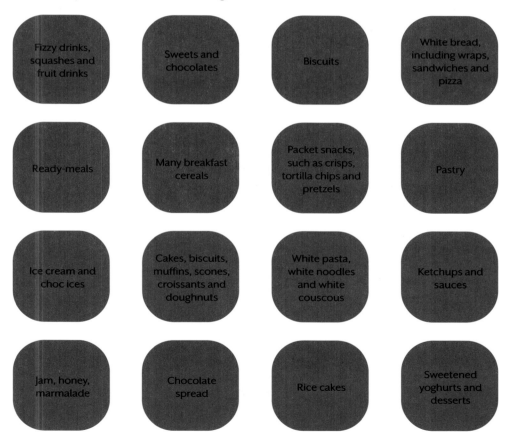

Fizzy drinks, squashes and fruit drinks

Sweets and chocolates

Biscuits

White bread, including wraps, sandwiches and pizza

Ready-meals

Many breakfast cereals

Packet snacks, such as crisps, tortilla chips and pretzels

Pastry

Ice cream and choc ices

Cakes, biscuits, muffins, scones, croissants and doughnuts

White pasta, white noodles and white couscous

Ketchups and sauces

Jam, honey, marmalade

Chocolate spread

Rice cakes

Sweetened yoghurts and desserts

WHAT'S WRONG WITH REFINED CARBS?

The fact that refined carbs offer little in the way of nutrition or goodness is a huge problem; the more of them we eat, the more high-fibre whole foods are elbowed out of our diets. But this is just the beginning. The next, even more insidious issue is that our bodies digest refined carbs really fast. This is because they are often finely ground (as in the case of flours, starches and white sugars) or even dissolved in liquid (as in fizzy drinks and concentrated squashes).

In effect, a lot of the work of breaking down these carbs has already been done by a machine. Foods based purely, or mostly, on refined carbs are therefore absorbed by our bodies much more quickly than fibre-rich whole foods would be. As Dr Giles Yeo has explained (see page 31), their calories are just 'too available'.

That is bad news because, after this swift digestion, our blood sugar shoots up. That stimulates a corresponding surge in the hormone insulin, which brings the blood sugar plummeting back down but can very quickly leave us feeling hungry again.

In other words, even though they are usually packed with calories, refined carbs don't fill us up and can actually drive recurring spikes of hunger, leading us to consume yet more. And when we get caught in this cycle, it's very easy to gain weight.

Refined carbs and excess body weight

Body weight should not be the sole means by which we measure our health, but it is really important. Being overweight or obese increases the risk of many very serious illnesses, including several types of cancer as well as type 2 diabetes, stroke, heart disease and dementia. Being obese can reduce life expectancy by anything between 3 and 10 years. And, crucially, carrying excess weight can rob us of healthy years while we are alive – it could be the thing that compromises our health at the age of 60, rather than, say, 70 or 80.

Reaching and maintaining a healthy weight is one of the most profound ways in which you can safeguard your health. The very last things we need are foods that make that difficult – foods loaded with refined carbs. Just as the latest science on healthy eating is clustering around consensus on the value of wholeness and variety in our foods, it's also concurring on the damage being done by refined carbs.

Professor Christopher Gardner, at Stanford University in the US, ran a year-long programme involving over 600 people aged 18–50 years, trialling a low-fat/high-carb versus a low-carb/high-fat diet. He wanted to find out whether a person's genetic make-up would predispose them to lose weight on one, or other, regime. But in both cases, the participants were also instructed to choose high-quality whole foods as the backbone of their diet.

As it turned out, it wasn't possible to predict who would do well on which diet and neither low-fat or low-carb came out 'on top' overall. But people did lose weight, lots of it – some up to 60lb over the year. Professor Gardner and his team suggested that the healthy eating pattern itself was the success story here. 'In my work, I see three factors come up again and again when it comes to successful weight loss,' he said. 'Get rid of added sugar, get rid of refined grain and eat as many vegetables as you can.'

Refined carbs and other health issues

The link to weight gain is probably one reason why diets high in refined carbohydrate can be associated with an increased risk of cancer, stroke, type 2 diabetes and heart disease. Refined carbs can also raise triglycerides (fats in the blood), cholesterol and blood pressure. They are a key component of what is now called a 'pro-inflammatory' dietary pattern; and inflammation in the body is linked to many diseases.

Refined carbs have also been identified as a risk factor for something called insulin resistance. This is when the body stops responding to insulin, even when there are high levels of it in the blood (a bit like someone shouting at you so much that you stop listening), and consequently, blood sugar stays dangerously high. Insulin resistance is a key driver for type 2 diabetes.

Professor Frank Hu, an expert on diet and obesity at Harvard Medical School, has also pinpointed refined carbs as one of the key problems in our modern diet. He has written about the foolhardiness of trying to strip fat out of our diet only to replace it with refined carbs. 'That doesn't reduce our risk of chronic disease,' he says, 'it does the opposite – and people who are overweight seem to be most vulnerable to the effects of refined carbs because they probably already have a level of insulin resistance.'

'The obesity epidemic and growing intake of refined carbohydrates have created a "perfect storm" for the development of cardiometabolic disorders, such as diabetes, heart disease and stroke,' says Professor Hu. 'Reducing refined carbohydrate intake should be a top public health priority.'

Isn't it great when top scientists can not only agree, but boil down their complex findings to such clear, achievable advice?

REDUCING SUGAR INTAKE

We need to cut back on sugar. White, 'golden', brown and 'unrefined' (which is still highly processed and in no way 'whole'), as well as syrups like maple and agave, honey and additives like glucose, dextrose and fructose – it's all sugar!

Sugary drinks in particular have been directly linked to weight gain and associated health problems (see pages 136–8). And there is evidence that the more sugar you eat (or drink), the more calories you eat overall – in other words, when we eat sugar, we tend not to compensate by eating less of anything else. This is because refined carbs don't satisfy us, and often lead to cravings. The government and the World Health Organization tell us we should be getting no more than 5% of our energy each day from added sugar. British adults actually get around 12%, and British teenagers an alarming 15%. Those numbers need to come down.

We can help that to happen by reducing our taste for sugar – by adding less of it to our food, and buying fewer sugar-added processed foods. We can still enjoy the natural sweetness of foods like nuts and dried fruits – though always in moderation. More on this shortly.

It's not just about sugar

Demonising sugar on its own won't solve our refined carb problem. It's helpful to group refined carbs together. They act in a similar way on our bodies. They are all bad news. Cutting out sugar but continuing to load up on white bread, white rice and corn chips doesn't make much sense.

The rather hackneyed adage, 'there are no bad foods, just bad diets' doesn't really hold up – and provides a spurious cover for the junk-food industry. I think highly refined carbs actually *are* bad foods – unnatural formulations that our bodies cannot process in a healthy way. They offer empty calories, carrying little in the way of nutrients and comprehensively failing to fill us up or make us feel satisfied. They drive hunger and overeating, play havoc with our blood sugar and energy levels, and they're linked with increasing rates of serious illness. It's outrageous to blame people for making 'bad choices' when the choices offered by the food industry are so often so bad.

But we shouldn't be cutting out carbohydrate *per se*. The quality of the carbs we eat is what matters. We should become much more carb-*selective*, eating a fibre-rich, whole food diet that includes healthy carbs – fruits, vegetables, whole grains and pulses – in their natural, nutrient-packed form.

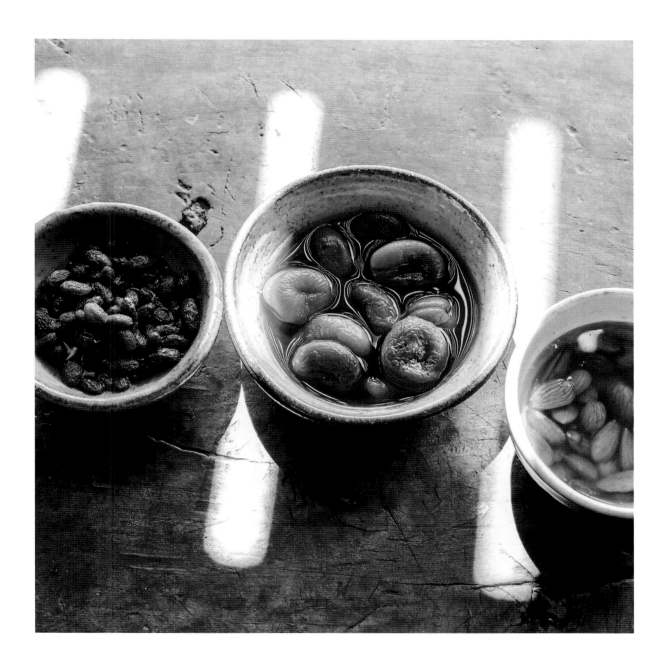

WHY ARE REFINED CARBS OMNIPRESENT?

Refined carbohydrates are ubiquitous. They've have got their sticky, floury little claws into endless different products, even those you might not expect: yoghurts, 'healthy' protein bars, veggie burgers, stock cubes, baby food...

Is this because they are nutritious, delicious or sustaining? No. They are omnipresent for two overwhelming reasons. Firstly, due to a combination of huge subsidies for the crops from which they are derived and industrial processing on a massive scale, they are cheap. And secondly, because their nature renders them extremely malleable, so they make the role of processed food manufacturers easier. Refined carbohydrates bind, thicken, glue and sweeten; they stabilise, moisten, firm and crisp. They blend with other highly processed ingredients to produce uniform food units that are easy to package, transport and store; and also easy to buy, cook and eat. It's all very convenient. But refined carbs are bad for us – really bad for us.

THE BLISS POINT

Let me tell you about the 'bliss point'. Sounds pretty sexy, doesn't it? In a way it is – certainly if you're a chocolate bar manufacturer. The 'bliss point' refers to the precise quantities of sugar, fat and salt within any one product that makes us metaphorically swoon with pleasure, then go right back for more. It is the holy grail of snack food designers. Nailing the bliss point means a food will trigger the reward centres in our brains in a way no natural food ever could. That is why you'll never get the same buzz from an apple that you would from a Mars bar. It's the reason that, no matter how much we know about healthy eating, we find highly processed foods, full of sugar and fat, so hard to resist – and it's why I'm focusing on them in particular when I talk about the tough issue of how we simply say 'no' to food sometimes.

The fat-sugar combo

Recent evidence shows that not only do we love to eat foods that contain both sugar (or other refined carbohydrate) and fat, but that we often find it almost impossible to *stop* eating them. We have inbuilt instincts that limit our intake of sugars and fats when eaten separately (imagine trying to eat a jar of sugar or a packet of butter) – but when these two are combined, those instincts are by-passed. Scientists believe that, because the sugar-fat combo barely exists in nature, we have not evolved mechanisms to deal with it. Our bodies and brains do not have an off-switch for it. So we find sugary, fatty foods like ice cream, biscuits, cakes, chocolate bars and doughnuts all too easy to eat in large quantity. And carby, fatty, salty combos, like crisps and nachos, get us too.

The food processing industry has human biology working for it. In our distant past, when food was scarce, largely plant-based and unpredictable, it was essential to our survival to take in sugar and fat whenever we could. A find of honey or a haul of sweet, ripe fruit or oil-rich nuts was a great boost, because it offered relatively high energy for relatively little effort. Now, of course, high-energy foods are the opposite of scarce. They are everywhere, and most of them are based on refined carbs and fat. But our animal instincts haven't had time to catch up. Our bodies and brains still have a strong sense that sugar and fat are things we need to eat whenever we find them. Our reward centres are still telling us they are a great find, even when they are doing us profound harm.

Time to get angry!

The thing that makes me angry (and hopefully you too) is that food manufacturers know all this. They know it and they exploit it cynically. And because their irresistible, bliss-pointed products sell well, retailers push them right under our noses too. Big business is peddling these harmful foods in the full knowledge of the damage they are doing. The prevailing view among health experts is that the ubiquitous availability of foods that are built mainly from highly refined carbs – most of our drinks, snacks, sweets and takeaways – is at the very heart of the global obesity crisis.

We need to resist. That doesn't mean pledging to never eat a chocolate bar, a bag of crisps or a takeaway again. But it does mean recognising these foods for what they are: intrinsically unsuited to helping us be well. So, if we do eat them from time to time (because, like anyone, we are susceptible to that bliss-point temptation and the short hit of pleasure it provides) then we should do so with the commitment that they will be our exception and not our rule. And that our rule, which will offset these occasional indulgences, is to make real, whole and healthy foods the mainstay of our daily eating.

While we are on the subject of getting angry, here's something that makes me positively incandescent: these obesogenic, damaging, sugar-heavy foods are targeted most ruthlessly at those with the least ability to resist them – our children. TV advertising, highly sophisticated marketing campaigns, promotional toys and gifts, branding with favourite cartoon characters – all of these things are designed to lure our children into consuming sugary, salty processed foods every day, as a matter of course.

The shocking result of this is that, despite the fact that we understand more about it than ever before, feeding our children well is becoming harder, not easier. Perhaps alarmed by the threat that better understanding of healthy eating poses to their bottom line, the food industry seems to have been doubling down on the aggressive marketing of junk food to kids. Product design gets smarter, the advertising spend gets bigger and the message that all this junk is really just fine for our kids settles deeper into the collective psyche. The pressure on parents is relentless. Saying no and policing our kids' food becomes exhausting.

And so it's a very welcome, if long overdue, development, that our government has recognised the seriousness of this problem, and resolved to take action. Curtailing the advertising of junk food on TV before the 9pm watershed is one central policy plank that will undoubtedly make a difference. Using cartoon characters to sell unhealthy foods to children also has to stop. And as so much of children's media is now consumed online, restrictions will need to be applied there to.

It will be some time before we see if the government action on obesity is robust enough to make a difference. And in the end the only difference it can bring is to help us make better choices. I don't underestimate how vital that support is. But until it kicks in (and frankly even when it does) our own vigilance and resolve, informed by good science and improving knowledge of what healthy eating really is, will need to see us through.

And we might want to reflect on whether the very idea of 'kids' food' is wrong-headed. We all need more or less the same kind of food – healthy, varied and whole.

A note on salt

Too much salt is bad for us. It increases the risk of high blood pressure and the associated risk of stroke and heart disease. If you have high blood pressure, there is clear evidence that cutting back on salt can help to lower it.

The maximum salt intake for an adult should be around 1 tsp (6g) a day – and note, that's meant to be the maximum, not a daily requirement. The target healthy intake is actually just 3g a day. On average, British adults are eating around 8g of salt a day – nearly triple that target. Our salt intake has actually reduced in the last decade or so, but clearly we still need to cut back.

We get around 75% of the salt in our diet from processed foods, including ready-made sauces, ready-meals, takeaways, bread products, processed meats and cheese, as well as salty snack foods like crisps and salted nuts. The best way to reduce your salt intake is to cut back on these over-salted processed foods.

We also need to be more restrained in seasoning our own cooking with salt, and that's something I have certainly done over the last few years.

CUTTING BACK ON REFINED CARBS

So much of the refined carbohydrate we eat is hidden in processed foods. To consume less of it, it helps to be able to see it. So it's a good idea to look at the back of the pack as well as the front. Ingredients are listed in order of amount, so if sugar or flour is the first item in an ingredients list, you know it is a major constituent of what you're holding in your hand. You don't have to put it in your shopping trolley!

Learn the label lingo

It certainly helps to get to grips with the terminology: sugar is not always called sugar. It is also found in the form of syrups, fruit juice concentrates and additives ending in 'ose' (maltose, dextrose, glucose, fructose etc.). Under these various guises, it is in everything from 'diet' yoghurts to cooking sauces, cereal bars to soft drinks. And in addition to the 'wheat flour' that goes to make bread, cakes, biscuits and pastries, are refined starches such as wheat starch, modified maize starch and maltodextrin. You'll find them in everything from chicken nuggets to chocolate mousse, salad cream to instant soup.

The sugar content of all manufactured foods is shown on labels as the number of grams of sugar per 100g of the product. It's not straightforward, as this figure includes naturally occurring sugars (for example in dried fruits) as well as added refined sugars. But you can cross-refer to the ingredients list to see what refined sugars are present. I'd say that any product that has more than 10g sugar per 100g should give you pause, and anything over 20g per 100g should be ringing alarm bells.

This doesn't just apply to products that you would expect to contain added sugar; you need to be vigilant with so-called 'savoury' products too. Frozen ready-meals, jarred sauces and pickles, including onions and gherkins, can often have alarming amounts of sugar. Check those labels.

Many packs now feature coloured traffic light labels – these are genuinely useful. Reds and oranges for sugar content are always worth a pause. We can expect to find red for sugar on biscuits, cakes and sweet treats – which is a good reason not to pick them up in the first place! But when choosing, say, breakfast cereals or yoghurts, I think we should have zero tolerance for red (which signifies more than 22.5g sugar per 100g). Orange merits a check on the actual amount of sugar, as it covers a wide range, from a relatively untroubling 5g sugar per 100g to the 22g threshold for red.

This traffic light labelling remains voluntary and some manufacturers are still putting the info on the pack without colour-coding it. So, don't let a row of benign-looking black and white numbers fool you – check what they actually mean!

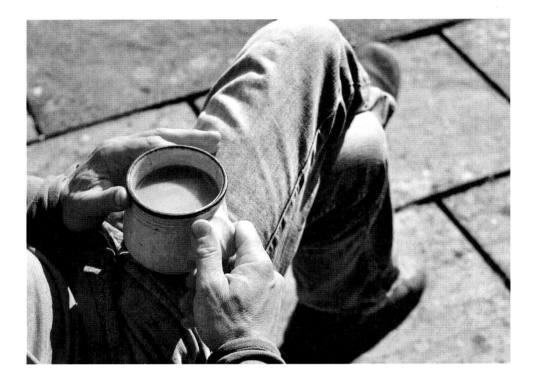

Retrain your sweet tooth

If, like me, you *know* you have a sweet tooth, then training it to get the same satisfaction from (ultimately much) less sugar is an excellent idea. Systematic reduction over time is the key – and it doesn't actually take long.

Reducing sugar in hot drinks is a relatively easy win and a great place to start. If you take even one spoonful of sugar in your cuppa, and you have only, say, four cups a day, then that's 20g of sugar. Over a week, it's 140g sugar (weigh that out and have a look at it – it's more than you'd get from a whopping 200g bar of chocolate). Over a year, it's more than 7kg sugar! If you take two or even three spoonfuls in your hot beverages, and you drink several a day, that's kilos and kilos of sugar going into your system over a year that you really don't need (and that definitely won't do you any good).

For years I took sugar in my hot drinks and I thought I would never be able to stop. Even (especially) when I got it down to one spoon per cup, I was convinced I'd hit my sweet-toothed limit, and would leave it there for life. Whenever I tried to go sugar-free, the attempt would run aground within a week. I just found my sugarless tea and coffee unsatisfying. Then a friend told me quite categorically, 'A week isn't enough, it takes two!' She was right – for me at any rate! After *two* weeks of drinking tea and coffee without sugar, I was quite content. My undeniable sweet tooth was starting to adapt, becoming more sensitive so I could appreciate the trace of sweetness that comes with the dash of milk, and it was all I needed. It's all I need today.

And it's not just about the tea and coffee. I'm convinced those sugary cuppas were supporting and fostering a sweet tooth that wasn't doing me any favours. I've always liked sweet things and I'm sure I always will. But now I know I can get the same pleasure from less sugar, and it's helped me dial down the sweetness in a lot of my cooking. And, of course, it's much better for my teeth!

Some people will succeed by going cold turkey when moving to sugar-free hot drinks, others may find a gradual reduction over a few weeks works for them. But I promise that once you are accustomed to unsweetened tea and coffee, you won't go back. In fact, adding sugar will make them taste horrible to you!

There's much more that you can do, of course, to retrain a sweet tooth. Cutting out sugary drinks (page 138) will help massively. Developing a 'sugar antenna' and avoiding oversweetened foods and dishes (however 'artisan' they may be), and scaling the sugar right back when you cook, is the way to go. And try to take your family with you, even (or especially) when it comes to the family's favourite treats, sweets and cakes...

Take control of the cake tin

Most of us like a sweet treat now and then, and most of our kids do too. But shop-bought biscuits and cakes almost invariably carry a heavy cargo: refined carbs, notably sugar and flour (along with saturated fat – often palm oil). They're not good news. Homemade biscuits and cakes can be rich in those things too. And no one actually needs cake in their life. So, if you're not a big fan of muffins and millefeuilles, then that is fantastic news for your health. Give yourself a massive high-five and move on to the next page. But if, like me, you are not quite prepared for a life without cake, read on.

I love home baking, for and with my family, and I'm not about to give it up any time soon. So, I've developed a form of better baking. I haven't found a way to make great cakes without any sugar at all, but I have found lots of ways to make our home-baked goods a whole lot 'wholer'.

A home-baked Victoria sponge, made from just flour, butter, sugar and eggs, is already a better, tastier option than a shop-bought version laden with a bunch of unhealthy ingredients and additives. But we can do way better than that. Our home-baked treats were transformed initially by one critical swap: I stopped buying plain white flour and started using wholemeal instead. The best type for general home-baking is fine wholemeal flour, which also goes under various other labels – wholemeal cake flour, wholemeal pastry flour etc. In all cases, the pack should tell you that it's intended for cakes, biscuits and pastries rather than bread. This is the flour that goes into all the cakes, scones, crumbles, pancakes and biscuits that we now make at home.

The next tweak is that I usually reduce the sugar in recipes by at least 20%. I promise you, no one even notices. I favour (and love devising) recipes for treats that include nuts, seeds, dried fruits, fresh berries and even grated veg. You'll find a run of such recipes on pages 384–395 that have become some of our family favourites. They prove deliciously that Going Whole does not mean missing out on the joys of home-baking.

Having said that, taking control of the biscuit tin also means leaving it in the cupboard sometimes. As with alcohol (coming up in Chapter 6), sweet treats are not something to make a daily, dependent habit of. So once in a while, when the biscuit tin calls, just note the moment has occurred – and make a beeline for the fruit bowl instead.

Having my cake and eating it?

I've been writing cookbooks for more than 25 years, and during that time I've published plenty of recipes containing refined carbs: cakes and desserts based on white flour and sugar, and dishes that I suggest serving with white pasta, white rice or white bread. My tune has changed. I can do better, and we can all do better.

These days I ask myself whether the new recipes I'm devising need any refined carbs at all. Can I make them as delicious as possible with only whole food ingredients? Or, when sugar is needed, how little can do the job?

I'm not going to disown my older recipes for cakes, treats and puds. But if you have any of my cookbooks on your shelf, I would actively encourage you to tweak some of those recipes where you see the chance to make them 'wholer'. This is what I've been doing at home quite systematically for a few years now, reducing sugar quantities, swapping in wholegrain flours, and switching white for brown with rice, pasta and bread. It's an overhaul I heartily recommend.

Healthier snacking

In principle, you can apply the same approach to seeking out healthier ready-made snacks and treats: look for less added sugar, more fibre from wholegrain cereals, more dried fruit and nuts. You'll have noticed there's a huge range of so-called 'healthy' snack bars that are promising they've done just that… but we need to be cautious.

When we pick up such treats off the shelf, rather than making them at home, we are no longer in charge of the ingredients. And these clusters of cereals, nuts and dried fruits

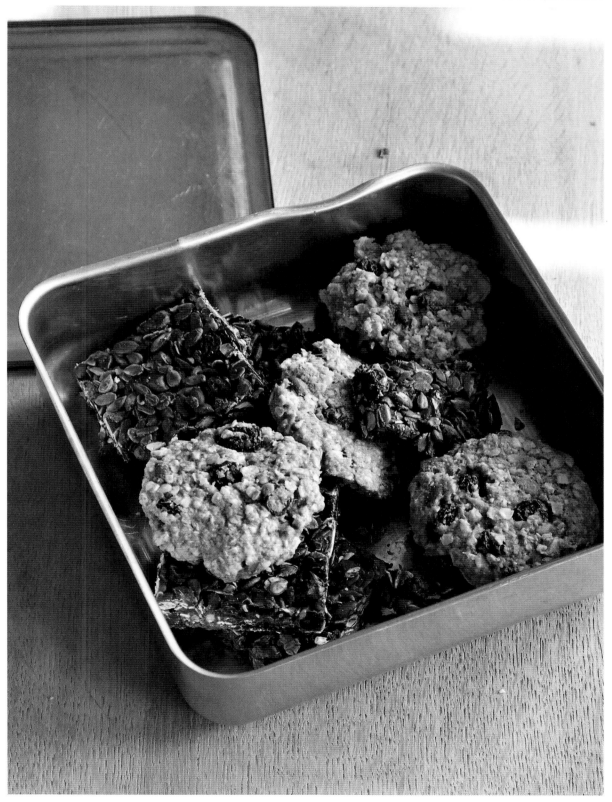

are often glued together with alarming amounts of refined sugar, notably glucose. These 'healthy' snack bars also seem to be homing in on the idea that 'protein' (often blazoned in giant capital letters on the packaging) is some kind of miracle food, that we might be in danger of missing out on. Or that it's the 'antidote' to carbs. Protein is an important food group, and nuts, seeds and pulses are great sources of it. But if you use them generously in your cooking, along with other whole foods, you really don't need them squashed into a fist-friendly rectangle by an industrial machine.

In the end, if you are looking for healthier snacks built around nuts, seeds and dried fruits, then it has to be worth asking yourself: Why not simply eat nuts, seeds and dried fruits? Buy the ones you like the best, mix them up yourself, and take them with you in a little reusable snack box. That way you can dodge the unnecessary plastic as well as the unnecessary sugar. And if you want to make up an even treatier trail mix (see page 84), add a little chocolate too. But make it the good stuff…

In the end, the best reason to recalibrate your sugar susceptibility is not only to reduce your exposure to a potentially harmful food that has few upsides. It's to enhance your pleasure in the very healthiest of foods. Almost all plants – not just fruits and roots, but leaves and shoots and nuts and seeds – contain abundant natural sugars. And as you wean yourself off (or at least significantly reduce) your taste for added sugars, you will increasingly relish the subtle (and sometimes outrageous) sweetness of those that are built in to whole foods. And that will make you feel so much better.

Check your chocolate

Chocolate is a pretty powerful symbol of what's gone wrong with our food system. At its core is a powerful natural ingredient – cocoa – rich in nutrients, dark and bitter, that has been valued for centuries as a health-giving food. Now, it is utterly fetishised yet utterly debased, the cocoa solids themselves often a mere vehicle for sugar and fat. Most milk chocolate is engineered to perfectly elicit that bliss-point response, making it almost impossible to have just a little bit and very easy to eat to the point of nausea.

Chocolate lovers, we need to return to true chocolate – to chocolate that's full of actual cocoa, with its antioxidants, minerals and even fibre. Nutritionally speaking, the darker the better (the flavanols in cocoa seem to be good for our all-important gut bacteria.

So, if you don't want to chuck in the choc, wean yourself on to a darker bar. Look for lower sugar bars too: say 20–25% sugar (there are dark chocolates out there with 50% sugar, more than some milk chocolate!). Eat a scant square at a time, letting it linger in the mouth and relishing every complex flavour note. Partner it if you like (as suggested above) with the natural and complementary sweetness of whole nuts and dried fruits.

There are also environmental and ethical issues in the farming of cocoa. Taking this into account too, I'd say the best possible way to reboot your relationship with chocolate, making it both healthier and happier, is to go dark, go Fair Trade and, ideally, go organic.

Not so daily bread

Bread is the bedrock (bread-rock?) of the Western diet. It's easy to eat, most of us love it and most of us tuck into it several times a day, both as part of a meal, and as a quick-fix snack. According to the National Association of British and Irish Millers (NABIM), the equivalent of nearly 11 million loaves are sold each day in the UK. Between 60% and 70% are made with refined white flour, which is digested quickly, sending up the blood sugar yet scarcely nourishing the body.

White bread can easily become a major contributor to our refined carb intake, and that's not a good thing. However, if you opt for bread made with unrefined wholegrain flour, its status changes: it becomes a contributor to our wholegrain intake and a source of fibre. And that's a much better thing.

It's true that, to some schools of thought, all bread is problematic. Some modern diet plans, notably Paleo, cut out bread and other grain-based foods altogether, reasoning that grains would not have been part of our ancestors' diets, and therefore we haven't evolved to digest them well.

These anti-bread arguments may have elements of truth to them. Obviously, our ancestors weren't roaming the plains of Africa foraging for bagels or baguettes. And it's clear that even in recent history, the grain we make our bread from has changed. Modern types of wheat are different from those that were eaten even 50 years ago. But there's not sound evidence that all bread is bad for all people.

Having read and thought about it quite a lot, I have decided not to banish bread from my diet. Instead, recognising that some breads are a lot more problematic than others, I have resolved to reduce my bread habit, and only to eat better bread. I no longer eat bread every day. In fact, I don't eat bread if it doesn't pass a couple of tests. First, I want to know, is it made with at least 50% wholemeal flours and minimal additives (ideally only yeast, water, salt and maybe a dash of oil)? Second, is it going to be delicious? If I can't get two yesses, I'll pass on it.

In the end, eating less, and better bread can be a big part of the balancing act that dials down refined carbs, making way for more whole foods, that do us *so* much more good.

ACTION POINT RECAP

1 Be carb-selective: recognise and replace refined with whole

Unrefined carbs from whole, high-fibre foods are good for us; they help us feel satisfied and energised, and they aid good digestion – and elimination! Refined carbs are the opposite – the good stuff is stripped out, leaving an over-available pile of empty calories. So know the difference, and act on it: cut right back on foods that are denatured, processed and packaged, and replace them with foods that are natural and whole.

2 Reduce your taste for sugar

Obviously sugar is not the only refined carb but it is the most pernicious – and the easiest to spot. Reducing the visible sugar in your diet is a good move. Get rid of the sugar bowl, if you have one, and wean yourself off adding sugar to breakfast cereals and hot drinks. Use it sparingly to make healthy foods (like rhubarb!) taste more delicious. And work steadily on recalibrating your sweet tooth by avoiding over-sweetened foods and removing or reducing the added sugar in your cooking.

3 Un-refine your treats

Factory-made confectionery, biscuits, cakes, waffles, muffins and pastries are some of the most obvious sources of refined carbs in our Western diet – and unfortunately the most popular. Many of them contain very little *except* refined carbs! We don't need them. That doesn't mean we should *never* have them – but let's see them for what they are: packets of pleasure, not goodness. If you use these foods for sustenance, rather than fun, the lack of goodness will soon take the edge off the enjoyment. Learn to take pleasure in treats that do you good, like dried fruits, raw nuts and a bit of dark chocolate. And when you do want to indulge in something baked, why not make it yourself? You can avoid the worst ingredients and tailor the recipe to be 'wholer' and healthier.

4 Eat less and better (wholer) bread

Too many of us lean too hard on bread. We eat too much, too white, too often. If that's you, it's time for a change. Eat less bread... and better bread, ideally wholegrain. The 10:1 carbs-to-fibre rule is really useful on packaged bread, so check the 'nutritional data' panel: if there is at least 1g of fibre for every 10g carbohydrate, you're on to a good thing. And don't stress if the bread runs out: it doesn't have to be daily.

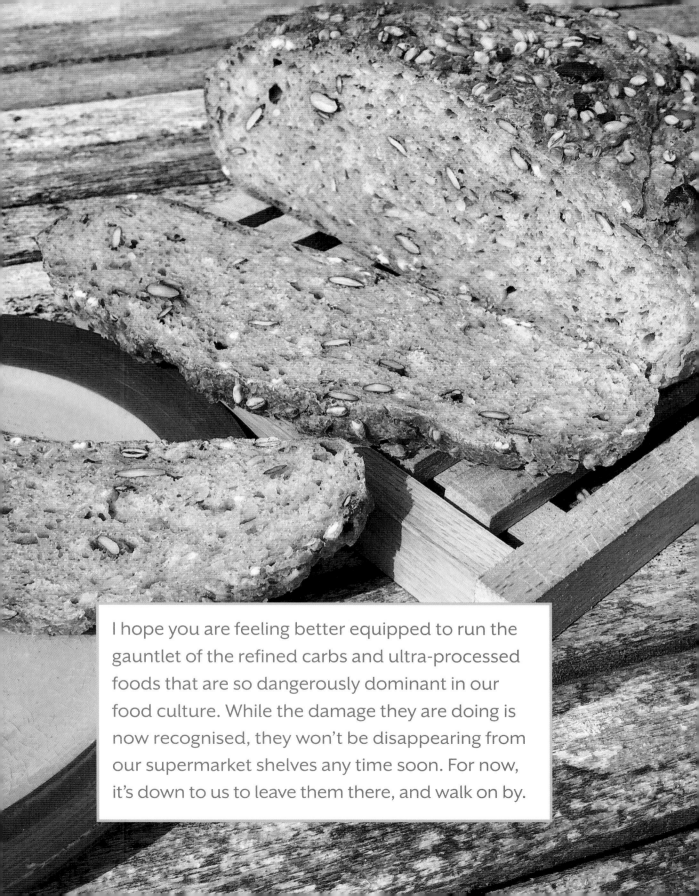

I hope you are feeling better equipped to run the gauntlet of the refined carbs and ultra-processed foods that are so dangerously dominant in our food culture. While the damage they are doing is now recognised, they won't be disappearing from our supermarket shelves any time soon. For now, it's down to us to leave them there, and walk on by.

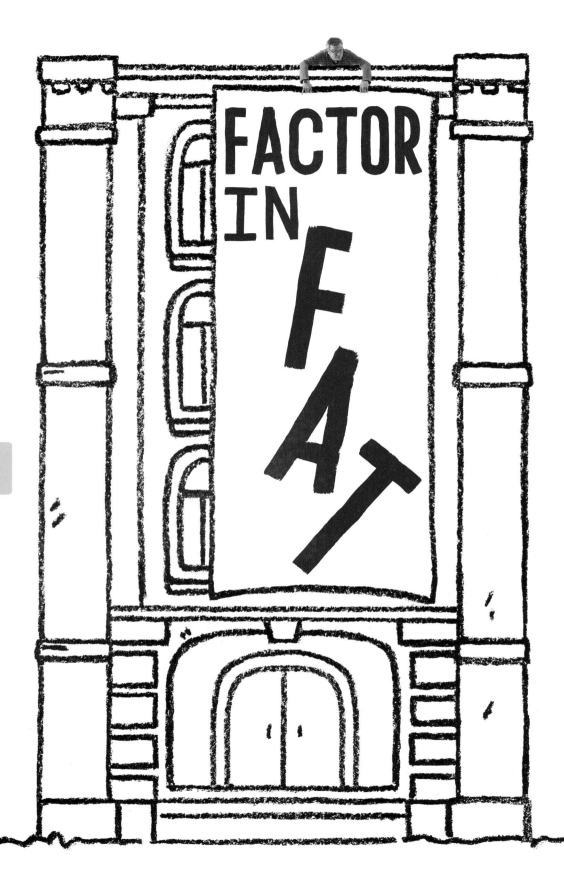

We need healthy fats in our diet. Yet for decades now, describing a food as 'low-fat' has been the same as calling it 'good for you' – implying fats are intrinsically bad. That's a misconception – a deception even. And it's one peddled by the diet-food industry to make a fortune out of selling us products that proclaim they are 'less than 2% fat', '97% fat free', or even '0% fat'. Let's get some perspective.

There are lots of different fats (and oils); some are good for us, most are fine in moderation, and a few are best avoided. The right amounts of the right fats are not only good in themselves, they can help make other healthy foods even more delicious. And that's a great virtue.

DON'T FEAR FAT

Fat is a weighty word, freighted with guilt, shame and confusion. For too long, fat – all fat – was portrayed as the dietary devil, thickening our waistlines and clogging up our arteries. We need to be smarter than this.

Fat is essential to humans, as it is to almost all animals. It provides energy, and is vital for the functioning of many cells within the body, including brain and nerve cells, and for moving the fat-soluble vitamins E, D, A and K around our bodies in the bloodstream. The World Health Organization tells us that adults need at least 15% of their daily energy to come from fat – an approximate minimum of 30g a day for women and 40g a day for men. If we are active and not trying to lose weight we can consume around double that.

Fat is also a great carrier of flavour, which makes it incredibly useful in creating delicious meals. This is so important. If 'healthy eating' becomes an ascetic act of self-denial,

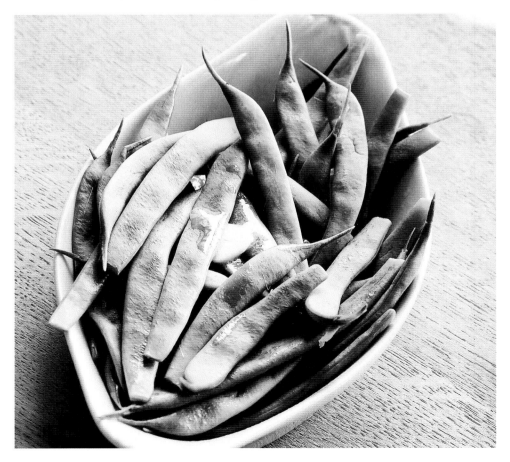

restricting us purely to 'virtuous' foods we don't actually enjoy, then we are all going to fail at it. I for one would be glum to give up the nut of butter I put on the first pick of peas or beans. A fat-free diet would be bad for our health and bad for our morale.

These vital truths about fat need to be factored in and the scaremongering weeded out. Let's start by recognising when refined fats are being used in combination with other refined carbs (see the previous chapter!) to make hard-to-resist foods that are not good for us. Know them, cut back on them or better still avoid them. Meanwhile, use the good fats well to make healthy food more delicious. Keep them where you can see them – the olive oil on the shelf, the butter and cheese in the fridge. Once again, wholeness (and the absence of industrial meddling) is the key.

THE FAT FURORE

Our fraught relationship with fat can be traced in part to a moment in 1983 when, in the midst of a rising tide of coronary heart disease, the National Advisory Committee on Nutrition Education released a report that suggested we reduce overall fat consumption to no more than 30% of total energy intake, and our saturated fat to a mere 10%. A key factor behind that advice was the belief that a diet high in saturated fat increases the risk of heart disease. And our consumption of saturated fat certainly was too high at that point, being about double the recommended level.

Deriving 30% of energy from fat is not particularly low – certainly not what you would call a 'low-fat' diet. But in the 1970s we were eating about 40% fat, around half of which was saturated, so the advice represented a significant reduction at the time, and was enough to light the blue touch-paper on a low-fat craze that swept the Western world.

That set the tone for the next 30 years of dietary advice in Britain, and it also shaped and fostered our processed food industry. Fat, including saturated fat, occurs naturally in many foods, so manufacturers started to develop ways of taking it out. But since fat is the source of some of the pleasure of eating, they had to find things to replace it with that would also be pleasurable. Foremost among those were refined carbs, starches, sugar, salt, emulsifiers and flavourings, all deployed to make foods more immediately appealing to our palates. Our diet certainly changed with the 'reduce fat' advice of the 1980s, but not necessarily for the better.

Was the advice simply wrong? The answer is: not exactly. But by isolating fat as the single 'baddie' in our diets, and demonising all forms of it, we have thrown out the baby with the bathwater. Not only that, but we've replaced fats in our diets with foods that are mostly no better for us, and often considerably worse.

UNDERSTANDING DIFFERENT TYPES OF FAT

Fat comes in three basic forms – saturated, monounsaturated and polyunsaturated. Saturated is the dominant type in animal-derived fats such as butter, cream, cheese, fatty meats and processed meats. It's also the main fat in some plant oils, including coconut oil and the palm oil found in many shop-bought cakes, biscuits and chocolates. To give you a brief scientific description, saturated fats have a dense, well-bonded chemical structure. Their molecules include a maximum number of hydrogen atoms – i.e. they are 'saturated' with hydrogen. That means they are usually solid at room temperature and are very stable – or resistant to oxidisation – which is why they keep well, and are so useful in food manufacturing.

Mono- and poly-unsaturated fats have a different, more flexible chemical structure, with fewer hydrogen atoms, making them usually liquid at room temperature. They are also less chemically stable and can oxidise more easily, which is why you might find the odd rancid nut in a bag (nuts being rich in monounsaturates), and also one reason why fish (rich in polyunsaturates) goes off so much more quickly than meat.

The evidence that has accumulated since the early 1980s has given us a rather more sophisticated understanding of fat in our diets. Optimum health requires the right *balance* of fats and other nutrients. But few people in the medical profession would dispute that too much saturated fat is bad for your heart. Most experts agree that eating a lot of saturated fat can raise 'bad' LDL cholesterol. (LDL stands for 'low-density lipoprotein'; this is the harmful type of cholesterol that gets deposited and narrows our arteries.) The other kind of cholesterol, HDL, or 'high-density lipoprotein' is actually heart-protective and we *don't* want to lower levels of that. In addition, too much saturated fat is also linked to *other* risk factors for heart disease (and indeed other major diseases), including chronic inflammation and insulin resistance, a key driver of type 2 diabetes.

QUESTIONING THE ROLE OF SATURATED FAT

There is a small but highly vocal contingent of doctors and dietitians who have questioned the role of saturated fat in heart disease – and this has caused huge media noise. One headline-grabbing analysis, published in 2015 in the British Medical Journal, concluded that the anti-fat guidelines of 1983 were not backed up by decent evidence (although there has been more good evidence since). In addition, there are one or two recent studies that could not find a clear link between saturated fat intake and heart disease. However, the group who deny the saturated-fat/heart-disease link have been roundly criticised by others in the health profession for cherry-picking evidence to suit their arguments and for using misleading data. The majority of the experts stand by the belief that too much saturated fat is bad for our hearts. But that doesn't mean we have to avoid eating saturated fat altogether. And we must remember that some other forms of fat are actively good for us! In fact, some are essential to our health.

It's really important to note that virtually all foods that contain fat contain *all three types* – saturated, monounsaturated and polyunsaturated. So, for example, while olive oil is around 75% monounsaturated fat, it is also 14% saturated fat, and 11% polyunsaturated. Lard, on the other hand, is about 40% saturated fat, about 50% monounsaturated and 10% polyunsaturated. Nature tends to give us a blend of all three fats, and eliminating any one of them from the diet is actually almost impossible. But that's okay, because we don't need to.

The reason we all get so confused about fat is that health messages have been over-simplified. In the media, different fats are consistently taken out of context and described as being purely good or purely bad. In addition, when a few commentators question the accepted wisdom on fat, they get so much media coverage that it looks as though the entire medical world is in disagreement. But it isn't really.

A HEALTHIER WAY FORWARD

The message on fat is actually pretty straightforward: a moderate fat diet, particularly a Mediterranean-style diet rich in mono- and polyunsaturated fat, is healthy. Saturated fat should be kept at low levels – but what's really important is what we replace it with. The most up-to-date and thorough analysis is in a report from the government's Scientific Advisory Committee on Nutrition, produced in 2019. It concludes that reducing saturated fat and replacing it with polyunsaturated fats reduces the risk of heart attacks and stroke, while replacing saturated fat with monounsaturated fat specifically lowers 'bad' LDL cholesterol – which further reduces the risk of heart disease. So clearly it's the 'polys' and 'monos' that are going to be the best source of healthy fats in our diets.

The debate on fat will probably continue to be a maelstrom – not least because it seems to make great news, or at least irresistible click-bait. But despite what the headlines sometimes suggest, no doctor, dietitian, researcher or scientist, no matter their position in the debate, is arguing that you can blame fat (or any other single nutrient) for ill health.

There is also a general consensus that fat is essential in our diets. And finally, *nobody* thinks highly refined ingredients are a good idea – and that certainly includes the refined fats that are used in many processed foods. More on these refined or 'altered' fats to come…

When you take these well-supported positions together, there actually is a pretty clear, commonsense path through the fat issue, and it's this: ditch the unhealthy fats found in processed foods, keep an eye on the saturated fats, and eat moderate amounts of poly- and monounstaurated fats, ideally from whole foods.

You can happily leave it there if you like. But if you want the nitty gritty, which might just help you see through the media smog on fats, read on:

ARTIFICIAL TRANS FATS

Just as the experts concur that it's best for our bodies if the fat we eat comes from natural, whole foods, there is universal agreement that the very worst type of fats are the artificial or altered 'trans fats' found in highly processed foods, including takeaways.

Small amounts of trans fats occur naturally in some animal foods, including dairy products, beef and lamb. They are things we have always eaten, and at low levels they are not a cause for concern.

Industrially produced trans fats are a different story. They are formed when liquid vegetable oils are subjected to a patented process called 'partial hydrogenation'. This is done by heating a liquid oil, combining it with a nickel catalyst, then adding hydrogen gas at high pressure. The result is essentially to force extra hydrogen atoms into the oil, thereby artificially 'saturating' it, and altering the molecular structure in a way that makes the fat solid at room temperature. It is very far from being a natural process.

This chemical transformation means that, like the natural saturated fats they are designed to (cheaply) replace, partially hydrogenated vegetable oils are firm, yet malleable, and have a long shelf life. This makes them very useful in food manufacture. Towards the end of the twentieth century, they became a major building block of processed foods, from margarines and spreads to pastries and cakes.

One consequence was that our consumption of trans fat rose to between 5 and 10g a day. That might not sound like a lot – but it's more than enough to be harmful.

It isn't understood exactly how altered trans fats act on our bodies and why they are so damaging. But in the 1990s, a clear link was made between eating trans fat and a significantly increased risk of coronary heart disease. A 2015 study found that a trans-fat intake of 6g a day compared to 2g a day increased the risk of heart attacks or strokes by about 40%.

Consequently, industrially produced trans fat are now banned in some countries. That does not include Britain, though over the last few years British manufacturers have voluntarily reduced their use of them in processed foods (often by replacing partially hydrogenated oils with palm oil – not so great for the planet). Our overall consumption of trans fat in the UK is now very low.

However, you will still find them in some products – notably those that list 'partially hydrogenated vegetable oils' among their ingredients. 'Mono- and diglycerides of fatty acids' (or E471) is another ingredient – still commonly used – that may be a source of some trans fat. It is used as an emulsifier and appears in many processed foods including margarines and spreads, cakes and cake mixes, hot chocolate mix, custard mix, pastries, breads and buns, ice cream and manufactured potato products such as crisps and croquettes.

Avoiding the bad trans fats

Takeaways and deep-fried food are major potential sources of dangerous trans fat in our diets. This is because they are still used in the manufacture of the kind of extruded potato products and crumb-coated items so popular as takeaways. But it's very hard to know if your takeaway chips or your chicken nuggets are trans-fatty or not – because you never get to see the labels. But even if they don't contain trans fats there is an additional issue here: fried takeaway food is often cooked in sunflower oil, or another polyunsaturated oil. Those oils are fine when used cold but there is now evidence that when heated to a very high temperature, they can oxidise and form toxic compounds called aldehydes (more on this on page 128).

Add to all of this the fact that take-out fast foods are often laden with salt and refined carbs, and you've got three good reasons for skipping them: it's going to be a win-win-win for your health. If takeaways are more than an occasional treat in your life, that's well worth addressing. Easier said than done, obviously, but achievable nonetheless.

One of the first things to consider is changing your routine. So often, bad habits are just that – habits. They can be altered. Something as simple as taking a different route home to avoid the chip shop can make a difference. Or replacing a regular takeaway with a different 'treat' – a trip to the cinema, for example (after a healthy meal at home).

One of the major appeals of take-out food is the total absence of effort it requires from you. One great way to be prepared for those evenings when you simply do not have the energy to cook is to have something homemade and healthy stashed in the freezer. Take your portion of veg curry out in the morning and it will be defrosted by the time you get back from work. Veggie soups can be defrosted directly in a warm pan in the same time it takes for a kebab to be delivered. And it's worth keeping a few potatoes or sweet potatoes on standby to bake and eat (skin and all!) with salad, hummus or tinned mackerel – or trickled with my pestomega (page 278), which takes no time to make in a food processor.

The recipes in the book are designed to help you swap out the takeaways for easy, healthy home-cooking.

SATURATED FATS

The latest available figures from the National Diet and Nutrition Survey (covering the years 2014–2016) show that Britons get 33–36% of their energy from fat, which is just about okay. But within that, we are still getting up to 16% of our energy from saturated fat, and that is too high. Foods rich in saturated fats include full-fat dairy products, fatty red meat, coconut oil – and also palm oil, which is used in many processed foods and is one reason why these are often a rich source of saturated fat.

We needn't banish saturated fat from our lives, we just need to keep it down, as dietitian Dr Michelle Harvie confirms. 'I advise people to get no more than 10% of their energy each day from saturated fat,' she told me. 'In real terms that's no more than 30g for men and 20g for women each day.'

Actually, that's not too stingy: purely as an illustration, 30g saturated fat is the total you'd get from a small steak, plus 60g Cheddar and 1 tbsp of butter. That doesn't mean we should all eat a cheesy buttered steak every day. But it does suggest we don't have to be overanxious about saturated fat in order to eat a healthy diet.

The fact is that if you follow a whole food diet with lots of vegetables, fruits, whole grains, nuts and seeds, it's pretty easy to keep your level of saturated fat low without having to think about it too much. If you eat moderate portions, you're active, you keep your weight down, you don't smoke and you reduce the stress in your life (see pages 202–3), then a small amount of saturated fat from whole foods is not something you need to worry about (unless you have been told otherwise by your doctor).

But keeping saturated fat at low levels in your diet is a good way to protect your heart – so be on the lookout for ways to both dial it down, and swap it out for preferable fats.

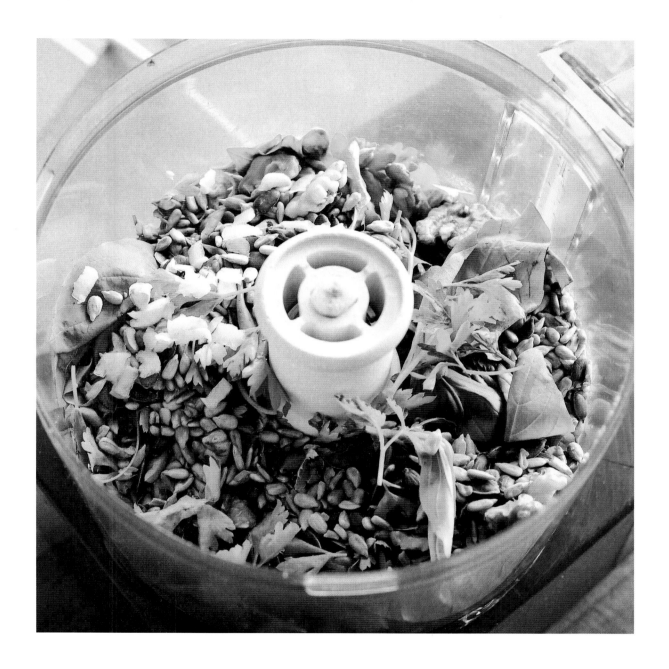

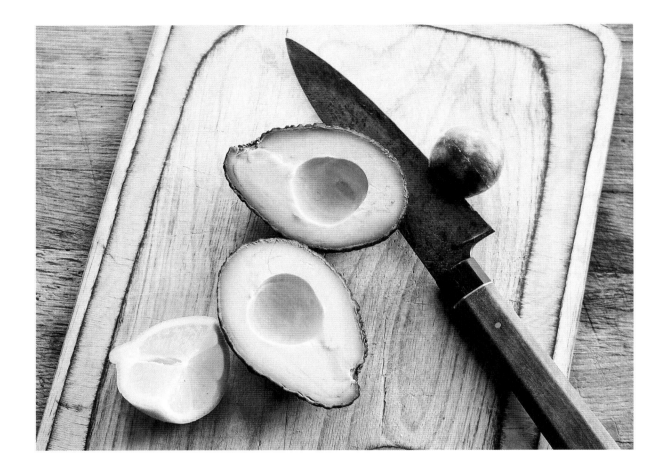

Easy ways to cut back on saturated fats

Butter swaps... Trickle your breakfast toast with extra virgin olive oil and top with tomatoes or spread with a little nut butter and sprinkle with fresh berries (see page 233). Hummus or bashed avocado (see page 233), or any veg blitz trickled with a little oil, are other tasty toast toppings that negate the need for butter. If you like butter on your cooked veg, try using a splash of cold-pressed rapeseed, olive, hemp or walnut oil instead, or at least ring the changes.

Cream swaps... Creaminess is a desirable quality in so many dishes – but it doesn't always have to come from cream! Blitzed-up nuts and seeds are a great alternative. Plain unsalted cashew nuts or almonds, soaked in water, can be blitzed into soups and sauces (see my dairy-free gratin on page 347). Smooth nut butters like peanut or almond can do a similar job of 'creaming' dishes and are particularly good in curries.

Cheese swaps... The savoury, umami richness of cheese is very good at bringing a dish together, but thick blankets of bubbling cheese carry a lot of saturated fat with them. One tip is to use highly flavoured cheeses, such as Parmesan (or a vegetarian alternative) or mature Cheddar, of which you only need a small amount to make a big difference to the flavour.

Alternatively, whole nuts, lightly toasted then roughly bashed, are a good alternative sprinkled on top of bakes or soups, or tossed through salads. A touch of something rich and salty, such as olives or anchovies, or my tamari-roasted pumpkin seeds (see page 281), can also hit the umami savoury spot. Just be restrained with quantities.

Meat moderation... For omnivores, reducing the saturated fats that come with meat is more about moderation than swaps. It starts with simply eating less meat – especially processed meats like sausages and salamis. And it extends to trimming the fat off steaks and chops, and skimming it from the top of meaty stews.

Curbing my enthusiasm for crisps

I love a crisp. But who ever eats just one? For millions of us, crisps and an almost infinite range of other fried, bagged snacks hit the bull's eye of the carb/fat intersection – the 'bliss point' described on page 100 – and leave us craving more.

A regular 25g bag of crisps will have 7–8g fat. A 50g 'grab bag' will have around 16g. That's close to a quarter of your daily allowance. Foods with this much fat in them – not to mention loads of salt – just shouldn't be everyday foods.

I have suggested some healthier swaps – raw nuts and dried fruits, for example (on page 108). But reducing our consumption of crisps and the like isn't just about finding alternatives. It's about recognising their nature and setting limits. Yes, they give us pleasure. But that's all they give us.

When the pleasing crunch, teasing mouth-feel and momentarily satisfying swallow is gone, they travel down into our stomachs, where they can do nothing good for us, and they may actually do us harm. That's what I tell myself every time the snacks trolley on the train approaches. And I'm much, much better at letting it roll on by.

Has this oft-repeated note-to-self enabled me to eliminate crisps from my life? Not entirely but, as part of a more mindful approach to eating (of which more in Chapter 7), it has helped me curb my careless consumption and I've got my crisp habit down to a bag a week... two at the absolute most.

MONOUNSATURATED FATS

Monounsaturated fats are the fun ones to talk about, as they include some of the most delicious and useful culinary oils, some lovely nuts and seeds, and they are good for us. We know that they help to lower artery-narrowing 'bad' LDL cholesterol. Prevalent among them are olive oil, rapeseed oil (including generic 'vegetable oil', which is usually refined rapeseed) and most nut oils, as well as avocados and whole nuts, sesame and pumpkin seeds, and nut butters and tahini (sesame seed paste).

In Spain, in the early 2000s, the PREDIMED study put three groups of people who were at high risk of heart problems (due to factors such as smoking, obesity or family history) on test diets for a five-year stretch. One was a Mediterranean-style diet supplemented with extra virgin olive oil, one was a Mediterranean diet supplemented with nuts, and one was a reduced-fat diet. At the end of the study, the two groups following the Mediterranean diets had suffered fewer 'cardiovascular events' such as heart attacks or strokes than those following the low-fat plan. In short, the Mediterranean diets, generous in their allowance of monounsaturated fats, seemed to have a protective effect on heart health – a result that backed up previous findings.

The classic Mediterranean diet model, rich in vegetables, fruits, whole grains, nuts and olive oil, and relatively low in dairy and red meat, is moderate fat, not low fat. But the fat comes largely from olive oil and/or seeds and nuts – both rich sources of monounsaturates. Of course, this fat can't be the only explanation for the heart-healthy effects of the diet. The PREDIMED study authors themselves theorise about a 'synergy' (that word again!) amongst the various nutrient-rich foods in the Mediterranean diet that reduces health risks. But this study is cited by many experts from different fields as good evidence that a traditional Mediterranean style diet is about the best possible option there is for most of us.

So, I would advise using plain (non-virgin) olive oil or generic 'vegetable oil' as your main oils for cooking, and virgin/cold-pressed olive or rapeseed for trickling over dishes and for making dressings.

POLYUNSATURATED FATS

Polyunsaturated fats are a good replacement for saturated fat but we need to think a little bit about the type of polyunsaturated fats we're choosing. The richest sources are vegetable oils such as sunflower and corn oils. The particular type of polyunsaturated fat they contain – called omega-6 – is abundant in the Western diet. We do need omega-6, but we also need omega-3 – the other kind of polyunsaturated fat, of which we eat far too little. Omega-3 is vital in the diet as it has anti-inflammatory effects in the body. Diets with a higher omega-3 content have been linked to lower blood pressure and triglycerides (circulating fats in the blood), and a lower risk of heart disease, stroke and some cancers, including breast cancer. Omega-3 may also have a role in reducing depression, and in improving muscle health as we age. So the ideal is to shift the current balance more towards 3 than 6.

Recent research suggests that taking omega-3 isolated in a supplement (fish or krill oils, for example, often not sustainably sourced) is of little or no benefit, which underlines the value of an overall healthy diet versus the ramping up of one particular nutrient. Simply taking omega-3 supplements won't 'overcome' a bad diet, particularly if that diet is high in pro-inflammatory saturated fat.

The best sources of omega-3 are oily fish such as mackerel, sardines, herring, salmon, trout and tuna. The last three on that list raise considerable issues of sustainability, so my preference is very much for the first three. Shellfish such as mussels and oysters also deliver a decent dose. The omega-3 in all these seafoods is also of the type most readily absorbed by the body. It's good to eat at least one portion of oily fish a week (though no more than two for pregnant or breastfeeding women) and in our house I try to make it two or three. If you are struggling to keep omega-3 oils on your radar, then it's really worth resolving to change that. Here's how…

Simple ways to get more omega-3 oils into your life

Mackerel is my favourite fish. One medium-sized mackerel is a perfect one-person serving; a big one will feed two. It's an easy fish to prepare, and mackerel fillets are, of course, even easier. Try the lovely, easy recipe for fresh mackerel on page 356.

Tinned, preserved and smoked fish – tinned mackerel, smoked mackerel, kippers, rollmops, anchovies etc. – are a convenient and tasty way to get some omega-3. These processed forms of fish often contain quite a lot of salt, so use them judiciously – a couple of times a month is fine. See recipes on page 264 and 268.

Fresh mussels are a great source of omega-3; they're sustainably produced and easy to cook (see recipe on page 320).

If you don't eat fish, you can get omega-3 from walnuts, chia seeds, rapeseed oil and walnut oil, flax seeds (aka linseed), hemp seeds and hemp oil (see my recipe for pestomega on page 278). You'll also get some omega-3 from leafy green veg.

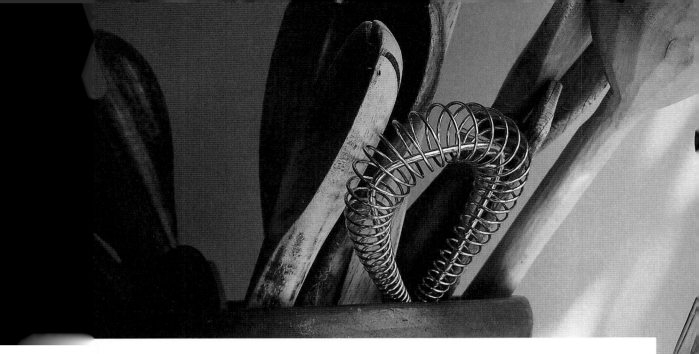

FATS AT-A-GLANCE

Here is a low-down on the different fats and their uses, increasing in virtue as we move from left to right across the chart. Note that all fats are equally calorific, providing about 9 calories per gram.

TYPE OF FAT	Trans fats	Saturated fats	Polyunsaturated omega-6
MAIN SOURCES	Less common now but still found in some processed foods; also in partially hydrogenated vegetable oil. Deep-fried foods and foods containing the emulsifier E471 may be a source too	Animal fats: butter, lard, cheese, cream; some vegetable fats: coconut oil, palm oil	Most sunflower, corn and soybean oils
PROS	None	Very stable when heated; solid at room temperature	Heart-healthy
CONS	Linked to an increased risk of heart disease	Can raise 'bad' LDL cholesterol	Not very stable when heated
BEST WAYS TO USE	Ideally never!	As a treat in your cooking (cakes, puddings, bacon sandwiches etc.)	Use unheated; i.e. on salads

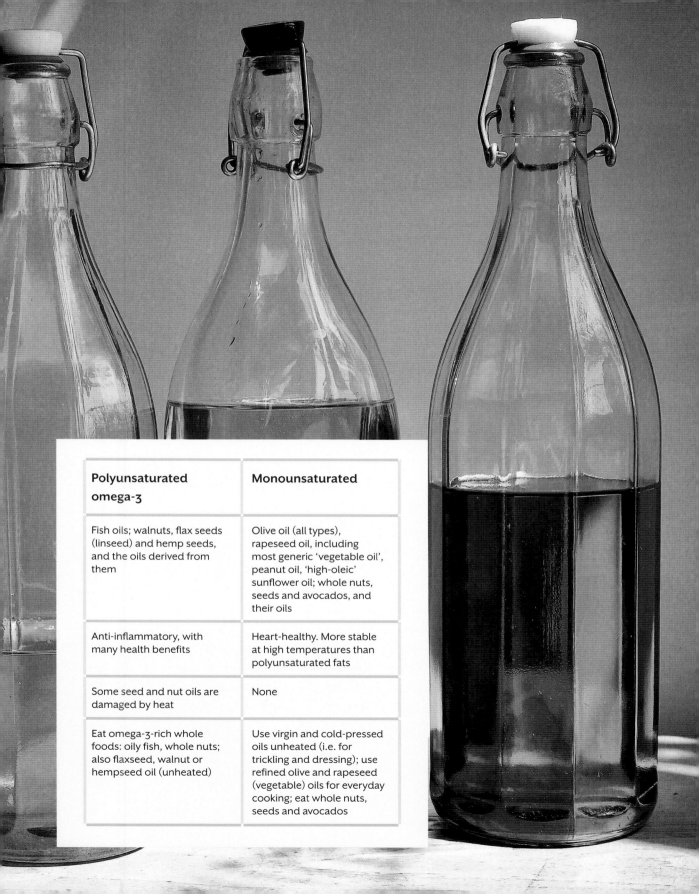

Polyunsaturated omega-3	Monounsaturated
Fish oils; walnuts, flax seeds (linseed) and hemp seeds, and the oils derived from them	Olive oil (all types), rapeseed oil, including most generic 'vegetable oil', peanut oil, 'high-oleic' sunflower oil; whole nuts, seeds and avocados, and their oils
Anti-inflammatory, with many health benefits	Heart-healthy. More stable at high temperatures than polyunsaturated fats
Some seed and nut oils are damaged by heat	None
Eat omega-3-rich whole foods: oily fish, whole nuts; also flaxseed, walnut or hempseed oil (unheated)	Use virgin and cold-pressed oils unheated (i.e. for trickling and dressing); use refined olive and rapeseed (vegetable) oils for everyday cooking; eat whole nuts, seeds and avocados

OILS: WHAT TO COOK WITH

Oil can be extracted from many different fruits, seeds and nuts, using widely varying methods. At the most basic and traditional end of the spectrum there is simple 'cold' mechanical pressing of the kind used to produce extra virgin olive oil. Oils produced in this way tend to retain all their natural, variable flavour, and are often distinctive and delicious. They also retain antioxidants and cholesterol-blocking substances called sterols and stanols.

The opposite to cold-pressed and relatively 'whole' oils are refined oils. These undergo a much more intensive industrial process, being heated, treated with a chemical solvent, bleached and deodorised; they emerge bland and almost flavourless.

My preference is for cold-pressed oils wherever possible, particularly extra virgin olive oil, cold-pressed rapeseed oil and cold-pressed hemp oil. They're simply more natural foods, and they are the ones I use for unheated applications such as dressing salads, trickling over soups or just dipping.

However, by removing particles and impurities, the refining process does make oils more stable when heated, and less likely to oxidise and form harmful substances. So plain old 'olive oil', which is refined, and refined rapeseed oil – usually labelled as generic 'vegetable oil' – are my usual options for everyday cooking. In any case, I think it's a bit of a waste to use extra virgin or cold-pressed oils for cooking because they are more expensive and their wonderful flavours get lost.

When it comes to really high temperature cooking, like deep-frying, it is best to use refined rapeseed (vegetable) oil or refined groundnut (peanut) oil. These oils have high 'smoke points' and are fairly resistant to oxidisation so they won't be damaged until they reach a very high temperature. Of course, as we've established, deep-fried foods should only be an occasional treat anyway.

Sunflower and other polyunsaturated oils have traditionally been used for high temperature frying but, as I have mentioned, there is now good evidence that when heated, they can oxidise and form aldehydes (toxic substances that have been linked to cancer and dementia). This oxidisation occurs before these oils reach smoke point, i.e. you can't see it happening. So, these oils are not safe for frying.

'High-oleic' sunflower oil (sometimes labelled 'sunflower frying oil') has a higher proportion of monounsaturated fats, making it more stable when heated, and so is okay for frying. There are some good organic ones out there.

It's good to Go Varied with your oils, as with other whole foods…

Here's a summary of how different fats and oils get used in my kitchen:

For non-cook (unheated) trickling and dressing, I go 'raw': extra virgin olive oil, cold-pressed rapeseed oil, cold-pressed hemp oil.

For 'gentle' cooking, such as sweating veg for a soup, curry or stew, I use plain (refined) olive oil, vegetable oil (i.e. refined rapeseed), and occasionally coconut oil, butter or lard (leftover from roast pork).

For frying (shallow or deep) where I want things crispy or browned, I opt for high-oleic 'sunflower frying oil', or occasionally refined veg (rapeseed) oil, or lard.

For roasting veg (which I do a lot), a good trickle (2 tbsp at most) of refined rapeseed or olive oil does the job. Toss the veg very thoroughly with the oil.

Frying lighter, and griddling

If you are frying a lot at home – especially deep-frying – you'll know how much cooking oil can be absorbed, particularly by anything potato-based or covered in breadcrumbs. I fry less than I used to, and when I do, I use less oil:

If I'm making pancakes, for example, I use just a drop of oil wiped around the pan with a piece of kitchen paper.

For a couple of fried eggs, I use just enough to coat the base of my smallest 2-egg pan with a fine film of oil. (That's about 2 tsp.)

And when frying a steak, a burger or a piece of fish, I often don't put any oil in the pan at all. Instead I lightly oil the to-be-fried food.

When I'm 'frying' veg I take the same approach. Take slices of courgette or fennel, wedges of cabbage and cauliflower 'steaks', for example. These all cook perfectly if you lightly brush them with oil before placing in a dry pan, or one wiped with the merest slick of oil.

You can also use one of those heavy, cast-iron griddle pans, with or without the stripe-imparting ridges, to 'barbecue' veg with no oil at all. The veg comes up nicely charred on the outside, vibrant and almost raw on the inside, and the oil – usually extra virgin olive or rapeseed – is sparingly trickled on afterwards, with perhaps a spritz of lemon or lime juice, and a pinch of salt and pepper.

A MODERATE-FAT DIET

Fat is high in calories. Most fats and oils have around 9 calories per gram (pure sugar has 4). So, clearly, if you eat a lot of fat, it can lead to weight gain. But as I've said, we do need some fat, it has important health-giving properties, and research suggests that the healthiest people in the world are *not* the ones eating the least fat.

In fact the right fats, used in the right way, far from harming us, will greatly enhance healthy eating. I've already mentioned that fat tastes good, and makes other things taste good too – including other really healthy things. Veg-lover that I am, even I would baulk at a bowl of raw salad served totally 'dry'. But trickle a little good oil over it, add a spritz of citrus juice or vinegar, and I'll devour it in minutes. A similar modest trickle of a more refined oil is transformative to a tray of to-be-roasted veg. The great thing is that you don't need a lot of fat to achieve this rather magical, taste-enhancing, satisfaction-boosting effect.

Another important thing to know about fat is that (like fibre) it helps you to feel full. So balanced cooking, with moderate amounts of fat, will help you feel satisfied by your meals and avoid those hunger spikes.

What is a moderate-fat diet? Eating around 70g total fat a day is about right for an active woman; the figure is around 80g for an active man. That's the equivalent of 4-5 tbsp olive oil – but this doesn't mean you should eat 4-5 tbsp oil a day! A lot of the fat we eat is contained in foods like meat, fish, eggs and dairy, nuts and even whole grains. In practice, the 'obvious' sources of fat, such as oils, butter and cream, or nut butters should be used sparingly – maybe 2–3 tbsp a day total (a bit less if you are trying to lose weight) – allowing us to enjoy moderate amounts of other healthy fat-containing foods such as oily fish, plain yoghurt, eggs, seeds and grains. And always alongside plenty of veg!

So choose natural fats, in moderation, and make them work for you. Discover how full-flavoured oils – like extra virgin olive oil, hemp or nut oils – enhance beans and pulses deliciously. Or how a bashed avocado makes a vegan chilli more luscious and tempting, and a smudge of peanut butter turns an oatcake into a treaty snack.

This is the truly healthy way to enjoy fat – not as part of a shop-bought pie, deep-fried takeaway or greasy doughnut, but as a dressing, topping or finishing touch that turns very healthy basic ingredients into very delicious meals. If you're trying to lose weight, cutting fat down to lower levels will help – but not if you replace that fat with sugar and refined carbs. Avoid processed 'diet' foods and swap in veg, fruit, pulses, eggs, low-fat unsweetened dairy and whole grains instead.

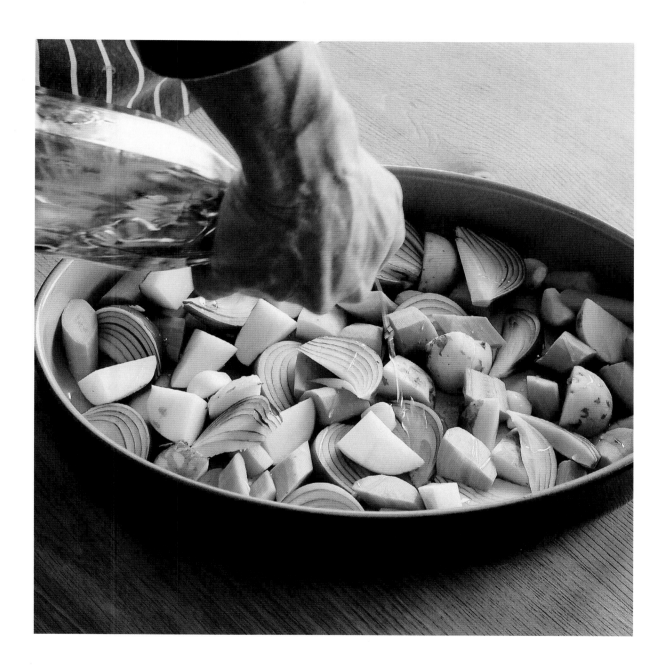

ACTION POINT RECAP

1 Up your omega-3s

Omega-3 polyunsaturated oils are one kind of fat most of us need more of, not less. Their anti-inflammatory properties make them helpful to our health – yet the average British diet is woefully lacking in them. So eat more oily fish, including mackerel, herring and sardines, and shellfish like mussels and oysters. Non-fish eaters, turn to nuts, seeds (and the cold-pressed oils thereof) as well as plenty of green veg. Be omega-3 positive and make sure you get your share.

2 Prioritise unsaturated fats for everyday use

Make the 'everyday' fats in your kitchen ones that also do you good. When it comes to cooking, go for moderate amounts of monounsaturated fat sources, such as refined olive and rapeseed (vegetable) oils. Even then, fry less, and use less oil when you fry. For dipping, dressing and trickling, enjoy virgin and cold-pressed olive and rapeseed, as well as seed and nut oils like cold-pressed hempseed, walnut, hazelnut or sunflower oils. Eat plenty of nuts and use them (in moderation) along with nut butters and even mashed avocado as swaps for butter, cheese and cream.

3 Minimise saturated fat

You don't need to cut out saturated fat altogether, but do look after your heart by keeping it at low levels. Don't eat (or cook with) too much butter and cream, and go easy on fatty meats and processed meats like salamis and sausages. You can always trim some fat off your meat and skim the fat off stews. Cut back on (or cut out) snack foods and baked goods made with palm oil.

4 Avoid artificial fats like the plague

Steer clear of industrial trans fats (including hydrogenated vegetable oils), which are formed by certain kinds of food processing, and are known to be a danger to health. Remember, they have a clear link to heart disease, and are banned in some countries. Try to cut out foods that might contain trans fats, such as highly processed baked goods and deep-fried takeaways.

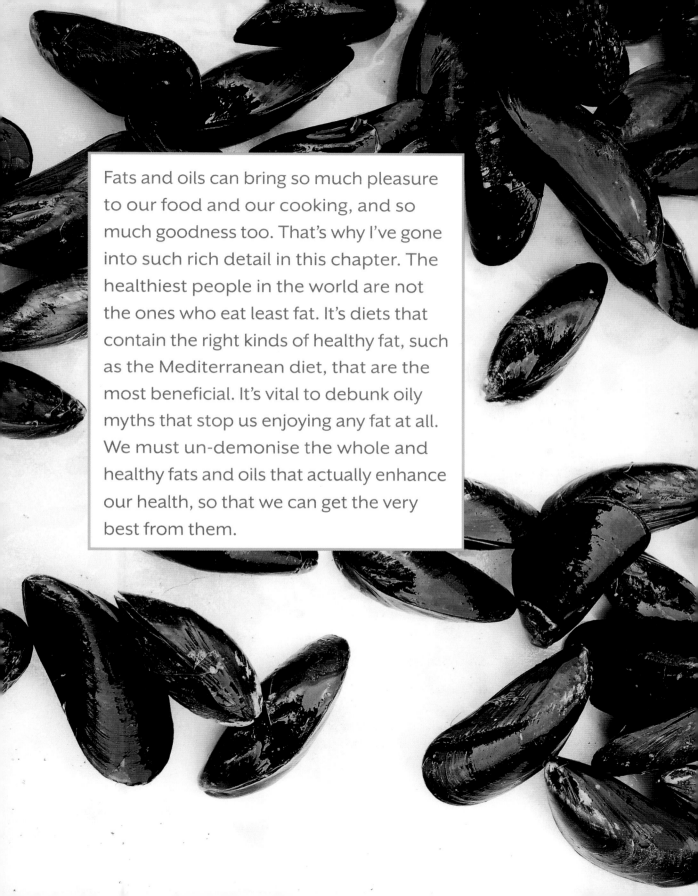

Fats and oils can bring so much pleasure to our food and our cooking, and so much goodness too. That's why I've gone into such rich detail in this chapter. The healthiest people in the world are not the ones who eat least fat. It's diets that contain the right kinds of healthy fat, such as the Mediterranean diet, that are the most beneficial. It's vital to debunk oily myths that stop us enjoying any fat at all. We must un-demonise the whole and healthy fats and oils that actually enhance our health, so that we can get the very best from them.

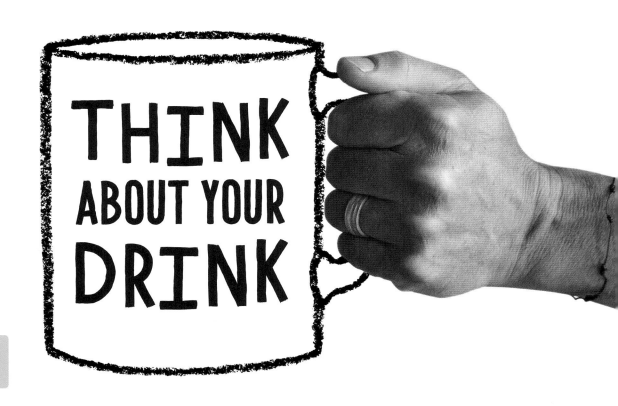

When it comes to a whole and healthy diet, what we drink is easy to overlook. We often think of our 'diet' as our solid food intake alone. But all those liquids we syphon into our systems through the day are just as significant as the plates of food we are eating. In fact, unless we are drinking plain water, or a simple infusion, then everything we drink *is food*.

Human beings, like all mammals, evolved to spend our first few months drinking only our mother's milk and, once weaned, to drink only water. Yet for most of us today, breast milk and water form a mere fraction of our liquid intake over our lifetimes. That's worth a pause for thought. It draws a huge question mark over all the other liquids we consume that are not one of those two things.

And we should be questioning them. On a day-to-day basis, it is very easy to go for 24 hours without drinking plain water at all, quenching our thirst instead with juices, squash, tea and coffee, milk, hot chocolate, fizzy colas and sodas, wine, beer and other alcoholic drinks. And we don't just drink because we're thirsty: often we choose to drink something because we need energy and stimulation, or because we crave the opposite – relaxation and comfort. Perhaps you have seen one of those mugs bearing the slogan 'coffee keeps me going until it's acceptable to start drinking wine'. For many of us, that quip is a bit near the knuckle.

All of these drinks – with the exception of herbal teas or black tea and coffee – are calorific. Some of them are highly calorific. Many are quite delicious too – hence their immense popularity! So, what's the problem? Well, there are a few...

CALORIFIC DRINKS: THE PITFALLS

The key thing to know is that our bodies do not recognise liquids as food in the same way they recognise solids as food. So, you can eat 200 calories and your brain will clock them and send out satiety signals: 'energy bank filled, stop eating.' If you drink those 200 calories, on the other hand, (a large, wholemilk cappuccino, say, or a pint of beer) your brain does not 'see' them in the same way: 'still hungry,' it thinks, 'eat more.' Liquid calories are sometimes described as 'stealth calories', which is apt: they creep up on you.

'When we chew food, we release hormones that tell our bodies we're eating,' confirms Dr Giles Yeo of Cambridge University's Department of Clinical Biochemistry. 'With drinks, there's no chewing, so your body doesn't release those hormones. Your brain doesn't know you're getting fuel, so it can't tell you. You don't feel full.' And so, you don't necessarily stop drinking. And you don't take actual eating off the agenda either!

Another way to look at it is that, generally speaking, the longer it takes something to pass through the digestive system, the more satisfying it is. And drinks, by their very nature, shoot through the system faster than you can say 'gulp', leaving behind calories without filling us up.

The result is that calorific drinks can play absolute havoc with our best intentions to eat a moderate diet. And that's why it's helpful to think of any drink that isn't water, herbal tea, black tea or coffee as food – a meal, or at the very least, a substantial snack. This is a mental shift to which I have recently committed myself. Consequently, I have almost completely stopped drinking fizzy drinks now, and rarely drink fruit juices either. More on the specifics of those two drinks in a bit.

Satisfaction delusion

This drink re-think wasn't an instant conversion for me: at first, I found it hard to think of these drinks as meals, because they don't really *feel* like meals. But when I flipped that idea around, it actually became quite motivating: most drinks don't feel like a meal because, beyond that very first hit of sweetness, they aren't really satisfying. So why am I drinking them anyway? The more I thought about it, the more I realised their hit of pleasure is fleeting – perhaps even illusory. I found that if I took time to notice this, even as I consumed a sweet fizzy drink, for example, I could actually discern the drink failing to satisfy me. I could sense the hope of satisfaction that came with the *pfffft* of the ring pull, or the unscrewed top, eluding me as the drink slipped down my gullet. And within seconds of the sweetness dissipating from my mouth I was thinking, 'well, that was a waste of time!'. Now I am satisfied that sugary drinks will never satisfy me. And I don't miss them at all.

Of course, there is a risk that the intrinsically unsatisfying nature of sugar-sweetened drinks leads us to keep trying, in the hope that the next swig, the next can or the next bottle may somehow offer up something that the last one failed to. And that's a cycle you really don't want to be caught in.

I'll be looking at the fraught issue of compulsive eating (and drinking) in the next chapter. But for now, let's just say if you can persuade yourself that you really don't need these liquids in your life, and you can cut them out for good, that's a job very well done. But not all drinks are demons. And I'm not advocating reverse evolution to the 'water only' days.

So, let's have a run-down of pretty much all the drinks we think we might want to consume – and work out a reasonable plan for approaching them in an enlightened way. It's well worth it. If we get it right it can make a *huge* difference to our well-being, and our morale. Let's start with those drinks that are no longer part of my life.

SSBS ARE NOT COOL

'Sugar-sweetened beverages' are known in the industry as SSBs (and it's always worth remembering that they *are* an industrial product). I think we should start calling them SSBs all the time – because it makes them sound so unappealing – and because it rhymes with WMDs (weapons of mass destruction). We are talking about fizzy drinks, colas, sports drinks and caffeinated 'energy' drinks, and also squashes, fruit-flavoured drinks and fruit-flavoured 'waters'. Together, these drinks are among the foremost sources of sugar in the modern diet. And researchers, doctors and dietitians are united in taking an extremely dark view of them.

In part, that's because of their ingredients: flavourings, colourings, preservatives, juice concentrates (sometimes) and really quite extraordinary amounts of sugar. A standard 330ml can of cola contains around 35g sugar – 7 teaspoonfuls – but even fruit-flavoured 'sparkling spring water' might have 20g. That is a ridiculous amount of sugar to pour down your throat in a few seconds, and it's going to do you no good at all.

The fact that it's dissolved in a liquid just compounds the harm it can do. 'Sugar,' says Giles Yeo, 'is probably the only major nutrient we can drink really fast. We can knock back literally hundreds of calories from a sugary drink in 5 minutes.' And then still ask what's for dinner...

Sugary drinks, then, are an efficient way to mainline refined carbohydrate into your system very fast, and below your body's radar – and all the bad news about refined carbs that I presented in Chapter 4 holds true here. Sugar spikes our insulin level, before bringing it crashing down again, leaving us feeling hungry. What's more, the fact that sugary liquids are less satisfying even than sugary food means we don't compensate for them by eating fewer calories from elsewhere. So, they offer a kind of double-whammy for weight gain: they don't fill us up and they can actually drive hunger. They are, in fact, perfectly designed to stimulate more drinking and more eating. In addition, sugar and sugary drinks are key components of the 'pro-inflammatory diet', which we now know is contributing to many chronic diseases.

Specifically, SSBs are associated with obesity, the accumulation of dangerous 'visceral fat' around internal organs, higher blood pressure and an increased risk of type 2 diabetes and heart disease. The message is clear: in the murky world of refined carbohydrates, sugar-sweetened beverages are the very worst option there is.

If they are a big part of your life, if you are drinking one or more every single day (as millions do) then I can't say I don't want to alarm you – because I do! But there's also a positive here – a great opportunity. Because if you can knock your SSB habit on the head, you will, for all the reasons above, be doing yourself a *massive* favour. Saying goodbye to them forever won't be easy, but there are lots of ways to do it.

Cutting SSBs

My first piece of advice is simple, yet potentially a total game changer: CARRY WATER. Unless you spend your working day within a few steps of a sink, then get yourself a reusable water bottle and fill it with clear cool tap water every day before you leave the house. More on water's qualities as a drink at the end of this section. For now, it's clear that simply having the option to quench your immediate thirst without having to go into a shop or café or even open a fridge is going to be a huge help in cutting out those SSBs.

Now with your trusty water bottle by your side, you can simply go cold turkey. This works best for some people, particularly if their SSB consumption is essentially a habit – same time(s), same place(s) even, almost every day.

If that's you, it's a good idea to identify all the times and occasions when you tend to feel the lure of a cold sweet drink and put some contingencies in place – distractions perhaps, like a (limited) session on your phone playing a game or sending messages, or physically moving to another place (going outside for some fresh air). Or set about a simple task that will bring you satisfaction. Then just go for it. You may be surprised how quickly you can kick the habit.

If cutting SSBs abruptly seems too daunting, there are more gradual methods:

When you feel the need for that SSB, drink a glass of water first anyway. It might quash the craving completely, or at least reduce the amount of the SSB you want.

———

Have a cup of (unsweetened) tea or plain coffee instead – it will give you the little energy boost that you might be craving from that can of cola, without the sugar. And the ritual of making it may be soothing in itself.

———

Get into herbal teas. If caffeine isn't really the issue, try a punchy infusion of herbs or ginger. Again, the making of it can feel like a pleasing act of self-care.

———

Switch to (moderate portions of) naturally fermented drinks like kombucha (page 244) or kefir (page 246), that are lower in sugar and have some good in them (see page 154).

———

Try gradual reduction by dilution. First, stop drinking 'by the can' (or bottle). Proceed by drinking 'servings' of your favourite soft drink (in a glass), increasingly diluted with plain cold water (or even soda water if you want to keep the fizz up). Use just a splash at first, then a little more each time, until you're at 50:50, then below. After a few weeks of your favourite SSBs diluted to 50% or more, I'm betting you will find undiluted SSBs unpalatably sweet. And that might just give you the confidence to ditch them altogether.

And if the idea of 'never again' seems too alarming, try reinventing SSBs as something you only drink in a very specific and occasional set of circumstances – for example when sitting outside in blazing sunshine, looking at the sea. But if you can enjoy that moment with a cup of tea or coffee (see pages 144–5), or even a glass of cool plain water, then you've got a lot to feel good about, besides the weather.

DIET DRINKS

If you can't have a nice cold fizzy drink with a load of sugar in it, then how about a nice cold fizzy drink *without* any sugar in it? That's the offer of the multi-billion-pound diet drinks business, and it's an invitation that many millions are accepting every day. It's hardly surprising. Diet drinks – also known as ASBs or 'artificially sweetened beverages' – seem to promise so much, particularly if you are beguiled by the prospect of zero calories. But the absence of calories doesn't equate to an absence of problems.

The sugar is replaced by artificial sweeteners, which ring their own alarm bells. There are emerging concerns that sweeteners like aspartame and sucralose might actually increase appetite in some people by messing with the brain's signals so it thinks it hasn't taken in enough calories, or by increasing our responsiveness to sweet tastes in food.

And something that really puts the nail in the coffin for me is the mounting evidence that sweeteners can sway the balance of our gut bacteria in a really unhealthy way. Studies in rodents have found that artificial sweeteners can increase the prevalence of types of bacteria that are associated with weight gain and obesity. So, diet drinks could be increasing the risk of diet-related diseases – how ironic is that?

At the very least, there is conflicting evidence over whether artificially sweetened drinks even help with weight control. A 2017 report co-authored by academics at Imperial College London concluded that there wasn't good evidence that these products helped people reach or maintain a healthy weight and recommended that they should not be promoted as part of a healthy diet.

It all amounts to a bunch of excellent reasons for giving ASBs as wide a berth as those SSBs. And I do.

FRUIT JUICE: THE COST OF FREE SUGARS

What about fresh fruit juice then, or pure fruit smoothies? These aren't full of nasties – many are indeed made from nothing but fruit. There's no added sugar, and don't we keep hearing that they count as part of our five-a-day?

Well, yes to all the above. But the latest advice is that even fresh pressed juices and homemade smoothies should be limited to no more than one 150ml serving a day (many single serving bottled juices and smoothies are larger than that, 250ml and 330ml being popular sizes). So, what's going on? Why the caution around portions of fruit that have been squeezed into juice or whizzed into smoothies?

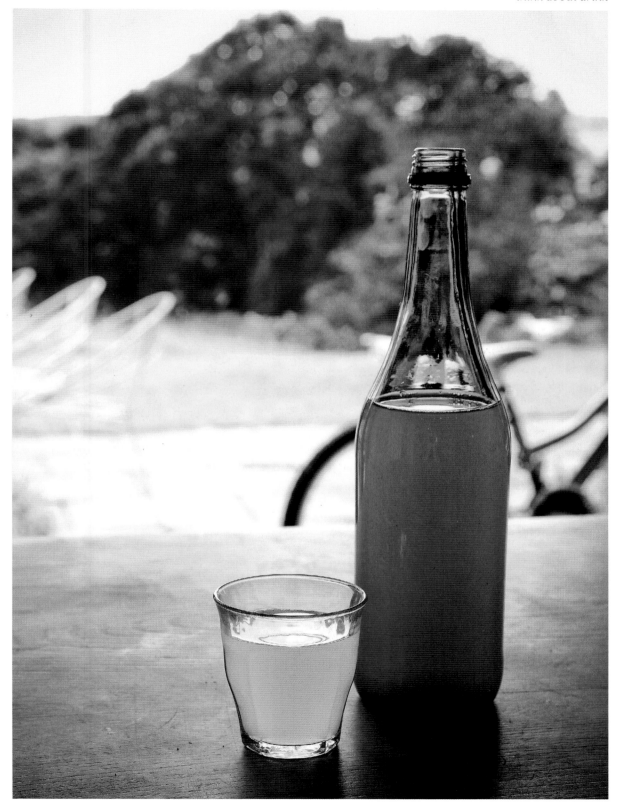

Well, the squeezing and whizzing is precisely the issue. These are processes that change the structure of the fruit (fairly obviously) and in so doing, they change the way our bodies respond to it. The natural sugars in the fruit (mainly fructose and glucose) when pressed and whizzed into juices and purées, become what are called 'free sugars'. And, unfortunately, they are then received and interpreted by our bodies in very much the same way as dissolved sugars, for example the added sugars in SSBs.

A free sugar is any sugar that has been unlocked from its natural source in a plant. That includes, fairly obviously, the refined sugar I've talked about in Chapter 4, that we buy in packets or find added to cakes and biscuits. And it includes the sugar in fizzy drinks. But it also includes the fruit sugars in juices and smoothies. That's because, even though some or all of the original plant is still present, the crushing, squeezing or puréeing 'frees' the sugar from the plant cells. That means our bodies can absorb it very quickly, just like refined carbs. I know it's irritating, and it has curbed my enthusiasm for juice.

There are a few reasons to be less negative about fresh juices, and especially smoothies, than SSBs. They do contain some of the goodness of the fruits they're made from. That is why modest portions are deemed acceptable. There will be vitamins and minerals. There may even be a small amount of fibre – but not much if the fruits are peeled, which they almost invariably are, and even less if the juices and purées are strained.

But if we glug fruit juice like it's going out of style (which, ironically, it kind of should be) then we will not only be setting the juice loose, but letting the free sugars run rampant. And the consequences can be similar to the over-consumption of those SSBs – weight gain, the accumulation of visceral fat etc. And while I'm wagging my free-sugary finger at you, free sugars are bad for your teeth too!

By the way, using honey to sweeten our drinks doesn't solve the sugar problem either. The sugar in honey is also 'free', because the bees have unlocked it from its original plant source. Only the sugar in *whole* fruits and vegetables, and milk, is not 'free'. It's bound up with fibre and other nutrients and is processed by the body more slowly.

A note on smoothies...

In light of the above, when I make a smoothie these days, from whole fruits, I like to leave it quite coarse – not over-blitzed. And for some fruits where the peel is palatable (apples and pears, for example) I'll leave it on. I also often add a handful of oats, which further ups the fibre and makes the smoothie a 'thickie', and sometimes yoghurt or kefir, for a bit of 'live'. When I pour this out of the blender, I admit that I'm not likely to measure it into a 150ml serving. But nor am I under any illusion that what I have in my glass is 'just a drink' – I know it is food. In fact, it's probably breakfast (see page 220).

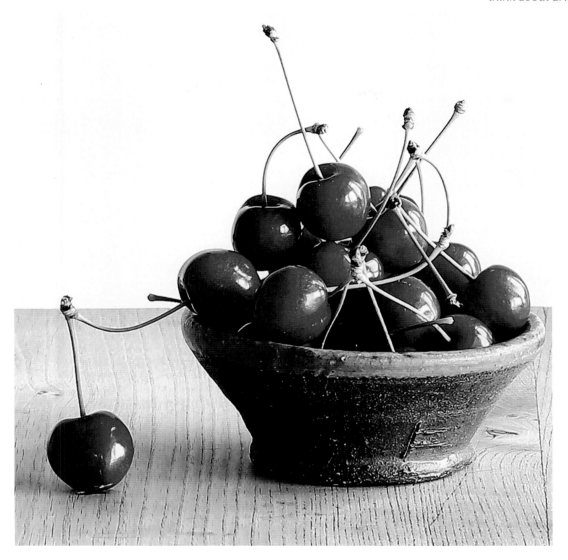

Think whole, again

One positive reaction to this accumulation of somewhat dispiriting news about juice is perhaps to remind oneself of the potentially refreshing nature of the whole fruits that the juicers started with. Might they just serve the purpose of refreshment, even when entirely *un*blitzed? Most fruits are upwards of 80% water – and come with their own natural flavourings! Apples, oranges, plums, cherries, raspberries and strawberries are particularly tangy and thirst-quenching and are all so much better for you than juice.

So just as it helps us to remember that drinks are all too often foods, once in a while, when we need them to be, let's remind ourselves that some of our most delicious whole foods can actually be wonderfully refreshing drinks.

A NICE CUPPA

I realise I have been doing some fairly major raining on parades here. It's hard to find much good to say about the sweet sugary drinks that have literally flooded our diets in recent decades. So, thank goodness for some better news about some other beloved beverages: tea and coffee. If you are fond of a cuppa, take heart because it certainly *can* be deployed as part of a healthy lifestyle.

Most of us know that the caffeine in tea and coffee, if we get too much of it, can disrupt sleep and increase anxiety, give you the jitters and make you feel 'wired'. For some people, caffeine has further risks – high levels can increase the risk of miscarriage, for example. But for healthy adults, caffeine in moderation definitely has its uses. It can dampen appetite and stave off hunger. A cup of coffee or tea can temporarily increase energy and alertness and boost your activity levels by reducing 'perceived effort'; for example, if you go for a jog after a cup of joe, you'll be able to push yourself a little harder. And, of course, these hot drinks are simple, everyday comforts – they can be the little treat that helps you through an afternoon slump – or indeed gets you past a craving for something sweet or carby. That's a useful trick to have up your sleeve.

In addition to caffeine, both coffee and tea contain a range of antioxidants – beneficial plant compounds that are associated with a decreased risk of chronic disease. A cup of coffee even contributes a tiny bit of fibre to your diet! There are many studies that link regular, moderate tea and coffee drinking to positive health outcomes. That doesn't mean that in order to be healthy you have to drink three americanos a day, or buy a mug with 'Keep Calm and Carry on Drinking Tea' written on it. If you're not a tea or coffee drinker, that's absolutely no cause for concern – there are countless other, much more significant, foods on which you can build your healthy diet. But if you are, and a cuppa or two really brightens your morning, you can feel good about it.

The general advice is that 400mg caffeine a day is a safe upper limit (roughly equivalent to 5 mugs of tea, 3 mugs of filter coffee or 4 double espressos). Pregnant women are advised to have no more than 200mg a day. But tolerance for caffeine varies a lot, and you probably know how much you can comfortably handle. It's wise to stay within your personal limit and to avoid caffeine in the evenings because it can play havoc with sleep.

There is, of course, a massive caveat (sorry!) to this positive appreciation of caffeinated beverages – and coffee in particular. And it's this: coffee is no longer *just* coffee. Time was when 'a coffee' meant a mugful of some scalding black brew – or perhaps Styrofoam cup of the same if you were out – softened by a splash of milk. End of story. If you were very with it (or arguably pretentious!), you might make your own espressos and take them black – but that was pretty recherché. How things have changed...

The coffee caveat

Britain's coffee shop economy, which wasn't even a thing 25 years ago, is sitting pretty on the crest of two decades of consistent and sustained growth. It is now worth over £10 billion a year. According to some research, we now prefer coffee-based drinks to the iconic cups of tea that are supposedly so integral to Britishness. Caffeine is available at every petrol station, department store and supermarket, and it sometimes feels like it's more unusual to see people walking the high street *without* those dreaded (and mostly non-recyclable) branded take-out cups clutched in their hands than with them. (Please get a keep-cup, coffee-lovers.)

Our flourishing café culture brings with it many issues – environmental, ethical and social. But let's stick to the health problem for now, which is that whereas an old-school cup of plain coffee with a little bit of milk contains 20–40 calories, a high-street latte (our favourite kind of take-out coffee, according to market research) contains maybe 100–200, depending on the type of milk used – i.e. up to 10 times as many. A big milky cappuccino can have over 200 calories, and a squirty cream-topped mocha can have well over 400! Come Halloween and Christmas the whole thing gets an extra dose of sugar and spice and a trickle of syrup on top, and you've passed the 500 mark! That is almost a quarter of the recommended daily calorie intake for a woman, in one 'hot drink'. Of course, as we now know, it isn't really a drink at all, it's a food – one perhaps best thought of as liquid cake.

If such sweet and creamy coffee-based concoctions are currently floating your boat, then it may be time to weigh anchor... by degrees if necessary (destination: macchiato, via cortado and skinny latte) or by cold turkey if you think you can do it. Why not row back to a simple, well-made cup of coffee, with a dash of milk? On pages 104–5 I talked about the simplicity and satisfaction of giving up sugar in my tea. Millions have done it, and never looked back. Millions more could cut out these coffee cocktails, and reap the same rewards.

For what it's worth, my daily hot drinks consumption is pretty consistent, and at the risk of irritating you, I'll spell it out: One cup of tea, with milk, on rising, and another an hour or two later. Very occasionally, a third – though that might be herbal. Mid-morning, a dacaff flat white. Occasionally another one before or after lunch. In the afternoon, either a cup of decaff tea, or a rooibos tea. Sometimes a second one. That's 4–7 hot drinks a day, all with milk (coffee sometimes with oat milk). I'm aware that on a 6 or 7 cup day that's about 250ml of milk, all in, which is not insignificant, *as food*. But it gets me through the day, *I'm aware* of what it is I'm consuming, and I think on balance it's reasonable.

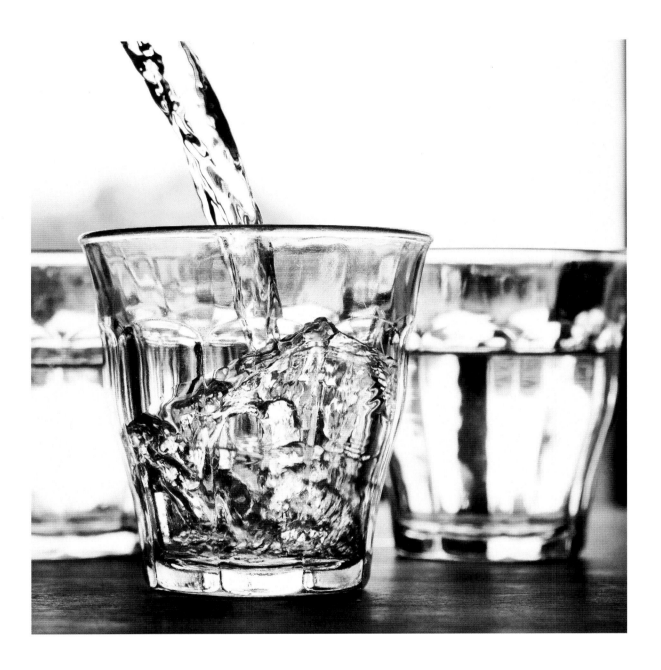

WATER WORKS

The best thing to drink for your health – the best thing to drink, full stop – is the number one choice of all living things: water. I realise that's not exactly breaking news, but it is important. It's the best because it hydrates you more effectively than any other drink. Its special status also comes from the fact that it promises (rather like doctors), first and foremost, to do no harm. And given the scale of the harm being done by some of the best-selling drinks on the planet, that counts for a lot.

However, the often-repeated advice that we need to drink a couple of litres of it a day is a little off the mark. Two litres of water a day is indeed a good amount, overall, for our bodies – but it does not need to come on top of everything else we eat and drink. We get a significant amount of water – 20–30% of our daily intake – from our food, particularly, if we so choose, from fresh fruit and veg! And we also get water from other drinks – including the tea and coffee we are generously allowing ourselves. This all counts towards our daily total.

So, in fact, drinking about 1.2 litres (2 pints) of *fluids* a day is fine (you might want more if the weather is hot, or you are exercising). And it doesn't all have to be plain water.

But for me, drinking at least some freshly drawn, good clean tap water every day feels like good practice. For a start, it reminds me what a pleasing drink it is and how that absence of negatives, even of flavours, can be a real positive. When you are properly thirsty, true satisfaction is in having your thirst quenched, not your mouth flavoured.

I don't measure my water intake – I don't feel I need to. I just build regular glasses of water into my day. I usually have a glass first thing in the morning, sometimes (but not always) a glass mid-morning or mid-afternoon, and usually one with each meal. But I'm really not counting.

Dr Michelle Harvie has the following advice: 'Don't let yourself get thirsty but don't feel you have to be constantly swilling back litres of water.' And she has one technical tip to add: 'The best guide to hydration is the colour of your urine – pale gold "straw-coloured" pee tells you you're adequately hydrated. If it's darker, tending towards orange, you should be drinking more water.' My translation is: If your wee looks more like Lucozade than white wine you should probably head for the tap – or put the kettle on. Not that I can remember what Lucozade looks like...

BOOZE: A BIG ISSUE

I couldn't write a chapter about drinking without, of course, talking about *drinking*. A normal part of life for millions of us, drinking alcohol has its pros and its cons. But it's clear that the cons can become pretty massive and that, if we are not in control of our drinking, it can be a very serious problem for our health.

Part of the problem is that alcohol is hard to avoid these days. It is woven into the fabric of our everyday lives. It's hard to go anywhere without passing off-licences, pubs or bars that are open all day. Booze can be bought in every corner shop and on trains and planes, at almost any hour. There are even online 24-hour delivery services. The practice of taking a tipple is no longer confined to certain places and certain hours, and the public conventions and boundaries around drinking have all but broken down.

According to the Institute of Alcohol Studies, alcohol consumption in Great Britain more than doubled between the mid-1950s and late 1990s, hitting a boozy peak in 2004. We have reined it in a little since then, but still, about 80% of adults in Britain drink alcohol. Beer and wine, in general, are much more affordable than they were 30 years ago, and the booze we get from supermarkets is particularly cheap – one reason why more of us choose to drink at home.

Drinking is not merely acceptable in our popular culture – it's desirable. The quaffing of wine, gin and trendy brands of beer and cider is feted everywhere in the media – models in adverts (and not just for alcohol), actors in soaps, TV dramas and major movies are seen clutching a glass in a reflected world where booze symbolises comfort, relaxation, reward, sophistication. But in reality, most of us are using it as a pretty standardised daily form of self-medication. That's not necessarily a disaster – there are upsides to the mood-enhancing effects of alcohol – but it has to be a flag for real caution in our approach to drinking.

Regular and frequent alcohol ingestion is so normalised in our culture that we can feel we barely have a choice as to whether to drink or not. So, the first point we must emphatically make about drinking comes in right here: drinking alcohol *isn't* compulsory, and drinking every day *isn't* normal – at least, not for our bodies. We *do* have a choice.

If we want to make alcoholic drinks a pleasurable but non-damaging part of our lives, then thoughtfully (or even *mindfully* – see the next chapter) exercising that choice can help us revisit those broken boundaries and reintroduce some well-considered conventions of our own. That will be most effectively done after absorbing some important information, and weighing up the pros and cons of drinking.

Alcohol: pros and cons

If you never (or only rarely) drink alcohol, by all means skip the rest of this section. It's pretty obvious that you can leave booze out of your diet and feel very good about it. Despite some evidence that moderate drinking can be part of a healthy lifestyle, there is certainly no good reason to *add* alcohol to your life if you don't already drink it.

If, however, you are fond of a regular glass or two (or currently a bit more than that) then here's food – or beverage – for thought. And since I'm a glass-half-full kind of guy, let's start with the pros.

The upside of drinking

The Blue Zones Project (see page 36) that studies long-lived communities worldwide, identifies moderate social drinking, ideally with food, as a potential contributor to a long and healthy life. This is to do with both psychological and physical factors – having a good time with our friends and family is good for our all-round health. But let's separate the two, and start with a look at the psychological plus side:

In moderate amounts the narcotic effect of alcohol, though it varies from person to person, helps us to feel relaxed. A beer or a glass of wine at the end of the day can take the edge off feelings of stress and help us 'reset'.

We often find the taste of alcoholic drinks quite delicious, and they can genuinely enhance our appreciation of food, helping us enjoy our meals more.

As social animals, the positive feelings we get from a drink are magnified through sharing – helping conversation and laughter to flow, and generally encouraging the notion that all might just be all right with the world.

On the physical side, there are potential benefits to *moderate* alcohol consumption, but these must be put in the context of the increased risk of other diseases, such as cancer:

Several studies have shown that moderate drinking can be beneficial for our heart; it is associated with a lower risk of some cardiovascular conditions including angina, heart failure and stroke. This may be because moderate levels of alcohol raise good HDL cholesterol, decrease blood-clotting and decrease insulin resistance – a risk factor for diabetes.

Abstaining from alcohol has been associated with an increased risk of dementia (but drinking more than a moderate amount is also linked with an increased risk).

There is evidence that the polyphenols (beneficial plant chemicals) in wine, cider and beer have a heart-protecting effect, and also that they can boost the numbers of good bacteria in our gut (see pages 84–5).

In terms of delivering these modest, possible health benefits of moderate drinking, red wine is probably a good choice. This is partly because it contains significantly higher quantities of polyphenols than white wine (or beer or cider). In studies into drinking and the development of dementia, moderate wine drinking in particular has an association with reduced risk.

It's worth noting that these health benefits don't apply equally to everybody. It seems to be people beyond middle age who show cardiovascular benefits from moderate alcohol consumption, for example, rather than younger people. There is medical consensus that pregnant women should avoid alcohol altogether. And many health conditions and medications are not compatible with drinking.

Crucially, any benefits related to consuming alcohol stop, or are reversed, *as soon as drinking goes above moderate levels*. Which leads us to…

The downside of drinking

Most drinkers know that too much alcohol can royally mess you up, both in the short term (by making you feel terrible) and in the long term (by damaging your health in all kinds of ways). If you want to kick the habit completely, there are websites including besober.co.uk and oneyearnobeer.com that can help. If you think you might be addicted to alcohol, or you already know it's making you ill, then you should seek help – either from your GP, or from one of the many organisations that offer help to people with a drink problem.

But even if you believe your drinking is moderate, there are clear points against it:

Alcoholic drinks are a rich source of calories and they can be a very significant contributor to weight gain. Undoubtedly, they are a real obstacle to weight loss. A large 250ml glass of wine and a pint of beer each carry around 200 calories. Swig for swig, that's in the same ballpark as those SSBs that we have already so roundly condemned.

Alcohol is very disinhibiting – it can skew your good intentions in all kinds of ways. Quite apart from leading you to do and say things you might later regret, it's very likely to lead you towards poorer food choices. I think most of us will recognise that having a drink in hand may make us more likely to polish off a bag of crisps before dinner, or (my own weakness) keep picking away at the food that's on the table (especially cheese!) at the end of a meal. There's a bunch of scientific evidence that drinking alcohol before or during a meal tends to make us eat more.

Alcohol is dehydrating, which can not only make us feel rough (as in the classic hangover) but can also make us tired, sometimes dizzy or light-headed and can affect our ability to concentrate and remember.

Alcohol can irritate the stomach and digestive tract, causing indigestion and heartburn, and aggravating other stomach complaints, such as ulcers.

Despite the fact that it may help you fall asleep initially, alcohol can disrupt sleep patterns and lead to poorer sleep. It can also exacerbate snoring.

Now here's the really serious stuff: Any more than a moderate level of drinking is a major risk factor in many diseases, and prolonged or excessive exposure to alcohol can shrink your brain, damage your heart and liver, and wreck your memory.

Alcohol causes some cancers. It is classed as a group 1 carcinogen and in 2015, around 12,000 cases of cancer in Britain were attributed to it. The cancers that have been causally linked to drinking include breast, bowel, liver, throat, stomach and oesophagus cancers. Even one drink a day can increase the risk of cancer to some extent; the more you drink, the greater your risk. In terms of cancer risk, the only completely safe level of drinking is none at all.

Moderation – the heart of the matter

I probably didn't need to tell you that regularly consuming too much alcohol can be horrendously damaging to your body. Yet despite this knowledge, millions of us, including myself, continue to drink alcoholic drinks on a regular basis.

If we are going to continue drinking, I think we should all be asking ourselves a vital question: how do we enjoy the modest but real benefits of drinking alcohol – emotional, social and physical – without harming ourselves? Or at least, while bringing the risks down to levels we are prepared to accept?

We've touched on the answer several times already, and frankly, we've probably heard it often enough: we should aim to be moderate in our drinking. But what is moderate drinking? Well, there is a technical answer to this, which the government has provided for us, based on a review of the latest science...

The current British guidelines state that moderate drinking means consuming no more than 14 units of alcohol a week. A unit is:

> One 25ml measure of spirits
>
> ―――
>
> A half pint of lower strength (3.6%) beer
>
> ―――
>
> About half a standard 175ml glass of lower strength (12%) wine

In real terms, if you're drinking more than a bottle and a half of wine, or six pints of beer, in a week, you are exceeding these limits.

But it's not just about how much alcohol you drink, overall. Your pattern of drinking is important too. Binging is definitely bad for you. But so is drinking every day. So, if you are pushing at the upper limit (or exceeding it), it's really important that your drinking is spread over several days (at least three, according to the guidelines), with no more than 4 units a day.

At the same time, it's important to have days without alcohol. Booze-free days can help you limit your overall intake, lower your tolerance for alcohol (which is a good thing as again it can help to reduce intake), and break the psychological dependence on that evening drink. And the consensus is that having the booze-free days consecutively maximises the benefits.

Remember that 14 units is an upper limit, not a recommended daily amount. And it's important to note that 'moderate' and 'excessive' are not absolute terms. We all metabolise alcohol differently. What's 'moderate' for one person may be 'excessive' for another. You'll know if one generous glass of wine is enough to see you sliding under the table. Or giggling at things that wouldn't normally strike you as amusing...

It's perhaps worth noting that these UK guidelines are stricter than in other countries – and stricter than they used to be here. But this is because we now know that even drinking at fairly low levels is a risk to our health. Most health professionals in the UK are strongly in favour of these revised guidelines.

Alcohol and you (and me)

So how do we translate all these limits, guidelines and warnings into a happy and (relatively) healthy personal plan for moderate drinking?

I feel I can only answer that in a personal way. I've enjoyed drinking with my friends for most of my adult life. I enjoy drinking good wine (or sometimes good beer or cider) with good food (and often before good food!). And I particularly enjoy sharing a drink with my wife at home when we are back together at the end of our working days. I must admit it's a bit of a struggle to imagine all these scenarios having quite the same appeal if alcohol were permanently removed from the equation.

So perhaps it's no surprise that I have often felt that I am drinking too much. Or rather, in terms of the official guidelines above, I have *known* I am drinking too much. But I've taken steps to adapt, improve and, crucially, *reduce* my drinking, so that I can feel more comfortable about it. And while I think I've been reasonably successful in this, I also plan to continue this journey, and make further positive changes. (I'm sure I'm not alone in being more concerned about my alcohol consumption as the years slip by.)

The key thing I have taken on board is the importance of alcohol-free days. I now aim for two a week, minimum. And I feel smug if I manage three. It's a commitment which has been hugely helpful in improving how I feel about my drinking. Psychologically, it helps me remember that I'm in control, and every drink is the consequence of a decision, not just a habit. That's reinforced by knowing that every alcohol-free day adjusts the alarming stats about alcohol and health outcomes in my favour.

If you, like me, are on a journey towards drinking less, and drinking smarter, or indeed hoping to begin such a journey, then you can probably relate to where I'm at, where I've been, and where I hope to get to. If you still drink every day, I would urge you to take that leap to a couple of alcohol-free days in your week. It's transformational.

If you are taking alcohol out of your plans for two or three evenings a week, you are probably going to miss it, at least to begin with. So it's really helpful to plan something else into those evenings that you can look forward to (going to the pub with your mates is not ideal). It could be that you make one of these evenings movie night, either at home (in which case it could also be box-set night – 2 episodes minimum, 3 max!) or at the cinema. For me, this is usually my Monday plan (family movie at home) and sometimes my Tuesday plan too (movie out, or sometimes theatre or concert, with my wife).

You could also make time for a new hobby, or evening class, or book yourself a treat, such as a massage. Or (and this is a really good one) you could regularly meet a friend, or small group of friends, who are also looking for a fun night away from the booze. It could be a book club or a board game session. Perhaps these things sound slightly nerdy – but don't dismiss them. You may find that socialising without alcohol is something of a revelation, especially if it's a commitment you've all made together.

Of course, you can also use this alcohol-free evening time for sport or exercise (of which more on pages 200–1). But I wouldn't make it all about that. It's helpful if your nights off alcohol have an element of treat about them.

Managing your alcohol supply

To start with I found it helpful on alcohol-free nights not to have delicious alcoholic drinks on ice and standing by. So, I used to take any cider, beer and white wine out of the fridge on a Sunday evening – and put it back in on Wednesday! This is pragmatic, but also symbolic. Pragmatic, because it removes temptation – I don't find warm cider, beer or white wine very appealing – and symbolic, because it reinforces my good intentions.

Of course, I could usually still lay my hands on a bottle of red at ideal room temperature. But given the steps that I've taken to get the best from not drinking, this would be blatant self-sabotage. I know where it is – but I can resist!

You can take this approach to the next level – if the way you shop supports it – and simply not keep alcohol in the house. You buy only what you plan to drink on the day you plan to drink it.

DRINK SUBSTITUTES

It's perfectly okay – useful in fact – if one thing you're looking forward to on your alcohol-free evenings is a delicious alcohol-free drink. And, of course, it's best – essential I'd say – if that drink is not heaving with sugar.

The market for no-alcohol, low-sugar drinks that are not laden with artificial sweeteners is pretty limited. But it is improving. Kombucha is a good call – and particularly satisfying if you have made it yourself (see page 244). It's good not just because it's live (with beneficial bacteria) and naturally low in calories (though note, some more than others), but also because it's quite 'dry' and 'tart'. To me these are important qualities that make my non-alcoholic drinks feel more grown-up, more sip-able, and basically more of a treat than those sweet, gluggable but ultimately unsatisfying SSBs.

There are plenty of branded 'grown-up' alcohol-free drinks out there that are worth a try. I have found a few alcohol-free (or less than 1%) beers that I like (they make a great 'shandy' with kombucha!). But I haven't found an alcohol-free 'wine' that I can get on with at all.

There are some fancy (and usually expensive) herbal 'brews' and 'botanicals' (and no doubt more on the way). But I reckon it's easy (and cheaper) to make more delicious versions yourself using herbs, citrus juice and zest, and even vinegar – a few favourites appear on pages 396–9. So, get your favourite non-boozy tipple chilled down in the fridge well ahead of your non-drinking evening.

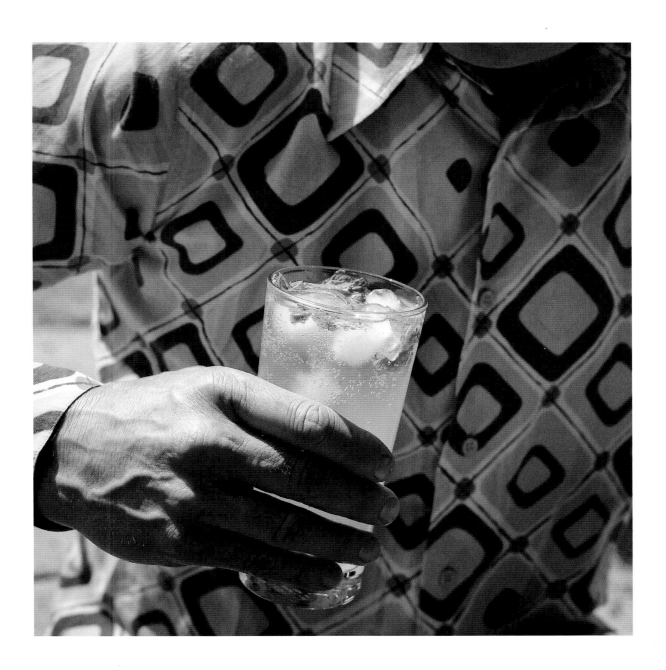

MORE MINDFUL DRINKING

Advance planning of your alcohol-free time – from arranging fun nights out (and in) to keeping a nice cold kombucha in the fridge – is largely about self-care. It's about keeping an eye out for your future self – the one who wants tomorrow's booze-free evening to be just as enjoyable as today's tipple-enhanced supper-time. And to be aware that you're doing this, to think about it *while* you are doing it, is an important way of drinking more mindfully.

A mindful approach to our eating and drinking can be very powerful, and I'm going to devote the whole of the next chapter to it.

Meanwhile, it can be helpful to learn something (or simply to admit a few obvious truths) about your own drinking behaviour. Do you instinctively feel you 'need' a drink when stressed? Or sad? Do you use alcohol to help you relax? Is that glass of wine a reward for getting through the day? I know those are all boxes I can tick from time to time. So are there other things you could do to help you manage these feelings, or that moment? Take a hot bath with a good soundtrack. Call a friend for a gossip – or to unload your sorrows, instead of drowning them.

I've noticed, for instance, that it's the end-of-the-day spot – work done, cooking to do – when alcohol calls loudest to me. Once I am past that (with the help of my glass of cold kombucha, and perhaps the Radio 4 6.30 comedy slot), and actually eating my supper (with a glass of water) I am pretty much 'over it'. And after supper, a movie, good book, or lively conversation happily gets me through to bedtime. I always feel good about going to bed under the influence of no alcohol, relishing a more natural, less boozy-woozy sleepiness. And I get my best sleep on these nights.

I hope some of these strategies – or your own, personalised versions of them – will prove useful. They may begin as distractions, but they should become welcome, healthy habits over time. Think about them as you set about them – and don't be afraid to acknowledge the occasional twitchiness along the way. It's okay to think, 'I could murder a drink!' – and brilliant when you decide not to in the end.

These are the first thoughtful, aware steps towards more mindful drinking, as opposed to mindless imbibing. And if you want to take further steps, it's worth knowing that there's a burgeoning mindful drinking movement in Britain now, fostered by people who want to drink at low levels, or not at all. There are websites, apps and books that can support your plan to drink more moderately and mindfully, or indeed to give up alcohol altogether – try joinclubsoda.co.uk or hellosundaymorning.com.

QUALITY OVER QUANTITY

I think it's important to remember that there are things other than alcohol in all alcoholic drinks (pure alcohol is a pretty lethal poison). The problem is, it is actually much harder to find out what ingredients are in industrially processed alcoholic drinks than it is to find out what's in processed foods. This is because, astonishingly, the makers of alcoholic drinks are under no obligation to reveal their ingredients. This is under review, and it seems likely the government may soon insist that calorie information, at least, is shown on the labels of alcoholic drinks. For now, the only additives they are compelled to declare are sulphites, which are widely used as preservatives and stabilisers in wine and cider (though they also occur naturally at low levels in fermented drinks).

The hidden additives

Other additives used in the drinks industry that you won't see listed on the bottle include concentrated grape syrups used to deepen the colour of red wine, tartaric acid to create acidity, tannins and commercial yeasts for flavour, and preservatives including dimethyl decarbonate (which is toxic in its natural state but breaks down once added to wine).

'Processing aids', which are not supposed to remain in the finished wine, include potassium ferrocyanide (which, to quote one paper, 'poses safety and environmental protection problems') to remove excess iron from white wines; copper sulphate, to correct off-flavours from sulphur compounds; lysozyme (derived from eggs) which is an antimicrobial agent, and fining or filtering agents which can be derived from fish, eggs or milk, as well as bentonite clay.

The exemption from declaring these and other additives applies to all alcoholic drinks. Booze bottles just don't have ingredients lists (for now). Sometimes ingredients are announced on the labels – the grape variety in a wine, a herb in a gin, the type of hops in a beer. But there's no mention of the additives that are used to make the product stable and taste the same every time.

This is wrong, of course, and it's amazing that the drinks industry gets away with it. Consumers are left in the dark and without the means to make the right choices: wines 'fined' with isinglass from fish are not suitable for vegetarians, for example.

There may be health issues too: given that we already know that sulphites cause allergic reactions in some people, I wonder what we don't yet understand about the possible effects of the other additives in alcoholic drinks?

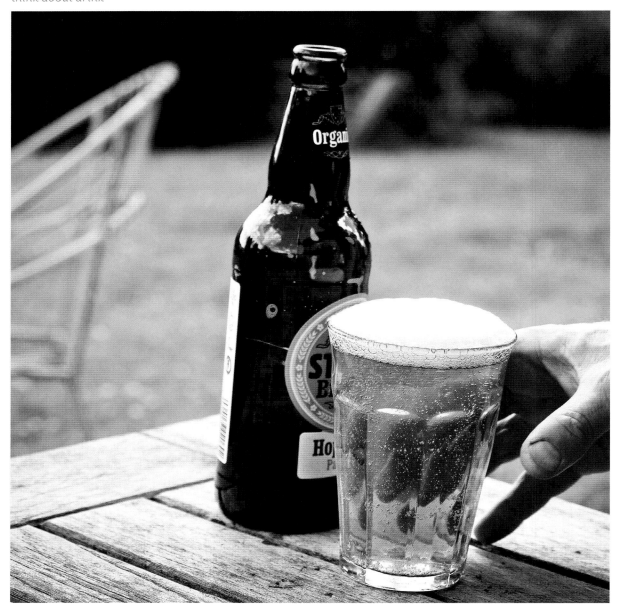

Seeking out better options

Avoiding the hidden additives is one reason why I choose 'organic' and 'biodynamic' wines. These are both legally defined and rigorously audited methods of viniculture, where far fewer additives, and only lower levels of sulphite preservatives, are allowed. I also occasionally buy 'low-intervention' or 'natural' wines. These do not currently have legally defined status, but are based on trust of the enthusiasts who make them, who are committed to working without chemical additives.

I also seek out 'craft' (which is not a legally defined term) and organic (which is) beers made from nothing but malted barley (or wheat, or rye), hops (and sometimes other plant-based flavourings) and water. And I am very enthusiastic about organic and 'artisanal' ciders (again, not a legal definition, but denoting local and small-scale production, often with apples from untreated, but not organically certified, orchards).

Buying these drinks also means avoiding residues of the agricultural chemicals used in the conventional production of wine grapes, barley for beer, and other fruits and grains used in alcoholic drinks. And, of course, it's better for the planet. The conventional, industrial agriculture of grapes for wine-making is heavily dependent on fossil fuels for both fertilisers and machinery, and the vines themselves are typically grown as an intense monoculture with zero tolerance of weeds, so they support very little biodiversity. By contrast, grapes for natural and organic wines are often grown with companion plants and complementary crops, which is a much more wildlife-friendly approach. If you're interested to find out more, there's a great (I so want to say grape) movie about natural wine-making in France called Wine Calling.

I should end this section by making it clear that there is no evidence that switching to organically produced alcohols confers health benefits or reduces the many risks of drinking alcohol. But it's a choice I've made on the precautionary principle that I would rather know what's in my alcoholic drinks – and reduce the risk that there's anything else in them, other than the alcohol, that might do me harm.

IN THE SPIRIT OF THINGS

So far, I've said next to nothing about spirits – gin, vodka, whisky, rum and tequila, for example. Suffice to say that served neat, they are at least twice as rich in calories as wine and they have the potential to intoxicate you with just a few sips. And, of course, the most popular way to serve them is with mixers, which are almost invariably SSBs (you know what we think of them!). Cocktails are another can of worms, bringing all the caveats of fruit juices into the mix, and sometimes SSBs and multiple shots of spirits too!

Of course, it would be disingenuous not to admit that a well-made gin and tonic, a top-drawer Bloody Mary, or a peaty single malt whisky with a dash of cold water (by all means swap in your own favourite spirit-based drinks) can have a certain appeal, at a certain time, in a certain place. I think it barely needs to be said that deciding to get by without such moments in one's life is a fine idea. And the next best thing (which is where I am at) is to aim for single figures of such moments in any given year. Let's make them enjoyable, and indeed mindful, moments when they happen.

ACTION POINT RECAP

1 Ditch the SSBs – and their artificially sweetened substitutes

There's nothing good to say about this band of beverages. Sugar-sweetened drinks are loaded with useless calories – and artificially sweetened versions are full of additives. Beyond briefly quenching your thirst and giving you a very temporary boost, these drinks have no benefits and can be actively harmful. Try to elbow them out of your diet, which will create more opportunity for you to…

2 Drink plenty of fresh, cool water

This is the one and only drink that really is just that – a drink. It's the perfect, 100% fit-for-purpose way to hydrate our bodies – without calories, additives, stimulants or anything else. Tap water is fine – plastic bottles are not needed – and a few big glasses a day are all you need.

3 Cut back on 'calorie-added' hot drinks

Research your favourite high-street coffee – most of the big chains provide nutritional info on their websites. How many calories are you consuming with your caffeine kick? The simplest coffees – americanos, espressos – are usually also the lightest. So, wean yourself off the 'recipe' coffees and treat yourself to some decent tea or fresh-ground coffee. Savour it with no sugar and just a splash of milk (or none at all). You'll soon relish it as much, or more, as any sugared-up, squirty-cream-topped coffee cocktail.

4 Dial down your alcoholic drinking

If you don't drink alcohol at all, good for you – keep it up! Those of us who do need to keep it moderate. Anything more than 1½ bottles of wine or 6 pints of beer per week and we're into the health-damaging stats. Booze-free days are the best way to cut back, so have at least two every week. For a 'treat' drink on your nights off alcohol, try something tart and zesty with minimal added sugar, like kombucha or an 'iced tea' type cocktail. There are lots of ways to reduce your drinking – and seeking support, or buddying up, to do so is plain sensible. Success is rewarding, as you join the ranks of those who report weight loss, better sleep, increased energy and a greater sense of fulfilment in their lives.

Liquid foods are just as significant as the solid ones. Water is essential; unadorned teas and coffees are a boost and a comfort; a small amount of juice is a healthy pleasure; and alcohol, thoughtfully managed, a relaxing treat. Most of the rest is best avoided. If that sounds radical, it's a measure of how wildly inappropriate and unhealthy our drinking behaviours have become. But the bright side of it is this: every time you feel thirsty, you have the opportunity to make a good choice. And those choices will add up, by the day, by the week, by the year, bolstering your morale and boosting your health and well-being.

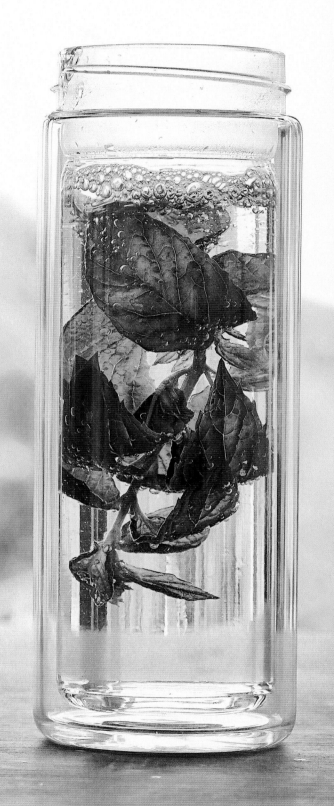

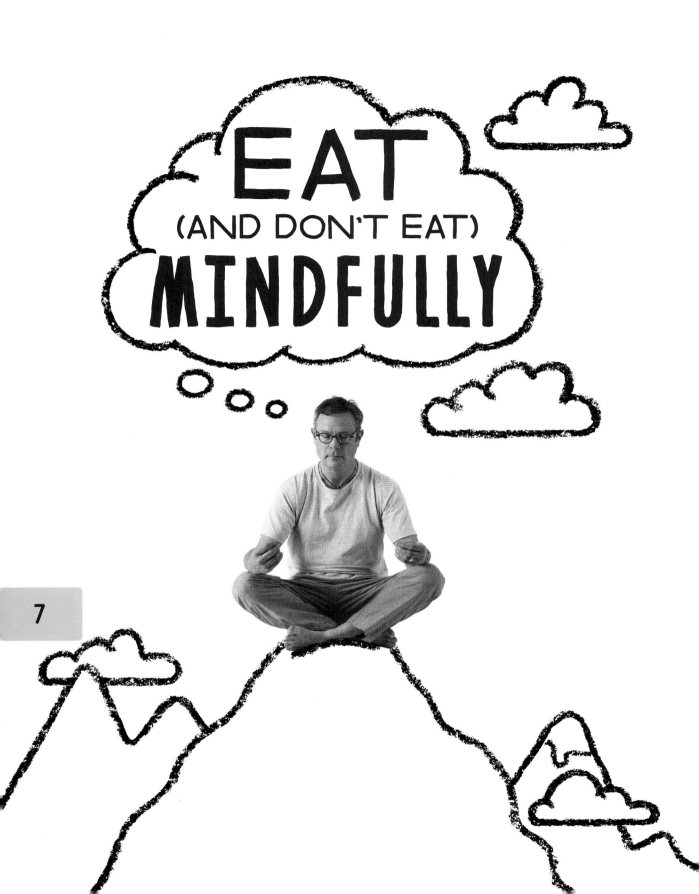

EAT
(AND DON'T EAT)
MINDFULLY

I've had plenty to say so far about what we eat (and drink). But just as important – perhaps more important – is how we eat. I don't just mean how in the physical sense, but how in a psychological sense: how we think (or don't think) when we eat.

Over the decades, the way we approach food – so often in a mindless rush – has changed as much as the food itself. It's easy to forget how much of our time is spent in the company of food, because so often we are thinking about something else: the bills, the box set or the bolshie boss. What if, every moment we connect with food – when we choose it, prepare it, cook it, share it and eat it – we stay with it? I think we can make all those moments good, by making them mindful.

The way that we eat now is characterised by foot-on-the-floor, pedal-to-the-metal acceleration: we eat more, we eat faster, we take risks (by consuming really unhealthy foods). We certainly aren't taking in the scenery. So, for most of us, most of the time, it wouldn't hurt to put the brakes on a bit.

This idea of not just eating better foods but eating in a better way, brings together everything else I've talked about in the previous six chapters. If we can bring moderation and reflection back to our eating – if we can simply pause, and actually *notice* that we are eating – then all that we've learned about what to eat will slot beautifully into place. We'll have the whole picture: we'll know what eating well in the fullest sense really means, and we will reap the widest possible benefits.

And talking of pausing, in this chapter I also want to discuss how *not* to eat. A lot of books have now been written about how refraining from food, or fasting, can help you lose weight and stay healthy. And from personal experience I am persuaded that it can indeed be a powerful tool. But, to me, fasting doesn't make sense as a single-fix solution – which is how it's so often presented. I want to put fasting in the context of everything that I've said so far, and frame it as part of an enlightened approach to *all* our eating.

So, how do we slow down and take a break from food in our crazy calorific culture of 24/7 eating, open-all-hours drinking and constant snacking? How can we eat better, eat less, eat with greater care and longer pauses, when we are perpetually being urged to consume more and more food, and to do it now, now, now? The answer is to use our heads, to think about what we are doing whenever we eat and drink. We need to be mindful.

MINDFULNESS: JUST A BUZZWORD?

Mindfulness may sound like a fad – a bit of trendy mind-yoga for those with plenty of time on their hands. Or it may seem like an excellent idea — but one that demands unrealistic levels of commitment. But please stick with me. You don't need to do a mindfulness course, or get an app, to eat more mindfully (though I certainly wouldn't hold you back from either). You can work towards it in gentle, incremental steps – a series of small changes and shifts in attitude. And it's really helpful.

Another way of framing it (popular in India, as it happens) is as a shift from unconscious to conscious eating: it starts with simply being aware that you are in fact chewing food. I like that. Too often these days we barely know we are eating, especially when we are also doing something else. (A study showed a 40% increase in crisp consumption when subjects were watching TV – we can all relate to that!)

Mindful eating is the healthy alternative to the kind of rushed, distracted, mindless overconsumption that has become normal for so many of us. Here's how to get started.

Mindful eating in practice

Mindful eating (mindful anything) takes practice, but only because in a way it *is* practice. One of the key tenets of mindfulness is non-judgement. So this is about noticing your thoughts and feelings, but not criticising or berating yourself for having them.

Start with a few questions. How hungry am I? Am I actually hungry at all or is it just my habitual time to eat? Am I eating because I am bored, restless or unhappy?

What do I want to eat? And don't judge yourself if the answer is 'ice cream and cookies' – just be aware. You don't have to choose the first foods you think of!

Put aside all distractions when you eat – the TV, your phone, headphones, even a book or newspaper. Focus on your food.

Notice the look, smell, texture and even sound of your food before you start. This is just as important if you are snacking on a biscuit as sitting down for a feast.

As you eat, notice how it feels – the heat or chill of what you are eating, how the first tastes arrive in your mouth, followed by more waves of flavour as your nose sends signals to your brain.

Slow down and chew more! It will help you notice your food – and digest it better (see page 170).

Relish the simple pleasure of eating, whatever the food is! If it's not giving you pleasure, ask yourself why that is?

Try to picture your food travelling down inside you, delivering nourishment and energy to your entire system.

Observe how your whole body feels as you eat, not just your mouth. When does the sensation of hunger pass, when do you feel satisfied? When do you start to feel over-full?

Put at least some of these into action at your next meal – you might be amazed at the sense of control it gives you. And look back at this list regularly over the coming weeks.

THE BENEFITS OF MINDFUL EATING

The happy fact is that food lends itself well to mindful thinking. For a start, it's something we come into contact with several times a day – giving us many opportunities to be mindful! And food engages all five of our senses, triggering all kinds of responses that we can choose to attend to with our thinking brains.

More mindful eating is something I'm backing from personal experience. It has increased my sense of joy around food. For someone who is easily excited by food, that's saying something! These changes have occurred, and endured, in part because more mindful eating helps me relish foods that are less obvious in the pleasure they deliver – and better for me – than ones that are designed and manufactured to push all my buttons. A dozen almonds, a small handful of raisins and a square or two of dark chocolate may not be a Picnic bar. But they are a satisfying treat when you eat the components one at a time, or in varying combinations, savouring their tastes and textures as you go.

This focus on what food really is, how it makes us feel right now (rather than how we hope it *might* make us feel, if we keep eating more of it) is at the heart of mindful eating. And while that focus is 'in the moment', it can ultimately lead to far-reaching change. It can help to dismantle an unhealthy, unhelpful relationship with food, and build a better one that allows us to enjoy delicious food without overeating. Two recent review studies have shown that mindful interventions are an effective way of changing eating behaviour over the long term, particularly when there's an emotional or compulsive component.

I can relate to that too, as I know this has been a factor in my own relationship with food, and in gaining weight too. I used to eat more, and make worse food choices (including that Picnic!) when I was stressed and anxious, especially about work. I began using mindful exercises (with the guidance of headspace.com) to address stress as I was approaching 50 and I was soon able to connect the benefits of 'calm noticing' of the world around me with the specifics of eating better food. Of course, I realise that some people are caught in an intense cycle of emotional eating, guilt and stress. If that's you, I believe this book, and this chapter in particular, can help you. But if you are feeling really stuck, and struggling to get started, then there are practitioners out there offering mindfulness therapy for emotional eating, both in person and online.

A broad, easy path

This will sound a bit 'touchy-feely' to some. But that's no reason for scepticism. Be assured that the concept of mindfulness supporting long-term behaviour change is backed up by the latest neuroscience.

The means by which this happens is sometimes called 'neuroplasticity'. Whenever we think, do or feel something, signals are sent along the neural pathways in our brains. When we think, do or feel the same things over and over, those pathways become well-worn, habitual, automatic. But because the brain is 'plastic' (not my favourite word, but let's stick with it), not fixed and unchangeable, it is always possible to create new pathways, over time, by doing things, or even thinking things, differently and repeatedly.

If you pick a new route through difficult terrain, treading the same route over time, even if it's narrow and difficult to start with, it *will* become broader and easier. Mindfulness can help make better eating (and other positive behaviours) a broader, easier path.

So, my 7th way is, in essence, to take a mindful approach to ways 1–6:

> You can be more mindful about the wholeness and goodness of the foods you are choosing. Think about the fibre in fresh veg and fruit when you buy and handle them. Keep in mind the vitamins, minerals, antioxidants and polyphenols that are bound up in them, and will be released when you eat them.

> Think about the rich variety of foods you are choosing, bringing you and your family goodness in so many different ways. Think about the health-enhancing synergies at work between those elements, delivered via so many amazing tastes and textures.

> As I suggested in Chapter 3, you can even ask yourself, 'Will my gut thank me for eating this?' I sometimes actually visualise gut-friendly foods such as fibrous raw veg and live ferments helping my gut bacteria do their vital work.

> Be more mindful (and pleased) about what you are not choosing too, allowing yourself a sense of calm satisfaction when you decide not to put refined carbs or ultra-processed snacks in your shopping basket.

> You can be more mindful of the fats and oils in your cooking, appreciating the vital roles they play in your metabolism, and thoughtfully acknowledging the ways in which they enhance the pleasure of eating – from the butter on your peas to the dressing on your salad.

> And I hope you will have come away from the last chapter about drink with a pretty clear sense that mindfulness is at the heart of a smarter, healthier relationship with our drinks and liquid foods, alcohol most especially.

So, as you can see, we have been thinking mindfully about food from the very first page.

MINDFUL FROM START TO FINISH

I hope it's becoming clear that being more mindful around food is a process that can kick in quite a while before you actually eat. It can – and should – start with your choice of ingredients: for example, I am now more mindful when I plan what I'm going to eat and when I buy, or sometimes grow, that food. I slow down when I'm choosing ingredients – fresh ingredients in particular – to enjoy thoughts like 'this garlic is still alive – if I planted it, it would grow!', or 'this beautiful cauliflower, with its creamy, curdy florets, was, just a few days ago, growing in a Cornish field with a thousand others, drawing up goodness from that rich West Country soil.'

Maybe not everyone will get quite so excited about a Cornish cauliflower (or a kohlrabi that looks like an alien baby, grown in the River Cottage veg garden). But if we slow down and notice the qualities of the foods we buy, and think a bit about where they have come from, then the process of mindful eating is already well under way.

It's a feeling we can then take with us into the kitchen, as we handle, wash, cut up and prepare our food. As we cleave through the grey-green skin of a squash with our best knife, we can marvel at the vibrant orange of the flesh inside. Approached mindfully, even the humblest of ingredients can deliver this sense of wonder. I am still awestruck by the layered beauty of every onion that I slice (and I've sliced a few) – not to mention the amazing smell that wafts through the kitchen when it's gently sizzling in the pan.

If anything about the business of shopping, preparing and cooking your food has become humdrum and routine, then a little mindfulness can re-engage the senses and unlock the magic once again.

And then, of course, there is the highlight – the enjoyment of eating itself. Here is where being more mindful is definitely most fun! If we take the time to sit down, at a table, away from distractions, screens put aside, and actually savour our food, then it's almost, I think, like getting to eat twice over. Your mind is engaged by the pleasures of the senses: the feel, look, smell and taste of the food can be noticed and relished, both separately and in combination. Your body reaps the satisfaction of having hunger sated and energy replenished; and there is a different but complementary kind of pleasure in having these most basic requirements met. Bring these two things mindfully together, and you have a more profound, more fulfilling experience of eating.

That said, being more mindful doesn't mean becoming some kind of food saint, never choosing anything that's less than perfectly wholesome. In fact, a mindful approach is very relevant to those foods and drinks we know are not exactly full of virtue – but which we are planning to consume anyway! I'm thinking particularly of things at the

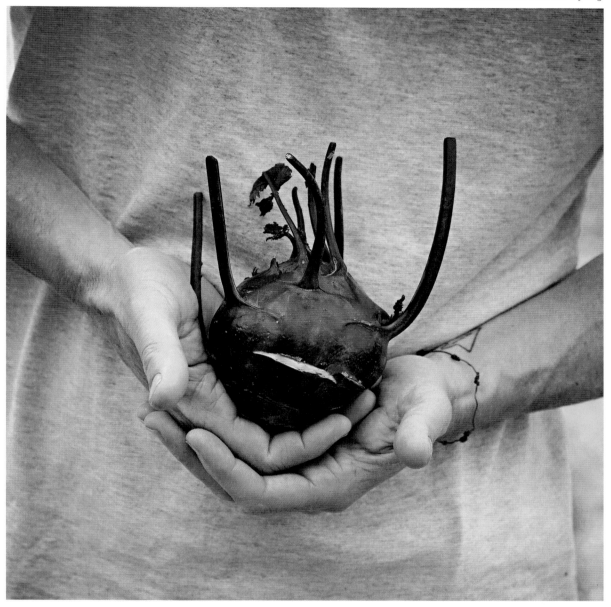

indulgent-baked-goods end of the food spectrum, and indeed, the boozy end. My tack is to be more mindful of just how deliciously chocolatey that brownie is, to fully marvel at the chilly tart-sweet creaminess of a raspberry ice cream, and to relish every slow and subtle sip of my deliciously complex red wine. If I do this, focusing my full attention on the pleasure they give, then at least I can say I have got the very best out of such treats. Indeed I believe mindfulness helps me to get a little more, from a little less of them. And getting more from less adds up – it can make a big difference to our health.

Something to chew on

Slowing down and chewing well – thoroughly and fairly slowly – isn't just a step towards more mindful eating. It also prepares your food better for digestion. It breaks it down into smaller and smaller pieces, which is obviously helpful, but it also mixes it with enzymes in your saliva and bacteria that are complementary to, but different from, those in your gut flora that will continue the digestive process. As you switch to a wholer way of eating, and a wider variety of foods, this is very important. It will help you get more of the good stuff out of the good stuff.

PORTIONING BLAME: SIZE MATTERS

We can begin to see how a more mindful approach to eating might help us with the very damaging problem of over-consumption. That's a huge deal, because one of the no-brainer causes of the Western world's current obesity crisis, and all the illness that comes with it, is this: too much of the time, we simply eat too much. The size of a 'regular' portion has, if you'll excuse the pun, mushroomed in recent decades. Our dinner plates themselves have expanded, our glasses have ballooned – and we

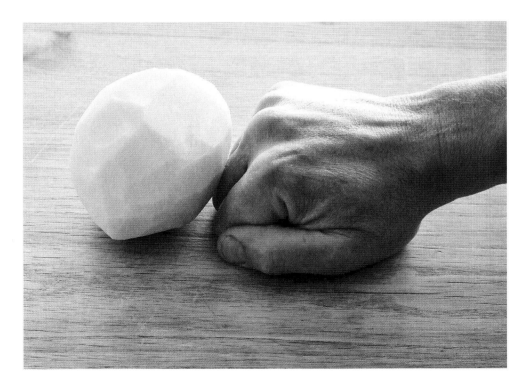

like to fill them. And, for the most part, we are filling them with the wrong things – if it was an excess of kale and celery we were eating, things wouldn't be quite so bad. But it's not. Too often, it's the carbs, the sauce and the meat.

As a basic exercise, it's definitely worth acquainting or reacquainting yourself with the recommended portion size of certain foods. Because for many of us, and with many familiar and habitual ingredients, portion size has grown wildly too big.

Here's a quick run-down of what a sensible healthy portion of a few popular foods should be – the lower figure being about average for a woman, the upper for a man:

Breakfast cereal: 30–40g – about 3 handfuls

Pasta: 60–75g uncooked – about 2 handfuls (or a tennis ball when cooked)

Bread: 1½–2 medium slices

Potato: 3–4 small new potatoes or 1 medium one – a baked spud or a portion of mash shouldn't be any bigger than your fist

Rice: 50–70g uncooked – about 2 handfuls (or a fist when cooked)

Cheese: 25–30g – about the size of two thumbs together

Meat: A piece about half the size of your hand, or 2 medium sausages

Dried fruit and nuts: 25–30g – a cupped hand, modestly filled

Chocolate: 20–25g – one fifth to one quarter of a 100g bar (not the whole bar!)

TIME FOR CHANGE

It's good to have these handy images relating to portion size at the back of your mind. But take time also to consider (mindfully) the way you fill your plate, and how you can do it in the most whole and healthy way.

One bad habit we should all aim to knock on the head, for starters, is the spreading of a carbohydrate 'base' over our plates – a thick blanket of rice, a pile of pasta, a cushion of mashed spuds – before we add sauce/vegetable/meat etc. We definitely need to rethink that.

Load your plate differently

Consider the simple idea of loading your plate first with vegetables, making *them* the substantial base, and adding carbs – even (and ideally) healthy wholegrain carbs – at the end. This is a great bit of behaviour change that can very quickly become a healthy habit. 'Seconds' are not necessarily verboten – but the carbs you thought you wanted more of may not call to you when you've already eaten some, and the best thing to have seconds of is the veg!

Cook a bit less or think leftovers

Being more mindful about portions may also mean simply cooking a bit less food to start with. Or, if you do cook more than you immediately need, do so thoughtfully, having a tasty leftovers recipe in mind for the next day. This means you need to make sure excess food gets saved, not scoffed. And one good way to do that is by putting the leftovers away *before* they are actually left over – perhaps before the first meal even begins. I do this all the time these days.

Be wary of pre-packed portions

Mindfully managing your food portions at home is one thing; but of course, over-consumption is enshrined in our flourishing food retail culture. And there's a particular challenge because it's the manufacturer, not you, who gets the first say on what a portion should be. Recent decades have seen a shocking 'up-creep' in the portion sizes of manufactured foods – ready-meals and snacks among the worst examples.

One study revealed, for example, that pre-packaged shepherd's pies on sale in 2013 were roughly twice the size of those sold 20 years previously in 1993. But once 'serves 1' is written on a pack, it's difficult to question it.

This is where a more mindful approach comes in – why it's vital, in fact. Because if we don't engage the questioning part of our brains when it comes to pack sizes then, as portion sizes of prepared foods grow, so will our calorie intake. And they've already grown far too much!

This amounts to another good reason to avoid pre-packed foods, ready-meals and snacks altogether. Doing so puts you firmly back in control of the amount you put on your plate. But if serving ready-meals suits your lifestyle, don't feel obliged to go along with the manufacturer's idea of portion control, as stated on the pack. That shepherd's pie for one might do very nicely for two (even if the second person is yourself, the next day) especially if served with a generous side order of veg.

Eating out: your rules, not theirs

Restaurant culture has to change too. In restaurants and cafés, diners and fast-food venues, value is increasingly associated with quantity. But that's a very short-term way of looking at things. A huge fry-up or a massive burger and fries, a 'bottomless' supply of fizzy drink or an 'all-you-can-eat' buffet may constitute a lot of bang for your buck – but what is that really worth if they also send you a little further down the road to type 2 diabetes? That's not a glib question – research has shown that people who eat out regularly are more likely to develop the disease.

We need to question all those givens that surround us when we enter a restaurant, café or take-out venue. To take one example, the very concept of the three-course meal is hard to justify when you apply a little thought to it: one of those courses might easily be sufficient for a meal on its own! For some time now, I have been reappraising restaurant menus with a mindful eye, and not feeling in the least obliged to follow the three-course pattern. I'm more likely to have two starters than a starter and a main. Or I might just share a main course with my wife – with a bit of extra veg on the side. Ordering a pud – also likely to be shared – is the exception not the rule.

The takeaway decision

And let's shed the assumption that takeaway food presented in a single serving, such as a burger, pasty, carton of chips, piece of battered fish, a pizza or soft drink, actually represents a sensible amount for one person. I mean, says who?? A mindful approach is most powerful when we fully own the decision about how much is enough.

Try the following more mindful approaches to help you limit portion sizes:

> If you're eating something that comes in a pack or tub, such as nuts or dried fruit (or treats like crisps or ice cream), portion them out into a small bowl before you start, and take a minute to register that you've served yourself this little meal. If you eat food blindly straight from the pack, it's much harder to stop – in fact you're very likely to finish the whole pack – and you won't appreciate it as much either.

> Reset portions for carbs such as rice, pasta or noodles, as the bit on the side rather than a hefty base to a meal. It's easier to do this – to start with at least, if you weigh out those starchy ingredients before you cook them. These foods are easy to over-serve because in their uncooked, dry form, they don't look like much. Most packs are pushing the idea of a 100g (dry weight) serving per person. It's far too much: 50–70g dry rice per person is plenty once it's cooked.

When you've got the urge to pile more on to your plate, try saying to yourself, 'this will do for now, I can always eat more later if I want to.' It's a lot gentler and easier than telling yourself a blunt '*No!*'. This 'deferral' trick can help to stop you over-serving or over-ordering, and you may well find that you don't want to eat more later on after all.

Slow down. Eating slowly and consciously gives your body time to register its fullness and helps you appreciate your food so that less feels like more.

When you've finished your main meal and find yourself reaching instinctively for something sweet, stop and take a breather. Leave it for 15 minutes, then ask yourself if you really do want that sweet treat after all. It takes 15 minutes for your body to really register fullness – give it a chance to tell you whether it's actually still hungry. And if it is, maybe a square or two of dark chocolate will do the job, rather than a fully fledged pud.

When you eat out, remember that no one *needs* three courses. This is a restaurant convention, but you don't have to stick to it – is it really what you need? You can still enjoy your meal: just skip the starter, or the pud, or ask for a second starter or a side dish instead of a main. Consider sharing a main course or a dessert – ask for an extra plate. Or leave food on your plate when you're full and ask for it to be packaged up to take home. Don't feel pressured by staff trying to 'up-sell' by asking if you want to 'go large' or 'have fries with that'. Restaurant culture pushes us into eating much more than we need. But we can push back.

A clear memory of what you've recently eaten can influence what and how much you eat next. A food journal – which can be helpful if you're trying to be more mindful about what you eat anyway (see pages 62–6) – will make you more aware of what you've already consumed, and can help you moderate your portions.

Mindfulness means acknowledging that, whenever and wherever we are eating, there must be limits; that we have to decide when our meal is over, and that it is helpful *not* to keep an open mind about whether you might go on grazing on the food that's on the table (or in the cupboard!). This may prove a little harder than bringing mindfulness to bear on the pleasure of eating itself. The trick is to focus on the positive: remind yourself that you will feel better, more energised, happier if you don't overeat, and that in any case, you need only wait a few hours before you can enjoy some more delicious food and drink. That is, unless you are planning an extended interval before your next meal – which may also prove to be a very good idea...

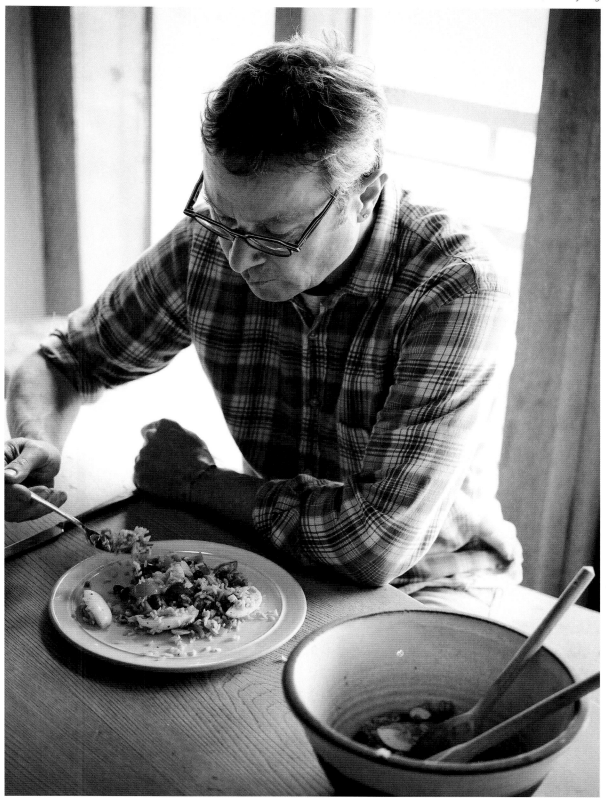

HEALTHY *NOT*-EATING

It may sound odd, given the thousands of words I've expended already talking about what we should be putting in our mouths, but I am convinced that, sometimes, the healthiest way to eat is simply not to eat at all for a while. I'm not talking about starvation or harsh dietary regimes; I mean simply stretching out the time when we are not eating a little bit more than most of us currently do.

The modern habit of mindlessly munching and grazing our way through the day is an understandable response to the ever-growing availability of food in all places and at all times. But it is at the very heart of what's wrong with our food culture, and it is why we have a global obesity crisis. And here, the application of a modicum of mindfulness can be highly significant – not just as an aid to healthy eating, but as a crucial way to support healthy *not*-eating. Let me explain...

A truly good diet, for me, means nutritious, healthy, delicious meals, certainly. It also means being conscious not only of the foods that are good for us, and those that do us harm, but also of *when* we eat (or don't eat) our food, and why that can make such a difference to our well-being.

Clearly, eating, snacking or consuming a calorie-loaded drink, six, seven or eight times a day can easily lead to weight gain and poor health. But there is compelling and still-mounting evidence that eating all the time is unhealthy in a much broader sense. The science is telling us that going for significant periods without food can bring us clear health benefits, aside from helping us to moderate the sheer amount we are eating.

I have incorporated this thinking into the way I eat for at least 7 years now. And, as with my commitment to whole foods, variety and the live fermented foods that I believe help my gut biome to thrive, I am convinced that committing to not eating from time to time, to a point where I recognise the sensations of being hungry, is good for me.

INTERMITTENT FASTING

You've probably heard of this approach. It's been widely disseminated in a host of diet books, including Michael Mosley and Mimi Spencer's compelling *The Fast Diet*, many of which have embraced the '5:2' concept, whereby you 'fast' by eating, usually, fewer than 600 calories for 2 days a week and try to eat 'normally' (and without overcompensating for those low-calorie days) for the remaining five.

The 5:2 pattern is largely based on pioneering studies done by Dr Michelle Harvie, this book's own resident nutrition expert, who published her own book, *The 2-Day Diet*, in 2013. Knowing that being overweight is a key risk factor for breast cancer, Michelle and her colleagues wanted to find a weight-loss diet that was simple and effective. They chose intermittent fasting, believing that people would find it relatively straightforward to cut their calories right back for two days if they didn't have to 'diet' the rest of the time. 'We wanted to restrict calorie intake by 25% overall, but in a way that was doable and, more importantly, sustainable,' explains Michelle. 'We didn't want our patients to go without eating anything at all for 24 hours, so our "fast" days allowed for 650 calories, which could be taken as one, two or three small meals a day.'

In her own studies, Michelle's diet proved extremely successful. Patients lost weight and kept it off. 'What was seriously interesting,' says Michelle, 'is that it seemed to improve overall eating patterns and food choices. We found patients reduced their calories by about 20% on their non-fast days. This way of eating makes people much more aware of when they are really hungry. It seems to change behaviour. For many people, we find the two-day diet is actually a really good way to promote an overall healthy diet.'

We can extrapolate from this, Michelle concludes, that intermittent fasting is actually helping many people to eat more *mindfully*. I'd second that – and for me it works the other way too: being more mindful helps me fast.

Fast talking

Before I go on, let's discuss the terminology. I'm using the word 'fast' throughout this section, because it is the simplest way to talk about eating very little – although not necessarily nothing. Diet scientists now employ the term 'fast' to describe days of not eating, but equally to describe days of reduced calorie intake – 650 calories or fewer.

Nevertheless, I'm aware that 'fasting' is a bit of a scary word. It can sound extreme, brutal and punishing, with connotations of religious penitence and self-denial. Long (or at least significant) periods of religious fasting were once the norm in many societies, and in some cultures they still are. But the notion of a lengthy period without food can seem pretty terrifying if it is unfamiliar.

I think it's okay to move with the times and allow the word 'fast' to mean what we need it to mean today, if it's going to help us to eat better. To me, it expresses the clear intention to abstain from food, or restrict your intake, voluntarily. Religion aside, there was a time when most people took a reasonably long pause between meals without eating anything at all. That time is long gone. The natural 'fasts' between meals are now largely undermined by our ingrained habit of snacking.

For most of us, only the overnight fast, the one while we are actually asleep (and which we traditionally end at 'break-fast') remains intact. And even that is under assault from late-night just-before-bed snacking and early morning lattes and croissants…

For reasons I'm about to explain, reinstating significant gaps between eating is a really good idea. And if we are looking for the motivation to achieve that (which at times we may well need, as fasting isn't always easy), I think it's best to frame that as conscious and well-planned self-care, *not* as any kind of fanatical self-deprivation.

What can fasting really do for us?

Many people first explore intermittent fasting as an aid to weight loss – and that includes me. I read the aforementioned *The Fast Diet*, and 'gave it a go' in the hope of losing a few pounds. It worked, helping me bring my weight down from 82kg to 77kg in just a few months. That was gratifying as it took my Body Mass Index from the 'overweight' category to within the normal range for my height (1.78 metres).

But there were other benefits. In fact, the whole thing was quite a revelation. As well as losing weight, my energy levels were lifted and I was increasingly free of the bouts of indigestion I used to suffer. I was converted and I've been using intermittent fasting ever since. Now, however, I fast primarily for well-being not for weight loss. Though, as you'll see at the end of this section, I also keep fasting in my back pocket for when I feel my weight may be nudging at the upper limit of where I'd like it to be.

Science is beginning to show that the benefits of intermittent fasting may go far beyond shifting a spare tyre. The work of Professor Mark Mattson, one of the world's leading authorities on fasting, along with other pioneers in this field, suggests that fasting initiates changes in the body that could have profound implications for our health.

Mattson's research has enabled him to describe in detail what happens on a cellular level when mammals don't eat – and the science is pretty complex. But his layperson's summary is really helpful: fasting is a form of mild stress on the body (just like exercise); and the body responds in all sorts of ways that have the effect of making it stronger and more resistant to injury and disease. With intermittent fasting, he believes, the whole body – even the brain – becomes more resilient.

For example, when fasting, our bodies produce less insulin – a hormone that promotes the growth and multiplication of our cells. Insulin-fuelled periods of growth are when cells are more likely to become damaged. When we don't eat, insulin drops and the body is more likely to actually clear out and recycle old or damaged cells. For me, this is perhaps the greatest appeal of fasting: that it can tip the body into 'repair mode', triggering a process of general maintenance and upkeep. This can occur in tissues throughout the body, including the brain. Studies in rodents show that fasting stimulates this process, and the exciting suggestion is that it could prevent or delay degenerative neurological conditions such as Alzheimer's.

Intermittent fasting, because it also reduces calorie intake, may reduce disease-causing inflammation in the body. And there's also evidence that people who have practised intermittent fasting have improved 'metabolic flexibility', which essentially describes the body's ability to switch between being fed and being unfed. It means we can efficiently metabolise larger meals when they come along, but also maintain good function in periods of low food intake too. This is a key marker for good health. Our bodies have evolved to cope well with these 'feast or famine' ups and downs, but modern patterns of near-constant grazing and snacking don't allow them to do so.

This is all new and developing research. There aren't a huge number of human studies to date: most fasting-linked benefits have been shown in studies on rats and mice, and this doesn't prove that fasting will have the same effect in people. But it does constitute emerging evidence that periods of fasting have the potential to extend healthy life. Certainly many people find intermittent fasting a good way of controlling their weight, and thereby reducing the risk of obesity-related conditions including type 2 diabetes, heart disease and cancer. But there are tantalising suggestions in the latest research that fasting in itself may provide additional protection against these killer diseases.

Mattson himself has been fasting regularly for 35 years now. In fact, plenty of the people who study the effects of fasting find themselves highly motivated to start doing it. For me, that's a pretty strong endorsement.

Is fasting just a fad?

The idea of letting yourself go hungry may sound a bit crackpot. Skipping breakfast or dinner, or even going for a whole day without food, flies in the face of the accepted wisdom about healthy eating. But despite popular belief, there is no evidence that eating every few hours is essential.

It's true that there have been some rather wild messages sent out about intermittent fasting: a lot of people have jumped on the 5:2 bandwagon – and the work produced is often a far cry from Mark's or Michelle's. Some of it – particularly the work packaged in glossy, quick-fix diet books – is approaching irresponsible, implying that it's okay to eat junk most of the time, as long as you fast once or twice a week. If there is a faddish face to fasting then unfortunately this is it.

But fasting itself is not a new concept. As I've mentioned, it's actually incredibly old. In fact, it's not even a concept. Going without food for hours or even days has been a completely normal fact of life for many mammals, including humans, for most of history. It's only in the last few hundred years that humans have come to regard three meals a day, every day, as some kind of cultural ideal. And only in the last few decades has constant eating become our really rather harmful human habit.

How I fast

Talking as I have to dozens of people who have dabbled with fasting, I know that many of us are impressed by the science, beguiled by the seeming simplicity, but come unstuck in the practice of intermittent fasting. I believe that this is mainly because, as I've said, it is so often sold as a kind of single-fix diet miracle that will sort out all our weight worries and food foibles.

That is simply the wrong way to look at it. It absolves us from thinking about some very important aspects of our eating, that we know can help us hugely to improve our health (and which we've explored in some depth in the previous 6 chapters of this book). And it also puts a massive burden of pressure on the success or failure of our individual endeavours in the challenging task of going without food for an extended period. It sets us up to fail, and to feel bad about failing. At which point, it's all too easy to throw up our hands and say, 'to hell with fasting' – and healthy eating.

This is why I advocate fasting as just one part of a blended, mindful approach to healthier eating. It immediately becomes both so much more achievable and so much more effective. You don't have to stick to a rigid 5:2 approach, and you certainly don't have to fast twice every single week, if that doesn't suit your life.

Rather I want to encourage you to anticipate good opportunities for fasting as they approach. Set a weekly plan if you like, but don't worry about adapting it if something (like a friend's birthday lunch) pops up. Resentment will not help you succeed.

I have developed my own way of fasting, slightly different to the 5:2, which still aims to reap all the potential benefits, without being particularly focused on weight loss (most of the time). It's based around having a minimum 12-hour break from food in almost every 24-hour period. I say almost, because there will always be compelling reasons that crop up once in a while (the 3am breakfast at the end of the wedding disco springs to mind) that make an exception to the rule.

But generally, every day, I try and eat nothing (and drink nothing but herbal tea or water) after 8pm and before 8am (or it might be 7pm–7am or 9pm–9am), thereby 'achieving' a 12-hour fast without any notable effort. And a couple of days a week (on average – sometimes it's 3 days, sometimes it just doesn't happen) I will extend that to 16 hours by eating nothing at all before 12am.

Once in a while (unlikely to be more than a couple of times a month), I might go all the way through the day, to 7pm supper-time with just a light lunch/snack – perhaps a couple of apples or a banana, or a couple of oatcakes, a little scrap of cheese and some kraut and kimchi (pages 282 and 284). This is my version of a fairly classic 'by the book' 5:2 fast day.

It's important to note that fasting does not mean letting nothing pass your lips. It's crucial to take on board fluids while you fast – lots of them. I like to keep my 16-hour fasts free of any food, including food masquerading as drinks (see the previous

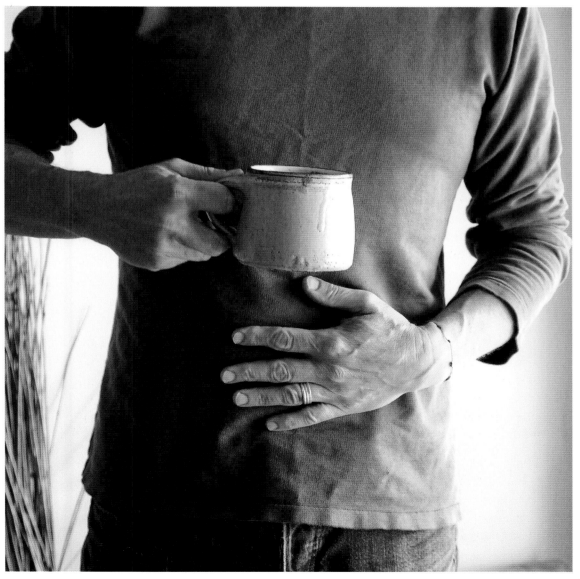

chapter!), but if you're finding it hard to begin with, you could take in a little very light food, such as a cup of vegetable broth, an apple or a raw carrot, a very small (150 ml) glass of juice or kombucha, or allow yourself a little milk in your coffee or tea.

Crucially (for me) this relatively light and I believe easily sustainable approach to fasting is not really pre-planned, but undertaken with a kind of mindful spontaneity. I decide when I wake up, based on the day ahead, and how I'm feeling, what seems sensible and achievable. If I have a hard day's filming ahead, or I'm going to be on my feet for some other reason, I'll have a normal-ish breakfast, around 8am, or pack a portable breakfast (for example, my overnight oats on page 227, or the grated root and fruit salad on page 222) to take with me on the train or in the car.

If I'm having a desk day, I will usually try and stretch the no-eating period well into the morning, ideally till lunchtime. This works best when I'm really in control of my time, and don't have to interact much with other people. The reverse may be true for others. Some people have told me they find it easier to fast when they are dashing about, working with colleagues, staying too busy to eat or think much about food.

How you might fast

Fasting patterns are personal: different things work for different people. But the following points represent a suggested gradual introduction to the practice of healthy not-eating, starting with simply leaving a clear break between your regular meals and extending to the idea of more committed fasts. I'm not suggesting this is a single track everyone should be on, and a lot of people won't want to attempt 'full-on' fasting. But even experimenting with the first couple of ideas here could be profoundly positive.

Snack less. A regular flow of mini-meals, including biscuits, crisps and sweets, wraps and sandwiches, milky coffees and fizzy drinks all add to our calorie intake. So start by skipping the snacks. You might find there's quite a lot of satisfaction to be had in it, leading to a rediscovery of the pleasure of being hungry when you sit down to a meal.

Give your gut a proper break overnight. As little as 12 hours (i.e. overnight) can be a significant duration for a fast. It takes roughly that time for the body to use up its stored glycogen (its instant energy reserve) and start burning fat instead, which seems to be the trigger for many of the beneficial effects emerging from the research. This 12/12 night/day pattern is a good place to start if you're curious about the notion of fasting. Maintain that for a few days and you could think about adding an hour to that overnight break sometimes – having dinner an hour earlier or breakfast an hour later.

Skip breakfast if it suits you. Some people struggle without an early meal, and children and teenagers should eat breakfast, but plenty of adults function perfectly well without it. That's really useful if you want to fast. If you can cope pretty well without fuel first thing, then the '16/8' pattern might work well for you, perhaps two or three times a week. It involves confining your eating to an 8-hour period during the day, such as 12 noon to 8pm. It's a simple way to build extended periods of non-eating into your life and it's the pattern favoured by Mark Mattson. Many others find it pretty doable and a few zealots do this every day. It's generally how I fast, though even when I manage a mere '14/10' I give myself a pat on the back.

Go further if you want to, if that works for you. To incorporate intermittent fasting as a regular thing, it is important to find what suits you and your lifestyle. If you're an all-or-nothing kind of person, the full 24-hour version, once or even twice a week, could be the ticket. You can achieve this by fasting between 7pm one day and 7pm the next, apart from the one light snack (ideally taken after at least 16 hours). And come 7pm you can still have (a sensible) supper!

If you can't face the idea of skipping meals, look at Michelle Harvie and Tony Howell's *2-Day Diet*, which allows for small meals, even on fast days. The more you experiment with fasting, the more your body – and perhaps more importantly, your mind! – adapts to it. Research suggests it takes 3–6 weeks for most people to get into the groove of intermittent fasting. I reckon my flexible approach optimises the chance of success.

The hunger gains

For many, fear of being hungry is a key reason – perhaps the only reason – not to try fasting. Hunger is something we are increasingly unaccustomed to; it is an unfamiliar and uncomfortable feeling and it makes us anxious. What's more, as food is available almost everywhere, almost all the time, we almost never *need* to sit with hunger – we simply snuff it out as soon as we can. And we've forgotten that hunger is not actually such a bad thing, when experienced for brief periods of time. This is where a mindful approach to fasting is so important. When viewed with clarity and calmness, hunger stops being scary. It can become neutral, even interesting.

And, at times, I can get pretty darned hungry during a fast day. People who tell you they fast and hardly notice it are probably not being entirely straight with you. Those pangs are our bodies' ancient way of spurring us into hunting, foraging or stealing our next meal! They are natural and healthy – but can be a bit alarming. If we want to sustain a fast for a few hours, we need to ride them out. The best way to do that, I find, is not to try and ignore them but quite the opposite. To be mindful of them, to pay attention to them – just not to act on them by eating food! (Though a cup of herbal tea helps.) So when I fast, I notice my hunger. I take a few minutes now and again to remind myself that while I am feeling that primal sensation, good things are going on inside me. My body is using this time to rest, regenerate and repair in a way it doesn't do while I am feeding it every few hours. That knowledge produces a feeling of positivity.

This more mindful approach undoubtedly helps fasting work for me. It makes it motivating and sustainable, rather than punishing. And, because I end a fast with a feeling of satisfaction, I don't then feel the urge to stuff myself with food. Fasting has helped me fall naturally into better eating patterns overall. And those patterns fall in with the variety of whole, nutrient-packed, fibre-rich foods I've been celebrating throughout the book. The content and form of my diet have both changed, undeniably for the better. And the whole thing feels sustainable, flexible, life-enhancing and right.

Is fasting for everyone?

Passionate convert that I am, the short answer is no, it's not for everyone. That's why I've placed it at the end of my 7 Ways, carefully in the context of mindful (not) eating, rather than promised it as miracle cure for all your food woes.

Michelle Harvie points out that there are still gaps in our knowledge of intermittent fasting. 'Most of the human research on it has been done with people who are overweight. We don't have hard evidence about the effects of fasting in people who aren't. Some data suggests a downside to fasting: for example, one study showed irritability and fatigue in women of normal weight. We also can't say exactly what the optimum pattern of fasting might be for people in the normal weight range.'

Some people just do not get on with fasting, and some people should not even attempt it. You *must* consult your doctor before you try fasting if you have any kind of health condition, including depression or diabetes, or are on any kind of medication. Some medications, including those for lowering blood sugar in diabetics, are not compatible with fasting.

Fasting is not okay for children and adolescents, the elderly or frail, pregnant or breastfeeding women, anyone underweight or with a history of eating disorders. There is also some evidence that intermittent fasting for normal-weight women could affect hormonal balance and fertility. This doesn't mean it's off the cards. But normal-weight women of reproductive age should go cautiously with fasting and try not to actually lose weight. You certainly should not fast if you are trying to conceive. If in any doubt talk to your doctor first.

ACTION POINT RECAP

1 Pause for thought

Slow down, separate yourself from distractions, and be more thoughtful and focused when you shop, cook and eat. It will increase your pleasure in food from start to finish. And it will also help you recognise your body's signals, to understand when you are actually hungry, and when there may be other triggers pushing you towards eating, such as stress or anxiety.

Pausing in such moments gives you a chance to make better, healthier choices, and for the right reasons – i.e. not out of fear, guilt or shame, but out of an active desire to nourish yourself with delicious, whole ingredients.

2 Scale down your servings

Be aware that portion sizes have crept up to an alarming degree over recent years – at home, in the supermarket and in restaurants. Notice how much you serve yourself: could you be satisfied with less – maybe much less? Is there scope to dial down the carb component on your plate, as you dial up the veg?

And question the portion size of food that is served to you by others – you are the judge of how much you need, not a big food brand or a fast-food chain, or even your mum! Remember that smaller portions leave you the option of eating more later if you need to; and also the chance to decide that, actually, perhaps you don't need to.

3 Try the fast track

Consider healthy *not-eating* as a way to enhance and augment everything else I've talked about in this book. That might mean simply ensuring that, as often as possible, you go for at least 12 hours overnight between dinner and breakfast. Or it could mean exploring how intermittent fasting works for you. Slot one or two '16/8' days in regularly every week if that is practical; or do it more spontaneously as you see the opportunity.

And reduce snacking and grazing through the day, opening up those pauses between food. Remember that not-eating gives your body the chance to switch into its all-important 'maintenance and repair mode'. It is a natural extension of mindful eating that can have far-reaching benefits for your health and well-being.

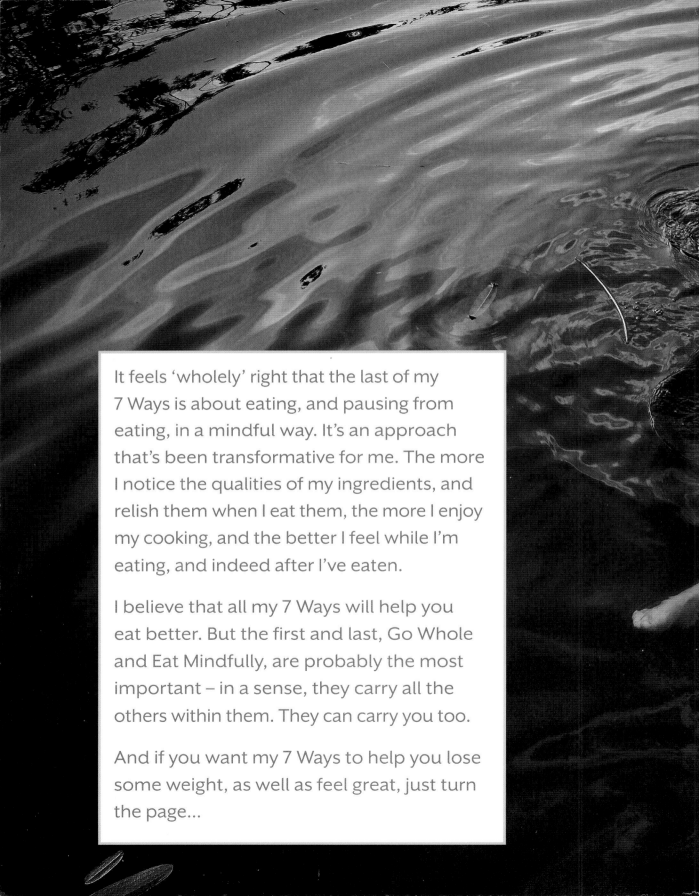

It feels 'wholely' right that the last of my 7 Ways is about eating, and pausing from eating, in a mindful way. It's an approach that's been transformative for me. The more I notice the qualities of my ingredients, and relish them when I eat them, the more I enjoy my cooking, and the better I feel while I'm eating, and indeed after I've eaten.

I believe that all my 7 Ways will help you eat better. But the first and last, Go Whole and Eat Mindfully, are probably the most important – in a sense, they carry all the others within them. They can carry you too.

And if you want my 7 Ways to help you lose some weight, as well as feel great, just turn the page...

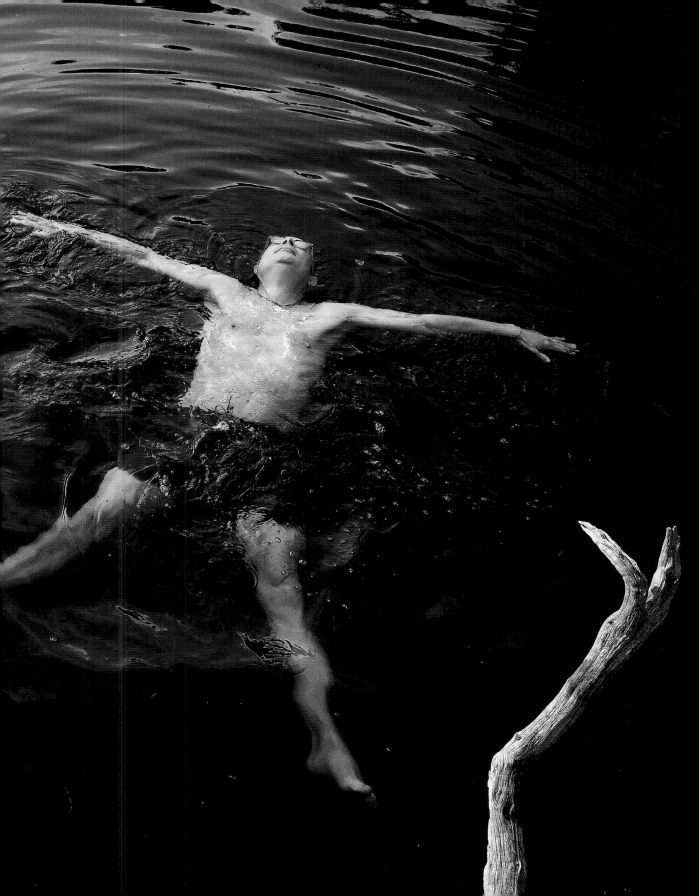

7 WAYS TO LOSE WEIGHT

First and foremost this book is about eating better to be well, and to stay well. It's for everyone who wants to eat in a way that keeps them healthy and resilient. But that doesn't mean you can't use this book as a tool to help you to lose weight. You absolutely can. And now I'm going to unpack that promise, before offering up the lovely recipes that will also help you to stay well (and to lose weight too, if you wish to do so).

If you are above a healthy weight, then taking steps to lose some weight is a really good idea. Put simply, every kilo you lose reduces your risk of suffering weight-related diseases, such as diabetes, cancer and heart disease. And we now know that it also reduces the risk of serious complications, and indeed fatality, from Covid-19.

If you are not sure where you stand weight-wise, then knowing your Body Mass Index, and whether it's in the healthy range for your age, is a good idea. There's an excellent calculator online: nhs.uk/live-well/healthy-weight/bmi-calculator. Another surprisingly good indicator (for the metrically minded!) is that your waist measurement should be within a couple of centimetres of half your height.

In truth, you probably already know whether it would be a good idea for you to lose weight. And the great news is that if you follow the advice and guidance in this book, it is likely that you will. My fantastic scientific and nutritional sounding board Dr Michelle Harvie and I have talked in depth about this, and she fully supports this statement.

But it's important to remember that although the reasons for gaining weight are many and complex, one aspect of the means by which it happens is constant. It happens when our bodies are taking in more energy (calories) than they can burn, and so what they cannot use gets stored as fat. (This is not *quite* the same as simply *consuming* more calories than we burn as some are 'less available' – see page 31 – but it's very closely related.)

If you choose a wide variety of whole foods, that give you the right balance of nutrients, that's going to make it easier to consume fewer calories overall (ideally without ever counting them). You will already be on the right path to improved general health and greater resilience to illness, to sustainable healthy weight loss, and ultimately to the holy grail of maintaining a healthy weight without it feeling like a constant struggle.

If weight loss is part of your goal in eating better, then I have a couple of approaches for you, and which you choose perhaps depends loosely on your personality type (don't worry, I'm not going to ask you to take a test).

One is, quite simply, to crack on with the 7 Ways and see what happens. Just go for it. The more wholeheartedly you commit, the better the chance that you will consume fewer calories overall. If that happens then healthy, moderately-paced, sustainable weight loss will very naturally follow (and you're going to feel a whole lot better too, both mentally and physically).

But much as I'd like to, I can't say that it's an absolute certainty that embracing the 7 Ways will result in fewer calories overall, and the weight coming off. It is possible to overeat even healthy foods. So, if you are someone who likes things nailed down, you might like to plan your eating ahead of time, and take up a more prescriptive approach, one that gently (without asking you to count calories) puts limits around your overall consumption.

If this appeals, then I have something coming up that's going to deliver exactly the prescription you need: a 7-day meal plan, based on the delicious recipes that are coming up in the second half of the book. But before you decide which approach is for you, I'm daring to think it might just be helpful to hear a bit more about…

…How I lost weight

Throughout my thirties and forties my weight went up and down between around 75 and 85 kilos – bouncing my BMI between 25 and 28 (which is firmly in the overweight category). The ups generally came with an increased and stressful workload – TV work, in particular. And I tended to be able to shed a few kilos over summer holidays, or when I was taking time out to write a book.

As I approached 50, the 'downs' were not really happening any more. My weight was stuck in the 80s (a bit like my taste in music). I knew there was an increasing chance, rising with my age, that my weight would have an impact on my health. I decided that I wanted to lose some weight *forever*, and I realised it was time to make some permanent adjustments.

Now personally, I'm not a meal-plan kind of person. I don't know what's for supper until I look in the fridge, scan the storecupboard and ideally have a wander round the veg patch. And I wanted to continue to eat 'spontaneously'. So, I knew I had to make a few clear-cut resolutions, to simply make better choices.

I started by addressing the areas where I could see obvious room for manoeuvre: the amount of alcohol I was drinking, the processed snacks I was eating between meals. Yes, I was a crisp fiend (see page 123) and a chocolate bar aficionado (I reckoned that

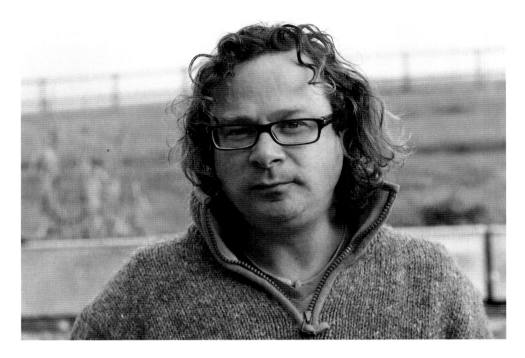

I preferred a Toffee Crisp to a Picnic and too often grasped the opportunity to remind myself why). And I was relaxing at the end of every day with several glasses of wine (or beer, or cider). So, I immediately put in a couple of alcohol-free days a week. I decided they could be transferable (if a good invite comes in), but not negotiable. I already ate plenty of fresh fruit and veg, but I decided to eat (and grow!) even more of them, and use them more, along with more nuts, seeds and dried fruits, to make lighter lunches and healthier snacks to replace the sandwiches, chocolate bars and biscuits I was often using to keep me going during the day.

I also reined in a bit on some of my favourite fatty foods – butter, cheese and ice cream for example – without giving any of them up. I resolved to fry food less often and to use less oil when I fried. And I made a big effort to use more pulses, nuts and seeds in my cooking, and to 'whole-up' my carbs. Rice was surprisingly significant. It took me a while to get the same enjoyment from brown as from white. Now I actually prefer the fuller, nuttier taste, and am content with a portion that's less than half of the white rice I used to spread right across my plate.

Finally, I embraced occasional intermittent fasting, increasing the periods between eating to include at least one, sometimes two, fasts of 14–16 hours each week. One thing

I noticed (and at first it was definitely more of an observation than a resolution) was that I was becoming much more conscious of my eating – what when and how (even how much I was chewing my food). As I was also beginning to read about meditation and mindfulness, I realised I was eating *more mindfully*. And I resolved to stick with that...

I never counted a calorie, but I did weigh myself, though generally not more often than weekly. I found it pretty motivating to see my weight come down, though it was rarely by more than half a kilo in a week. When it didn't shift at all, or even went up by a few hundred grams, I wasn't disheartened. I knew I was going in the right direction. The most motivating thing was how much better I felt.

I also began making *Britain's Fat Fight* for BBC1. It was both motivating and illuminating. And it gave me the opportunity to read books and articles by leading scientists, and to talk to many of them too – people like Tim Spector, Giles Yeo, Christopher Gardner, Susan Jebb, Corinna Hawkes, Kawther Hashem and, of course, my collaborator on this project, Michelle Harvie. They are not sponsored by the food industry, but motivated by a genuine desire to help people – and the whole world – move out of the grip of bad eating and obesity-related disease. They have been busting many of the old myths about diet, and converging on a consensus of what healthy eating really is. I have learned so much from them (you should look them up, they are an impressive bunch!).

And so, through some combination of improving self-knowledge, research, and a generous but healthy helping of good luck, I believe I have finally taught myself to eat better, forever. For a few years now my weight has never dropped below 74kg or risen above 77kg. Right now I weigh 75.4 kilos. My BMI is 24, just nudging the high end of normal for my age (55, since you ask). I still eat too much sometimes, and I drink too much once in while. The journey's not over. But I no longer worry about my weight – and I always think about what I'm eating.

...How you can lose weight

My 7 Ways are a distillation of what I believe to be the most useful knowledge to pass on to *anyone* who wants to eat better, but *especially* to those who also want to lose weight in a healthy and sustainable way, to improve their health and simply feel better for the rest of their lives.

If that's *you*, reading this *now*, then I *really* want to help you succeed. And so, I'd like you to walk through the 7 Ways with me one more time. This time, let's scrutinise them through the lens of sustainable, healthy weight loss. I think it's going to boost your confidence that this really will work for you.

1 Going Whole

Going whole means making sure that the primary building blocks of your meals are whole ingredients, not highly refined or processed foods. Every credible dietician and nutritionist agrees that a plant-rich diet centred on whole foods is the healthiest way to lose weight.

Whole foods are high in fibre and more filling than processed foods. Switching to whole foods enables you to feel more full having consumed less food. This is conducive to gradual, sustainable weight loss.

Remember also Dr Giles Yeo's sweetcorn (see page 31). All calories are not the same. When you eat whole, more fibrous foods, more of the calories consumed will pass through your system unmetabolised (and so they won't get stored as fat) than when you eat refined foods. So even if your calorie consumption remains the same, Going Whole will either lead to gradual weight loss or, if you have been gaining weight, at the very least slow the rate of gain.

2 Going Varied

Going Varied multiplies the benefits of Going Whole. Diverse combinations of whole foods are more than the sum of their parts, helping you achieve the 'constellation of protective nutrients' (see page 57) that is crucial to good digestion, a healthy and diverse gut flora, and a resilient immune system.

A varied diet is associated with improved mood, so ringing the changes with whole foods is a morale booster when you are trying to eat better and lose weight. It also increases the choices available that allow you to make healthy swaps. This can help you break bad habits and ditch the poor choices that you may be turning to when you feel stressed or anxious.

So even if variety does not guarantee you reduced calorific intake in and of itself, it will help to make the changes from bad eating to better both more achievable and more sustainable.

3 Going with Your Gut

There are not yet clear, repeatable studies establishing direct causal links between improving the diversity of gut bacteria and sustained weight loss. But there is growing consensus among gut health scientists that there may be a positive feedback loop acting on your diet when you choose foods that improve your gut biome.

Studies show that a healthy gut microbiome has positive effects on the levels of hormones and neurotransmitters that play a role in regulating your appetite. They increase your sense of satiety (fullness) and can therefore help you not to overeat. Splice that with the correlation between a diverse gut biome and improved general mood and mental health, and it's clear that better gut health over time can give you a better chance of sustained success in healthy eating and healthy weight loss.

4 Reducing Refined Carbs

Pretty much by definition, if you are dialling down refined carbs you are dialling down calories (unless you are replacing them with different refined carbs – let's not do that!).

When you reduce and replace foods that are mass-produced from refined carbs (for example, confectionery and biscuits, crisps and snacks) you are also reducing your vulnerability to the 'bliss point' effect (see page 100). Remember these highly processed foods (that cynically combine refined fats and refined carbs) are actually designed to excite the pleasure responses in your brain, releasing dopamine. They can override your sense of when you are full and when to stop eating, so avoiding them is a good way to avoid the temptation to overeat – and indeed to avoid actually overeating!

As you replace refined carbs with whole (white with brown), be mindful that whole food carbs (and pulses, which also make a great swap for refined carbs) offer you a great chance to feel fuller and more satisfied, with less food. That's an opportunity to savour (not an excuse to cut loose on) the wholemeal bread and brown rice – one that dovetails very nicely with a mindful consciousness of the foods you are choosing and eating.

5 Factoring in Fats

Fats are a vital and healthy component of our diet, essential for our cells, nerves, hormones, blood flow and much else besides. We literally can't live without them.

Fats are also very calorie-dense foods that can lead to weight gain if consumed in excess. By decoupling them from refined carbs (with which they are systematically and cynically combined in highly refined industrial foods, see previous page) you can improve the visibility of the fats you eat, understand them better, use them more appropriately, and consume them more moderately.

When you Factor in Fats, you harness them as a tool for successful, sustainable weight loss. You can use just enough in your cooking and eating to make all kinds of healthy whole foods, especially plants, even more palatable and delicious. You'll do this most effectively by using them less for frying and baking, and more for dressing and trickling. But when you do bake and fry, you can take more control: you can select your fats more appropriately and moderately than the industrial food brands do when they are frying and baking for you.

By avoiding trans fats and reducing saturated fats you will be consuming fewer calories, providing you replace them with smaller amounts of healthier fats.

6 Thinking about Your Drink

As soon as you recognise that many 'drinks' are, in fact, significantly calorific foods, you are empowered to reduce the amount of calories you consume through drinking. If you drink soft drinks (SSBs) or 'recipe' coffees regularly, replacing them with low- or no-calorie alternatives offers an opportunity for very significant calorie reduction.

When it comes to alcohol, if you are currently a daily drinker, putting in 2 or 3 (or more) alcohol-free days per week immediately reduces calorie consumption. It also reduces the number of mealtimes where the mild euphoria of alcohol may facilitate the stealthy or unconscious consumption of 'more' (the red wine and the cheeseboard...).

Switching to non-alcoholic alternatives that are also lower in calories – water, herbal infusions, sensible portions of fruit juice and kombucha – is an excellent weight loss strategy, provided you consume them in more moderate quantities than you would alcoholic drinks.

7 Eating (and not eating) Mindfully

Eating mindfully means being aware of whatever you are eating – not just when you are eating it, but even when you are buying it and preparing it (or ordering it in a restaurant). Its provenance, the goodness it contains (or doesn't), the pleasures of eating it (and the pitfalls of eating *too much* of it), can all be held in mind. This empowers good decision-making every time we choose, prepare and consume our foods.

Mindful eating is the antidote to mind*less* eating – we know we eat more when eating is an unthinking companion to other activities, like watching telly or driving. Less mindless eating means fewer calories for sure.

Mindful eating also brings two powerful tools into play. The first is portion reduction. The mindful self-instruction to 'fill half your plate with plants' (page 50), and keep your carbs not only whole, but moderate (the fist-sized spud, the brown rice on the side, not covering the plate) can become habits of mindful self-care that help you navigate every mealtime, consuming better food and fewer calories, day after day.

The second tool is intermittent fasting. For those who find it achievable and helpful, putting one or two 14–16 hour fasts into your week can gently accelerate the weight loss that will come with embracing most or all of the six other elements described above.

And the general rule of keeping 12 hours in every 24 (including your sleep) free of food, is a very healthy habit for all. It's not just 12 hours of uninterrupted maintenance and repair for your metabolism, it's 12 hours without calories too!

I hope you can see that these are not only 7 Ways to Eat Better, they are 7 Ways to Lose Weight healthily and sustainably too. If you feel ready to set about making them part of your life (perhaps you've already started) then please crack on. You can come back to the book whenever you want reminders and reassurance – and great healthy recipes.

If, on the other hand, you would like a little more hand-holding as you get started on my 7 Ways, then it's my absolute pleasure to oblige. What follows is a slightly more prescriptive (but no less delicious) route, with my recipes curated for you, and set out in a clear, easy-to-follow meal plan. Just turn the page...

7-DAY 7-WAYS MEAL-PLAN

This 7-Day plan offers you a balanced week of nicely varied, 7-Ways eating based on recipes in the book. Following the plan for 3–4 weeks will give you a feel for whole food cooking, healthier snacking and sensible portion sizes. As you get to week 3, feel relaxed about swapping in other recipes (especially from the same chapter). You can always add in one or two or three '16/8' fasts to this plan (to boost your weight loss), skipping the breakfast and mid-morning snack for example (see page 183). There will be days where life (or a nice invitation) takes you off-piste. Just start back on the plan the next day. After a while, go elsewhere in the recipe section for inspiration, and take in healthy, whole food recipes from other sources. You'll know when you're ready to take full control of your 7 Ways. But you can always come back to the meal plan if you have a little wobble.

	Mon	Tues	Wed
BREAKFAST	One of the fruit/nut/seed plates (pp.216–9)	Overnight oats (p.227) or Tea porridge (p.231)	Poached egg on toast with kimchi (p.238)
SNACK	Veg snack	Treat snack	Veg snack
LUNCH	Bashed bean pâté with crudités (p.274)	Oatcakes with cheese, apple & kraut (p.261)	Coronation chicken (p.265) or Mushroom, almond & olive blitz (p.273)
SUPPER	Brassicas, lentils & live dressing (p.296) plus Fruit snack	Baked fish & veg parcels (p.353) or Seared cabbage with hummus & dukka (p.348) plus Fruit snack	Spicy roast parsnips with barley, raisins & walnuts (p.298) plus Oaty seedy apple crumble (p.387)

Veg snack = About 100g cut-up raw veg (free pass on cucumber, celery, lettuce, fennel).

Fruit snack = 2 pieces fresh fruit and a small handful of seeds/nuts or one of the fruit/nut/seed plates on pp.216–9 (but not always the banana!).

Treat snack = A portion of one of the treats on pages 388–95 or fruit compote (page 224) with yoghurt.

Portions There are 3 portion sizes for the meal plan. The 'standard' portion size is for a man aiming to lose weight and a woman aiming to maintain weight. When a recipe says 'Serves 4' then a quarter of the made recipe is the correct standard portion. For a woman aiming to lose weight a slightly smaller portion of one-fifth is appropriate and for a man aiming to maintain weight it's slightly larger – one-third of the recipe. With breakfasts and lunchboxes most recipes are 'Per person' or 'Serves 1' with a low to high range of quantities for some ingredients: low is 'weight-loss woman' and high is 'maintenance man' with the standard portion in the middle. When it's 'Serves 2' then half is the standard portion, and you can nudge it down about 30% for weight-loss woman and up by 30% for maintenance man.

Thurs	Fri	Sat	Sun
Grated root & fruit salad (p.222)	One of the fruit/nut/seed plates (pp.216–9) or Tea porridge (p.231)	Fried egg omelette (p.237) or Toast for breakfast (p.232)	Half-baked granola (p.228)
Fruit or veg snack	Veg snack	Treat snack	Veg snack
Beans & greens summer soup (p 314)	Sardines & beans (p.268) or Cucumber, lettuce & cashews (p.267)	Beetroot, radicchio, plums, beans (p.254)	Omelette slaw (p.302)
Mackerel on roasted veg & fruit (p.356) or Roasted purple power (p.344) plus Fruit snack	Nutty beany beetroot curry (p.330) or Roasted veg & bashed chickpeas (p.332) plus Treat snack	Chunky beef chilli (p.376) or Asian hot pot (p.338) plus Fruit snack	Baked chicken & veg curry (p.374) or Yellow split pea soup with harissa & almonds (p.318) plus Treat snack

Drink plan Your drink of choice is water. You can also have 'normal' tea or coffee (no sugar, a dash of milk if you like) and one small glass (200ml) of juice or kombucha every day. In all cases, drink alcohol on no more than 4 nights this week, with a maximum of two units each night, i.e. one glass of wine or one pint of beer (see page 152).

KEEPING WELL TO EAT BETTER

I hope I've made a compelling case that the single-fix diet is a fatally flawed concept. My 7 Ways will bring you further-reaching and more sustainable health benefits – and weight loss if you so choose – and the very fact that it incorporates a variety of approaches is key to its success.

By extension, it's important to acknowledge that, while better eating can have a huge positive impact on your well-being, there is more to good health than what you put in your mouth. That might seem obvious. But less obvious, perhaps, is the way in which various small steps towards taking better care of yourself can come together to add tremendous potency to improved eating. In other words, if you eat better *and* live better, you will find that two plus two adds up to more than four!

Exercising regularly, reducing stress and giving yourself the best chance of good sleep are three of the most effective ways to support and enhance – maybe even accelerate – the real benefits of better eating. Each of these areas could be the subject for a book as long as this one (though not as much fun, I'm betting!). But actually, there's a lot of useful strategy and practical motivation that can be gained from a simple summary of the latest good science and smart thinking on these topics.

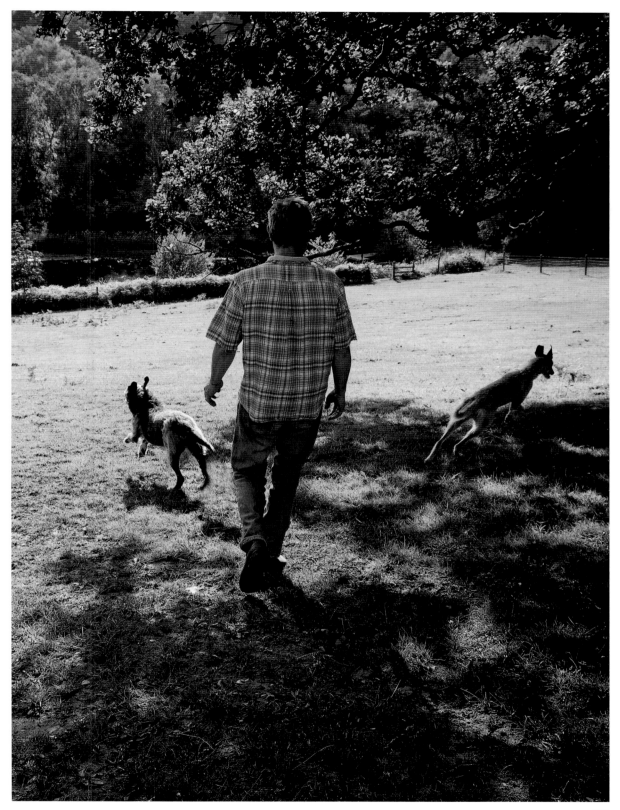

EXERCISE

It's a no-brainer, of course: we all know that being active is good for us. But do you know *how* good? Study after study and expert after expert agree that exercise is colossally important for all kinds of reasons:

It significantly reduces your risk of a whole spectrum of serious diseases, including heart disease, stroke, type 2 diabetes and cancer. It can literally add years to your life. But the more important thing is that it can add *healthy* years to your life.

Exercise reduces blood pressure, inflammation and triglyceride levels (fats in the blood). It increases levels of good (HDL) cholesterol, and also combats stress, anxiety and depression – all linked to physical as well as mental ill-health.

If you want to lose weight healthily, diet is the key (it's hard to shift pounds through activity alone). But if you exercise *and* eat well, you can turbo-boost weight loss.

Weight-bearing exercise, like walking, running, weight-training or dancing, builds bone strength when you're young and slows bone loss as you age. High-impact forms of exercise – like most racket sports – are particularly good for bone health.

Evidence suggests exercise may improve the balance of microbes in your gut.

As well as improving psychological well-being, physical activity can make you feel more energised.

Exercise can help improve sleep.

How much exercise makes a difference?

The simple answer is *any at all*. There is no minimum level below which exercise ceases to be worthwhile. Any exercise that's even moderately challenging, that increases the heart rate and strengthens the muscles, is helpful. And you'll get the greatest benefit from the first steps. Going from doing almost no exercise at all to doing even a bit – say, a brisk 10-minute walk every day – gives a huge boost to your health.

You don't need to exercise in long, punishing sessions. Short bursts of activity peppered through your day are highly beneficial, and if they become part of your routine, you are much more likely to stick with them. Cycling to work, getting off the bus one stop early, choosing the stairs instead of the escalator – those choices add up.

Whatever activity you choose, it shouldn't take too long to activate your body's built-in reward system. Your endorphins 'kicking in' is a real phenomenon; one recent survey found that it took, on average, only 10 minutes for people to start feeling a mood boost during physical activity.

Build exercise into your life

The best kind of exercise – the kind you will stick to – is the kind you enjoy. Keep an open mind as to what that could be; you might be surprised. No matter what your level of fitness is now, you can find a form of activity that suits you.

A few years ago, I went from being a complete non-runner to a regular 5k'er. My personal 'couch to 5k' (there are apps and online plans called exactly that) took about 4 months. I did it as part of a TV series, to show solidarity by running a 5k-course in Newcastle with a bunch of lovely people who were also transforming their lives through better eating and more exercise. I imagined I would hang up my running shoes as soon as the show was over, but I accidentally got hooked!

Now my Sunday run around the local Devon country lanes is a high point of my week. I don't measure my times – and I still walk up the really steep hills. But I do try to speed up on the flat and add new loops of lanes from time to time to increase my distance. If I can achieve that transformation, anyone can! Set your sights on something that really piques you.

Being active outdoors appears to bring particular gains; one scientific review concluded that exercising in natural environments was associated with feelings of greater energy and reduced tension, anger and depression. So, consider walking, gardening, running, climbing, football, netball, rowing, kayaking, body boarding or sea swimming – anything that gets you out in the fresh air.

Exercise isn't a test of character or ability, you don't have to measure scores and times. It's about self-care and protecting your health. And it can take any form that suits you. The first steps can be hard – I won't pretend otherwise. But every effort brings benefits, and makes the next session just a shade easier.

As you repeat those healthy behaviours, they will eventually become healthy habits. And they'll magnify every other healthy choice you make in your day-to-day life. You'll choose not to miss them, as you feel just how much good they are doing you.

DE-STRESS

I don't want to worry you, but stress is something we have to take very seriously. It can have real consequences for our physical health as well as our mental well-being. It may push us towards poorer choices (more sugar, more alcohol, less energy) that lead to weight gain and further cycles of negativity. Along with poor diet and lack of exercise, stress is the third point in a toxic triangle that keeps many people trapped in ill-health.

But stress is unavoidable, isn't it?

Modern life is stressful. No doubt about it. And we are conditioned to accept it, even to embrace it. Stress can be seen – along with being busy and working long hours – as a sign that we are good, conscientious people. But we've got to stop wearing our stressed-out demeanours as a badge of honour. Cutting down stress is just sensible – like cutting down on booze, sugar or takeaways.

What's the big deal about stress?

Stress in itself is a normal part of existence. For most animals, physical threats to survival, such as predators, are the things that cause stress. When faced with a 'stressor' like this, animals experience a fight-or-flight response that kicks their brains and bodies into high gear and enables them to deal with the problem. They then return to normal.

It was the same story for human beings until fairly recently in our history. But these days, stress is a very different experience for most people. Rarely is it about a sudden direct threat to our lives. Instead it comes from a prolonged and persistent series of 'worries' – about work, money, family, relationships or health, or social anxieties, phobias and fears. Rather than facing down one, big, scary beast and then returning to a state of calm stability, we experience a constant drip-feed of mid-level angst.

Stress is not merely psychological or emotional. Our bodies respond to it physically by releasing hormones like adrenaline and cortisol. They course through our blood into organs and tissues; our entire system can be bathed in stress chemicals at cellular level. So it's no surprise that stress can make us ill, impairing our immune system, increasing inflammation and contributing to heart disease, high blood pressure and strokes. Stress is also linked to obesity and type 2 diabetes, and not just because it drives us to eat fatty, sugary comfort foods. Studies show that prolonged exposure to cortisol can affect the way we store fat, and is often linked to a bigger waist measurement.

Tackling stress

As you can see, there's a compelling crop of reasons for reducing the stress in our lives. It's fortunate then, that there's a bunch of accessible, effective ways to do it:

Phone a friend. One of the simplest and most effective ways of managing stress is to spend time with people you like. Social support should be central in anyone's anti-stress strategy – in fact, in anyone's *life* strategy. Doctors know that people with social support have stronger immune systems, whereas isolation and loneliness actually increase our risk of heart problems, depression, dementia and early death.

—

Cut back. Get to the root of things and see if you can remove or reduce some of the factors that are stressing you. Are you trying to fit too much into your day? Can you pare back activities or chores that bring you no joy? Can you ask for help with things that put pressure on you? Stress often comes from activities that we feel we ought to be doing but we need to consider the effect they are having on our health.

—

Meditate. Practices such as mindfulness, meditation and yoga – along with relaxation techniques such as deep breathing and positive visualisation – can help to relieve stress. One recent study found that mindfulness meditation caused a measurable drop in stress hormones, while it seems yoga can increase levels of a neurotransmitter (GABA) which is associated with better mood and lower anxiety.

—

Do things you enjoy. Everyday activities such as walking, gardening, arts or crafts (including knitting, sewing and mending stuff) can also have a meditative quality about them and can massively improve your state of mind.

—

Be in nature. Walking, or even sitting calmly, in a green space (away from noise and traffic), brings down your stress levels. And observing the things that are living and growing around you can enhance the benefits of being out in the fresh air.

—

Exercise. Regular exercise is one of the best ways to de-stress. If you are not getting it, there's a case for putting it top of your de-stress programme – just avoid over-obsessing over goals or scores (which can actually add to stress levels).

—

Cold water. Surprising perhaps, eccentric even, but don't knock this one until you have tried it. A dose of cold water (for example 2–3 minutes on the coldest setting at the end of your morning shower) is certainly an exhilarating way to start the day. Studies indicate significant improvements in mood and reduced stress levels for many who've tried it. I've been doing it for 2 years now, and it's definitely helped me.

SLEEP BETTER

Lack of sleep can affect our health on many different levels – and we're not just talking about feeling a bit grumpy and craving caffeine. People with recurring poor sleep are much more likely to experience mental health problems, for a start, and the effects can also be profoundly physical. A recent report from Oxford University explained that 'there is now a wealth of evidence to conclude that lack of sleep and poor sleep are inherently bad for our health, being associated with a huge range of negative conditions including diabetes, depression, heart attack and cancer'.

Short or restricted sleep can even lead to weight gain because it reduces a hormone called leptin that tells our brain we're full and increases one called ghrelin that stimulates appetite: lack of sleep literally makes us more hungry.

Yet poor sleep is incredibly common. Hands up if you get at least 7 hours every night? In Britain, one in ten of us suffer with chronic insomnia and a recent study reported that a colossal 77% of British people fail to wake up feeling well rested, with men getting on average 28 minutes less sleep than they want on week nights, and women faring much worse with nearly an hour of lost sleep each night.

I feel all this personally. I have, at various times in my life, suffered from pretty severe and prolonged bouts of insomnia. This is usually when a combination of stress and excitement (often over a new project) get a grip on me. These things don't usually prevent me actually falling asleep but they do lead to me consistently waking in the small hours feeling 'wired' – buzzing with thoughts that I just can't seem to 'put to bed'.

Having difficulty sleeping can be absolutely exhausting and there have been times where my insomnia has felt way out of control, debilitating, and pretty scary. It's been a huge relief, therefore, to find there are things I can actually do to greatly improve my chances of a good night's sleep.

So how do we get those zzzzzs?

The first thing to say about improving your sleep is that good eating, regular exercise, and reduced stress levels – in other words everything we've covered so far – will all help. Emerging evidence suggests that a healthy diet can be an important tool in tackling sleep problems, with the foods that may support good sleep being exactly the same ones I've been championing throughout this book: high-fibre plant-based whole foods that nurture your gut and your immune system.

The sleep-supporting benefits of good food, more exercise and stress-reduction are increased when you make them part of a routine, along with other key aspects of self-care. 'A good night's sleep doesn't start when you go to bed,' says Professor Kevin Morgan, of Loughborough University's Clinical Sleep Research Unit, 'it starts well before that with a de-escalating, down-regulating, pre-sleep routine.' That routine should include at least some elements of what is commonly known as good 'sleep hygiene'.

Sleep hygiene

This is the set of positive habits that almost all researchers agree is likely to improve your sleep. Sleep hygiene lists vary in emphasis and different things work for different people. My list below is based on advice from Professor Morgan and other sleep experts but I've tweaked it a bit. I find it helps to categorise my sleep hygiene 'rules' into three groups:

1 Good consumption

Avoid caffeine for 4–6 hours before bedtime.

Don't eat too late in the day (ideally no food within 3 hours of bed).

Don't drink alcohol too late in the day, or every day. Booze may make you drowsy but it can also contribute to 'early waking' insomnia. Teetotallers get sleep problems too, but alcohol isn't helpful for many. I usually sleep better on alcohol-free nights, and on evenings when I have alcohol I try to stop drinking when I stop eating.

Don't drink too much 'sleepy tea'. A cup of herbal tea an hour or so before bed is fine, but if you are prone to getting up in the night for a pee, don't overdo it.

2 Good timing

Give yourself at least an hour's 'wind-down' time before bed, without work, homework, emails etc., when you can do something relaxing and enjoyable. This could be reading, chatting – maybe watching TV, but in the living room, *not* your bedroom, and not on a close-up screen (i.e. phone or tablet).

Go to bed and get up at roughly the same time, even at weekends: this will help to 'anchor' your body clock: 'Sleep loves routine,' as the saying goes.

Minimise daytime napping to short periods of no more than 20 minutes (maximum two in a day), and try to avoid napping after about 4pm.

3 Good habits

Exercise well, eat well, de-stress.

———

Keep your bedroom quiet, dark and cool and use it only for sleep (or sex!). This helps strengthen the association between your bedroom and your sleep.

———

Don't take your phone or laptop to bed with you, or watch TV in bed.

———

Get outside during the day if you possibly can. And expose yourself to plenty of light when you are awake, especially early in the morning – even artificial light in the winter. People exposed to greater amounts of light during morning hours fall asleep more quickly at night because light helps calibrate the body's internal 'circadian' clock. Exposure to sunlight can lead to an increase in melatonin, which can help us sleep.

Back-up plan: brain dump

Insomniacs often experience what is known as a 'racing brain'. Typically, this is when your mind is hopping and skipping from one concern to another, taking in anything from work and family anxieties, to shopping and to-do lists, or unanswered emails. Even things you know are trivial start to loom large and gather storm clouds around them if you are lying awake at night.

If that's your experience, try writing down anything that's worrying or preoccupying you before bed (ideally on paper, not your phone!). This can help take the 'waking power' out of negative or intrusive thoughts and also lessen your tendency to 'scan' for problems to worry about when you are trying to sleep. Making a pre-sleep worry list is sometimes called 'brain-dumping' and you can find various guides to it online.

Heard it all before?

For many people who experience occasional insomnia, taking some of these simple daily steps can be enough to restore regular restful nights. However if, like me, you are a long-term slave to sleep problems, you can do all these sensible things and still find that good-quality sleep eludes you. Where do you go from there?

Medication may be one answer to insomnia, in the short term – but it's definitely not a good permanent solution. Dependencies on sleep medication can develop quite rapidly and higher doses will be needed just to keep you where you are. It is also important to realise that a medicated night's sleep is not as restful or restorative as one your body has achieved naturally, or even a slightly 'humpy' night of unmedicated sleep. Herbal remedies said to promote sleep, such as lavender, chamomile and valerian, can work for some people. They don't have a lot of scientific evidence behind them but if they are part of a bedtime routine that works for you, then knock yourself out – literally.

There's a newer approach that tackles sleep problems in a more profound way, and has been proven to have lasting results. It's called CBT-i (cognitive behavioural therapy for insomnia). 'It's a very specialised form of CBT driven by an understanding of how sleep works,' explains Professor Morgan. 'It starts with the simple fact that the longer you've been awake, the more likely you are to sleep, so there's an initial sleep-restriction element. That then gives you a platform from which you can develop strategies for how you think about sleep and ways to deal with the kind of intrusive thinking that tends to keep people alert and awake. The system works.'

An outline of CBT-i

CBT-i basics include not napping during the day and not even getting into bed until you are really sleepy so that the pressure to sleep builds up.

In the initial stages, sleep may be restricted to as little as 5 hours a night, then slowly expanded.

Spending as little time as possible in bed but *not asleep* is also key. If you are awake, get up, even if it's 3am. Do not *try* to sleep, or lie there waiting for sleep to come to you. Not only is this self-defeating, it starts to create negative associations. 'You'll learn to hate your bed,' says Prof Morgan, 'you'll start to see it as a hostile environment.'

CBT-i also uses cognitive strategies to tackle the way we think about sleep, and what to do about intrusive pre-sleep thoughts.

You can find out more about CBT-i online, for example at sleepful.me, or sleepio.com. CBT-i has a proven track record of helping chronic insomniacs improve their sleep, but I know from personal experience that the restricted sleep regime of the initial stages can feel quite brutal and dispiriting. In the end the professional advice that has most helped me comes from sleep therapist Sasha Stephens, who has created the online course Sleep for Life (sleepforlife.com). It's a compassionate blend of sleep hygiene advice, CBT-i basics, relaxation techniques, and aspects of positive affirmation and visualisation. It's been absolutely transformative for me.

7 WAYS TO SUPPORT THE 7 WAYS

By taking exercise, de-stressing and sleep improvement together, it feels like we are settling on another 7 Ways – actions and resolutions that can enhance and magnify the benefits of healthy eating. They are all complementary: the more of these you can absorb into your daily life, the easier other healthy changes become, in a virtuous circle of eating better, living better and feeling better.

1 Build exercise into your life
Any at all makes a difference.

2 Tackle your sources of stress
It's more important than you think.

3 Go outside whenever you can
Fresh air, daylight and green spaces help everything.

4 Prioritise sleep
Really prioritise it!

5 Change is a challenge, so be kind to yourself
Reward and forgive yourself as you would a good friend...

6 Get support, give support
You might be helping others, just as they are helping you.

7 Practise relaxing
All of the above should help you to feel significantly calmer, but some form of mindfulness or meditation may well seal the deal.

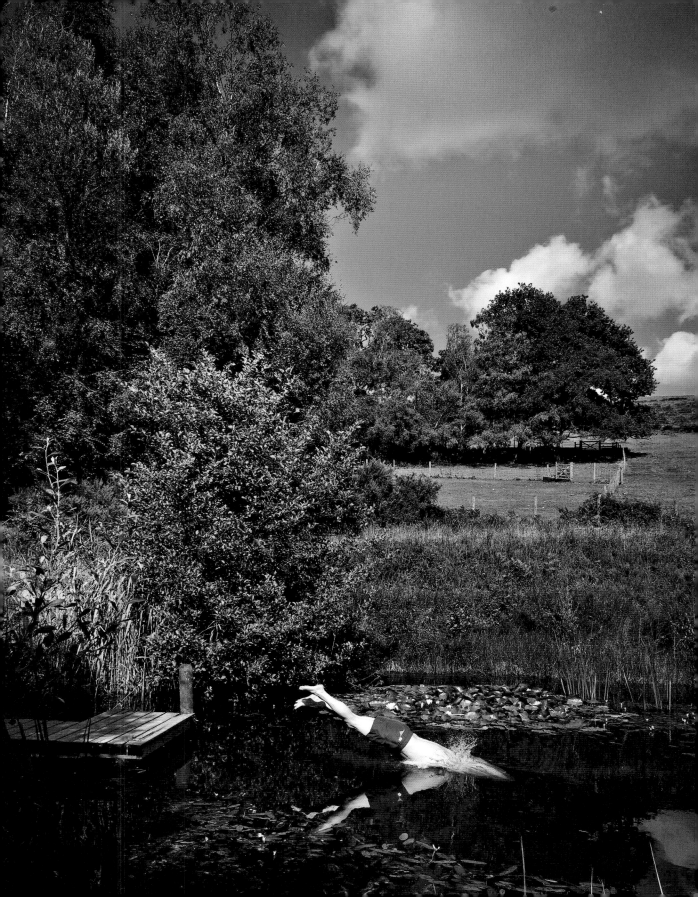

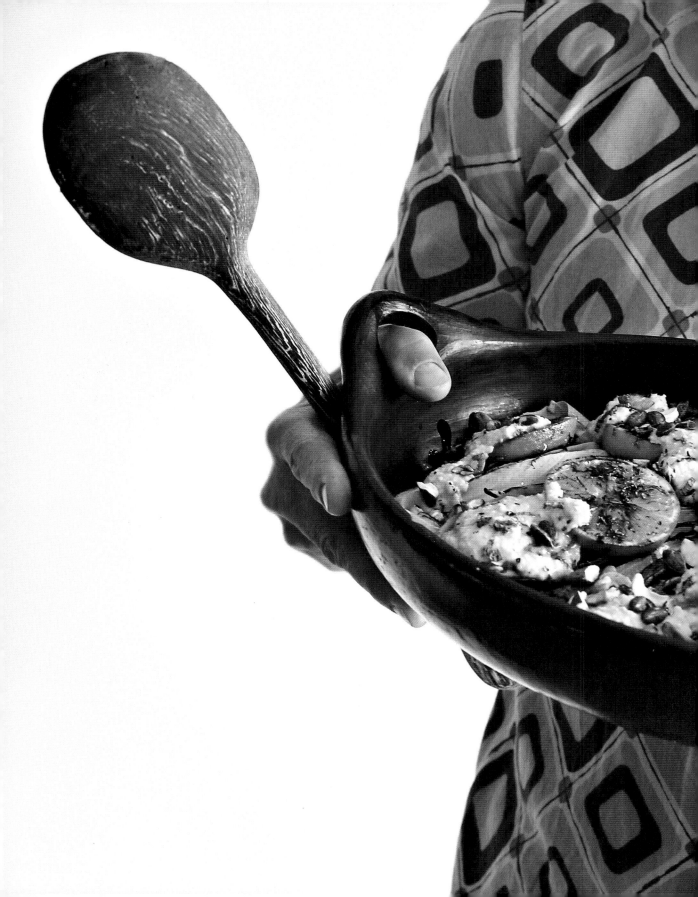

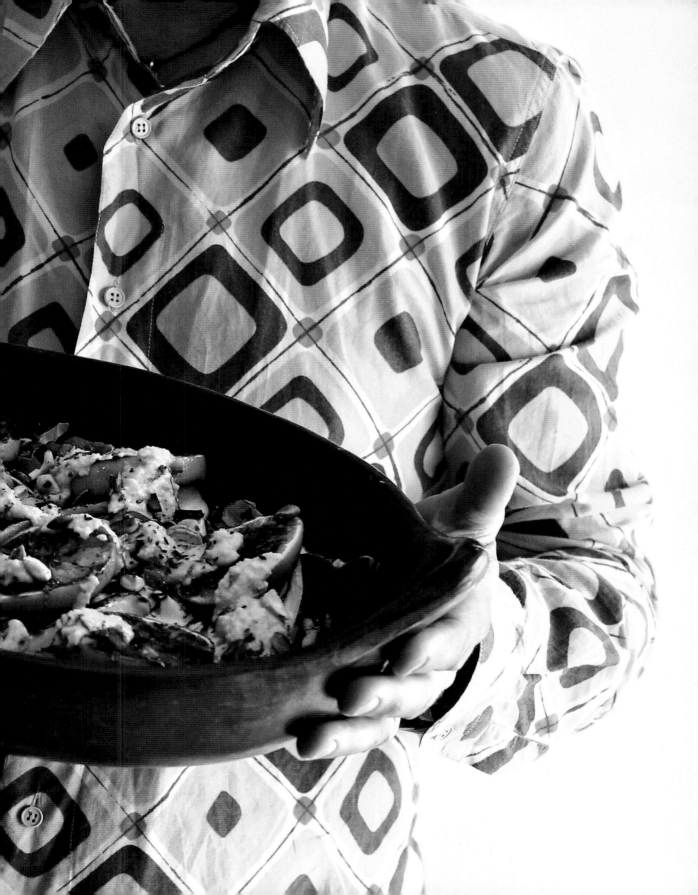

RECIPES

All of the 7 Ways that underpin this book are represented here, in dishes based on whole, high-fibre, gut-friendly ingredients, with healthy fats and minimal sugar, and a huge variety of different ingredients. You'll find the raw and the cooked, the cold and the hot, a lot of colour and every texture under the sun. They are the kind of recipes that will slot themselves easily into your routine, designed to become familiar, reliable favourites and smooth your path to eating better, every day.

There are satisfying breakfasts, brekkie dishes that work for lunch and simple healthy lunchbox ideas. I've given you a whole raft of hearty (and heart-healthy) mains, salads and soups substantial enough to serve as suppers. Plenty of the recipes freeze well. Good-for-your-gut ideas abound, including a couple of simple home ferments, and my own kombucha care and maintenance plan – SCOBY-doby-do! And there's even a range of virtuous sweet treats and alcohol-free tipples.

I'm offering easy recipes to address every challenge you might face on your journey towards better eating, and tackling head-on the unfamiliarity with ingredients, lack of time and dearth of inspiration that can hijack the most well-intentioned bid to be healthy. I've kept everything as simple and straightforward as possible, with minimal effort and time involved, and a very relaxed approach to ingredients. I never want you to feel you can't cook a recipe just because you're missing a particular vegetable or a certain kind of spice – and my variation ideas are there to ensure you never will.

I've already said that it's hard to eat healthily if you view the kitchen as a no-go zone. A modicum of prep and a little cooking will open up to you a whole world of delicious meals. But you don't need to be an experienced cook to make any of these dishes.

A note on adding salt and sugar

We know that too much salt is bad for us and most of us need to cut back on the amount that we consume (see page 102). I continue to use salt in the kitchen, but more consciously and carefully than I did in the past.

As a cook, I value salt for its unique seasoning action. It can bring the best out of fresh, whole, natural ingredients, especially vegetables, making them more pleasing to eat. So, a judicious use of salt can help you to really enjoy your food, as you set about upping the wholeness and diversity of your meals. However, salt is always optional in my recipes. If you prefer to avoid it, by all means leave it out – with the exception of the fermented veg recipes on pages 282–7, for which it is essential.

It is very easy to develop a taste for too much salt – it's happened to me in the past. This is something that can be reined in simply by reducing the amount you use in your cooking over time. Your taste-buds adjust and become more sensitive so you can detect the same amount of flavour with less salt. That's what I've been up to and it's working well, for me and my family. I've also stopped automatically putting salt on the table at meal times.

As to sugar, I have said plenty about the health problems associated with its use in processed foods, and as an added ingredient, in Chapter 4. It crops up in a few of the recipes because, as with salt, a little sugar (or honey) sometimes helps us eat more of the wonderful foods that can do us a power of good. Tart fruits like rhubarb and plums; grains and seeds in breakfast dishes and baked treats; dressings that can make salads irresistible: these are good reasons to deploy a light sprinkle of sugar or a tiny trickle of honey. As with salt, systematically reducing your taste for sugar is a really good idea (see pages 98 and 103–8).

Following the recipes

- All spoon measures are level unless otherwise stated: 1 tsp = 5ml spoon; 1 tbsp = 15ml spoon.
- All herbs are fresh unless otherwise suggested.
- Use freshly ground black pepper unless otherwise listed.
- All fruit and vegetables should be washed before you start cooking. Use organic fruit and veg if you possibly can.
- If using the zest of citrus fruit, choose unwaxed fruit.
- Oven timings are provided in the recipes for both conventional and fan-assisted ovens. As ovens vary, these are intended as guidelines, with a description of the desired final colour or texture of the dish as a further guide.

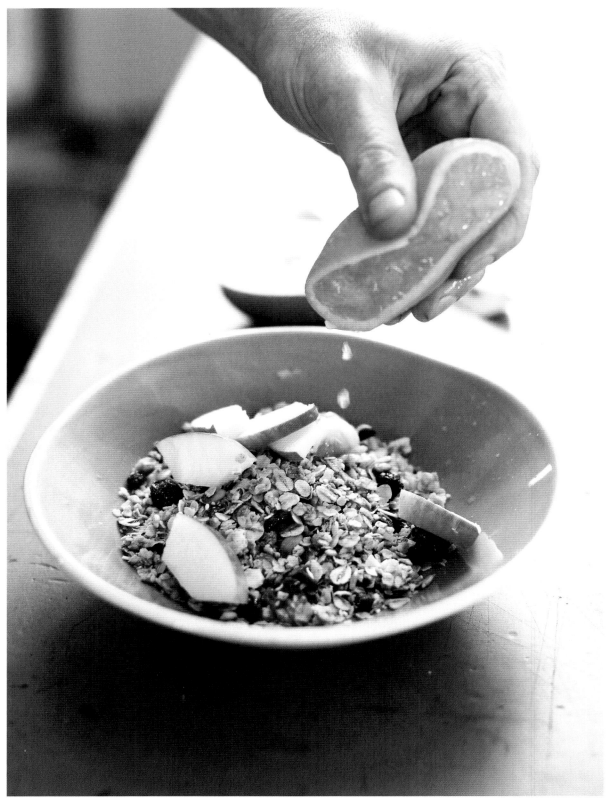

BRILLIANT BREAKFASTS

Breakfast offers a brilliant opportunity to build more variety into your diet – and plenty of fibre too – which are both so central to my 7 Ways to Eating Better Forever. Often, we eat the same brekkie every day of the week – something we wouldn't countenance at lunch or supper-time! Simply mixing and matching a few different breakfast dishes throughout the week is an easy way to significantly increase the variety in your diet – and that's before you even look at your other meals and snacks.

Another thing you can vary is the time you eat your breakfast. The first meal of the day it may be, but it needn't be at the break of dawn. While an early-ish meal is important for growing kids and teenagers, there's little evidence to suggest that it's essential for healthy adults. Push your breakfast back a bit – to mid-morning, late morning, lunchtime even – and you'll be extending that crucial 'rest and repair' time that seems to be so good for our internal systems (see Chapter 7). If I'm going for an '18/6' (see page 180), I won't eat anything until early afternoon, but I might still choose to break that fast with a dish from this chapter, rather than something that looks more like lunch.

The point is, these healthy-start-to-the-day dishes are all delicious no matter when you choose to eat them. They are simple too – quick to throw together in a few minutes, and in some cases easy to make the night before so you can tuck in, with zero prep required, the following day. I've built probiotic, gut-friendly elements into many of these recipes, because the first meal of the day is a particularly great time to be good to your gut. Fibre comes in the form of whole grains and seeds, fresh fruit and even veg. And there's protein too: eggs, natural yoghurt, kefir, nuts and seeds, which is satisfying and great for safeguarding your energy levels through the morning and helping to stave off the mid-morning, reach-for-the-biscuit-tin slump.

More days than not, the first thing I eat is fresh fruit. I love the natural sweetness and refreshing tang – and the pleasing, yielding textures. Sometimes I'm munching an apple or popping in some berries as I go. But If I can spare a few minutes, I love to prepare a simple plate of two or three fruits, cut up to make eating them, and combining them, a treat to myself (and sometimes my family!). Sometimes chilling the fruit makes it more refreshing, but actually you'll relish the natural sweetness and aromatics more at room temperature. I'm kicking off with a quartet of delightful fruit combinations – with a few nuts and seeds thrown in. I hope you will rapidly and enthusiastically experiment with combinations of your own.

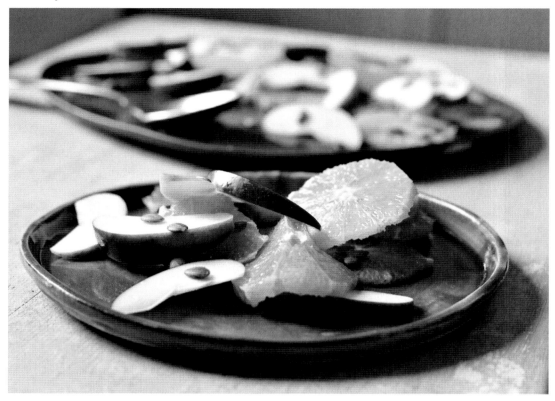

APPLE & ORANGE BREAKFAST

A perfect example of how a minimal bit of trimming and slicing can transform fresh fruit. Juicy slices of pith-less orange and thin wedges of apple are so much more appealing than a plain, whole fruit. The only dressing needed is the juice naturally released by the orange. Nuts and/or seeds boost the energy provided and add some welcome crunch.

Per person

1–2 oranges

1–2 crisp apples, such as a Cox or Katy

1–2 handfuls (15–30g) pumpkin seeds or nuts (optional), soaked overnight if you like

Using a sharp knife, slice the peel off the orange(s) on a board: first cut off the top and base, then work around the fruit, slicing off all the peel and pith in segments. Then turn the orange on its side and cut into 5mm–1cm slices. Arrange over a serving plate.

Quarter the apple(s), remove the core, then cut into nice, thin wedges. Scatter these over the orange slices. Tip any juice left on the board back over the fruit. Scatter over the seeds/nuts, if using, and the salad is ready to eat.

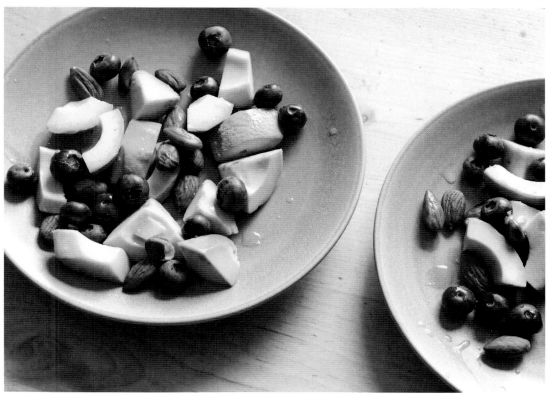

ALMOND, AVOCADO & BERRIES

This is a lovely, healthy way to start the day – a fantastic alternative to sugary, starchy cereal. The almonds give you texture and bite, the avocado provides creamy richness, the berries and honey lend sweetness – and every ingredient packs a nutritious punch! Get the almonds soaking a few hours ahead of time so they become nice and plump.

Serves 4

2 large or 3 medium ripe avocados

80g whole almonds, soaked in cold water for at least 2 hours

About 350g raspberries, strawberries or blueberries (or a mix)

A squeeze of lemon juice

1–2 tsp runny honey or soft brown sugar (optional)

Halve the avocados and remove their stones, then quarter them and peel away the skins. Slice each quarter thickly and divide between serving plates.

Drain the soaked almonds and scatter them over the avocado. If using strawberries, hull them and slice thickly. Arrange the berries over and around the avocado and nuts.

Give each salad a little squeeze of lemon juice and, if you like, a tiny trickle of honey, or a pinch of brown sugar and they're ready to serve.

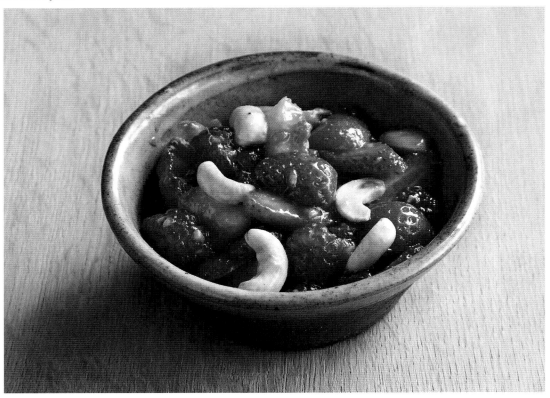

SUMMER BERRIES & CASHEWS

Raspberries and strawberries are often thought of as pudding (and jamming) fruits, but I love them raw, and early in the day. Soaking cashews makes them plump and tender – more so even than soaked almonds – so they become a creamy contrast to the sweet-sharp berries. You can slice and arrange the ingredients, or give them all a bit of a stir and squash, so the juices run. I usually choose the latter approach.

Per person

A dozen strawberries

1–2 ripe peaches or 3–4 ripe apricots (optional)

100g raspberries

30–50g cashew nuts, soaked overnight

Hull and slice the strawberries and cut up the peach (peeled if you like) or apricots, if using. Arrange all the fruits on a plate and scatter over the soaked cashews. Alternatively, put the prepared fruit and cashews into a bowl and stir to break them up a bit.

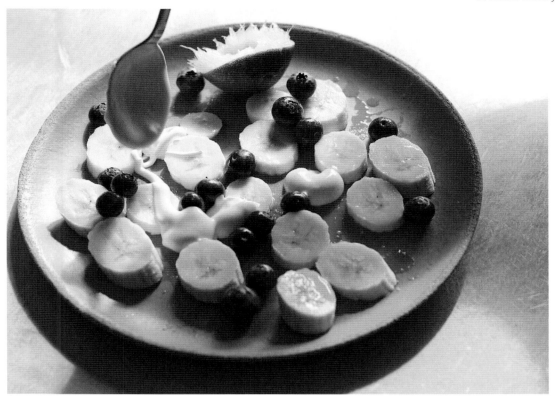

BANANA BREAKFAST

Again, this is barely a recipe – but I really do want to suggest how you might serve a banana for breakfast and make it irresistible. The point is that the simplest tweaks and additions – slicing on the diagonal, a squeeze of lime juice, some fresh berries and perhaps some nuts or seeds – can turn a plain bit of fruit into something really special.

Per person

1–2 not-too-ripe, medium bananas

1–2 handfuls of berries, such as blueberries, raspberries or redcurrants, or ½ apple or pear, cut into small chunks

½–1 lime or lemon

1–2 generous tbsp natural yoghurt or kefir (page 246), optional

1 tsp ground flaxseed, or a sprinkle of mixed seeds (optional)

A small handful (10–20g) of walnuts or whole almonds (optional), soaked overnight if you like, roughly chopped

Peel the banana(s) and cut into 1cm thick slices, slightly on the diagonal. Arrange the slices on a plate or in a shallow dish. Scatter over the berries or apple or pear pieces. Squeeze over some lime or lemon juice – this really enhances the sweet banana flavour.

Tuck in straight away or, to build up this fruity plateful a bit more, add a spoonful of yoghurt or kefir. A teaspoonful of ground flaxseed adds some valuable omega-3 fats or, for some texture (and fibre), you can add a handful of mixed seeds or roughly chopped nuts.

BANANA & BERRY THICKIE

A thickie is a bit like a smoothie but it includes yoghurt and oats, for texture and substance. This is also a kind of 'instant' version of the overnight oats. A banana and berry thickie is classic (and delicious) but you can get busy with those nuts and seeds too, if you like. Kefir is a good swap for yoghurt, and even richer in beneficial bacteria.

Serves 1–2

1 medium-ripe large banana, peeled and sliced

200ml fridge-cold natural yoghurt or kefir (page 246)

2 tbsp porridge oats

100g fresh or frozen berries, such as blueberries or raspberries, or chopped/grated apple

Put all the ingredients into a blender and give them a good whiz until smooth. You can add a splash of cold water if your thickie seems a touch too thick. Drink straight away, but not down in one! Sipping slowly will help you to digest this brilliant breakfast and get the best from it.

SEEDY/NUTTY VARIATIONS
To the above recipe you can add 1–2 tbsp seeds such as sunflower, pumpkin, flax or chia seeds. You can also add raw almonds (ideally soaked in cold water for a few hours first) or cashews, or 1–2 tsp of your favourite nut butter.

NO-BANANA VARIATION
Use a whole grated apple and a dollop of nut butter for a banana-free thickie that still blends nicely, and add 1 tsp honey if you like.

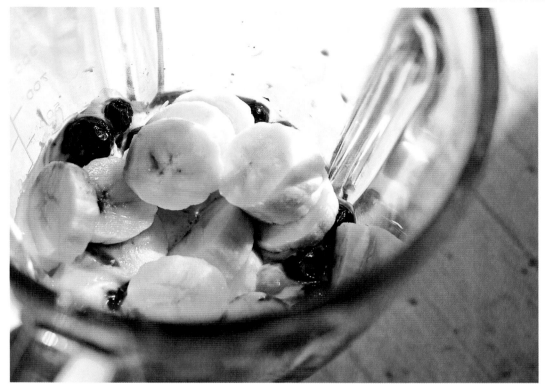

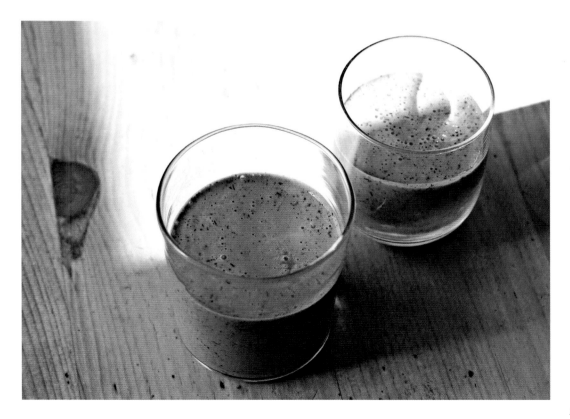

GRATED ROOT & FRUIT SALAD

A great way to get some plants into the first meal of the day, this simple fruit-and-veg breakfast salad is sweet and delicious. You can make it the night before, to save time in the morning. It makes a perfect portable snack pot too.

Per person

1–2 medium carrots

1 large, crisp apple, such as a Cox

A handful (15–25g) of raisins or 3–5 dried apricots, chopped prunes or dates

A handful (15–25g) of whole, skin-on almonds (optional), ideally soaked overnight

Juice (or flesh) of ½–1 orange or 1–2 clementines/easy peelers

A small piece of fresh ginger, finely grated (optional)

A little finely grated zest from the citrus fruit (optional)

Coarsely grate the carrot(s) and apple into a bowl (no need to peel the apple). Add the dried fruit, and almonds if using. Add the citrus juice (or chopped orange flesh), the ginger and/or citrus zest if using, and stir everything together really well.

You can eat this salad straight away, leave it for an hour to macerate, or even refrigerate it overnight – taking it out of the fridge about half an hour before you want to eat it, so it loses its chill.

NUTTY VARIATION

To take the overnight version up a notch, add 1–2 tbsp mixed seeds to the carrot and apple mixture before leaving it to soak. To serve, you can finish off with a spoonful of kefir (page 246) or natural yoghurt if you like.

BEETROOT VARIATION

If you like beetroot, a small raw one makes a luscious purple-tongued alternative to the carrot.

PEAR VARIATION

If you find yourself with a slightly crisp, under-ripe pear, it makes a great swap for the apple.

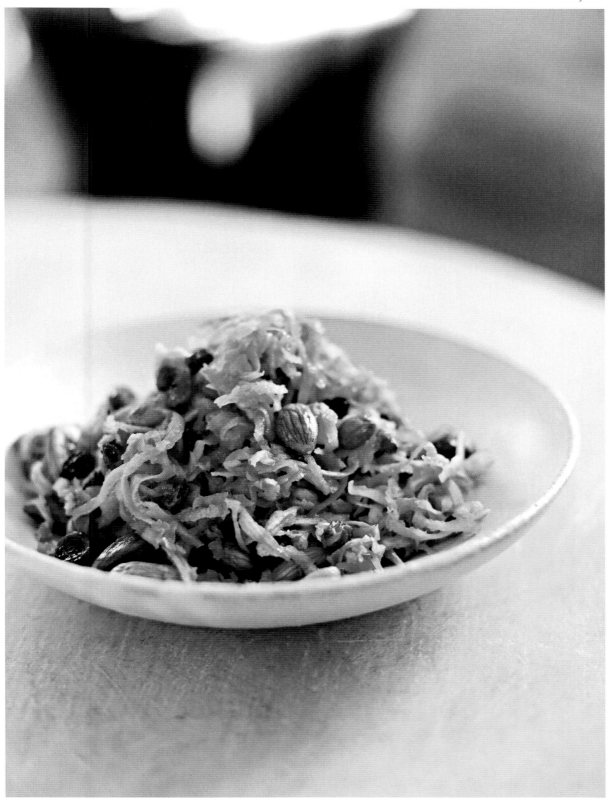

ROASTED PLUM COMPOTE

Roasting is a great way to intensify the lovely, sweet-sour flavour of plums. It also breaks them down into a sort of rough compote, which is delicious for breakfast. Eat plain, or add a dollop of natural yoghurt and/or a spoonful of half-baked granola (page 228) or seeds. Alternatively, pile them onto wholegrain toast, or serve with wholegrain pancakes (page 234), tea porridge (page 231) and other grainy breakfasts.

This recipe also works brilliantly with other stone fruits, such as greengages and apricots (halve and stone them, as for plums), or whole cherries (just nick them with a knife to let the juices run and de-stone after cooking). Outside of stone-fruit season (late summer to autumn), I like to roast rhubarb instead (see opposite).

Serves 4–6, with other things

About 1 kg ripe plums, halved and stoned

½ vanilla pod, 1 tsp vanilla extract or 2 star anise

1 orange

A little honey or brown sugar, to serve (optional)

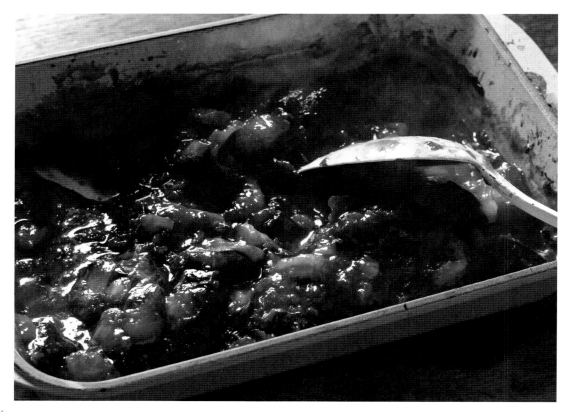

Preheat the oven to 180°C/Fan 160°C/Gas 4.

Place the halved plums, cut side up, in an oven dish. You want them to fit in relatively snugly to minimise the evaporation of their juice.

If using a vanilla pod, split it open lengthways, and scrape out the sticky black seeds with the tip of a sharp knife. Dot these as best you can over the plums. Cut the pod into 2 or 3 pieces and add it to the plums too. If you're using vanilla extract, just sprinkle it over the plums. If using star anise, break them up a bit and scatter over the plums.

Using a fine grater, grate the zest of the orange over the plums. Squeeze the juice of the orange over too. Transfer the dish to the oven and roast for 25–30 minutes, until the plums are really soft.

I like to give the hot fruit a gentle stir so it breaks down a bit, releases more juice and the flavour of the spice gets mingled in. But you can keep the fruit whole if you prefer. Either way, leave to cool then remove the coarser spices. If you're not serving straight away, transfer to a bowl or plastic tub and keep covered in the fridge.

Serve the plums warm or cold, tasting to appreciate their natural, fruity acidity before you decide whether or not to add a trickle of honey or a sprinkle of sugar. If the plums are sweet you may not need any. You can soon get accustomed to tart fruits with less or even no sugar, if you reduce it by degrees.

ROASTED RHUBARB VARIATION

Trim about 1kg rhubarb and cut it into roughly 5cm lengths. Put these into a small roasting tin or oven dish. Scatter over 2–3 tbsp (30–50g) soft brown sugar (or trickle over a similar amount of honey). Add the spice, orange zest and juice, as above. Roast at 150°C/Fan 140°C/Gas 2 for 25–45 minutes (this will depend on the age and toughness of the stalks), until the rhubarb is tender but still holding its shape. Leave to cool. The amount of sugar/honey should be enough to balance the sharpness of the rhubarb, but you can add another pinch (or trickle) if you really need it. Then aim to use a bit less next time...

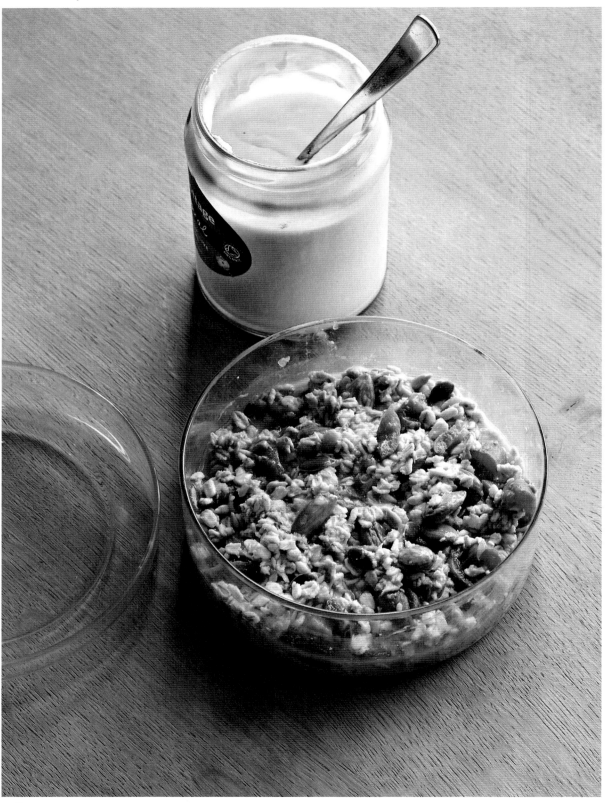

OVERNIGHT OATS

Soaking oats is a time-honoured route to a tender, tasty high-fibre breakfast – Bircher muesli is the classic example and 'overnight oats' the trendy interloper. This super-simple version uses jumbo oats, omega-rich seeds and skin-on almonds, which plump up and soften as they soak in orange juice and kombucha (or water). The result is juicy and mild, ready to be sweetened with a little fruit; I like a handful of raisins (which you can soak with the oats), or a grated apple – or both. If you include chia and/or flax seeds you'll get that distinctive slippery texture, which not everyone loves but I do!

Serves 4

120g (7–8 tbsp) jumbo oats (or porridge oats)

A generous handful (30g) of mixed nuts and seeds (such as almonds and pumpkin, sunflower, poppy, flax and chia seeds)

Juice of 1 large or 2 small oranges

A small glass (about 150ml) kombucha (page 244) or water

To serve

A handful of raisins, chopped dried apricots or other dried fruit (soaked with the oats if you like), and/or a handful of berries, or a sliced small banana, or an apple, chopped or coarsely grated

1–2 generous tbsp natural yoghurt or kefir (page 246), optional

Toasted buckwheat groats (optional)

Combine the oats, nuts and seeds in a breakfast bowl (adding some dried fruit if you like). Add the orange juice and the kombucha or water. Mix well.

Cover the bowl and place in the fridge or a cool place for 6–8 hours or overnight. If possible, take the soaked oats out of the fridge half an hour before you want to eat them, so they're not too chilly.

Serve with your chosen fruit. You could also add a spoonful or two of yoghurt or kefir and, to bring some crunch, a few toasted buckwheat groats.

HALF-BAKED GRANOLA

I call this 'half-baked' not because there's anything second-rate about it, but because it's only the oaty base that actually gets toasted in the oven. I like to keep the seeds and nuts raw, stirring them in later on. This granola is loose and sprinkle-able, rather than chunky and clustery, so as well as forming the base of your breakfast or brunch, it can easily be used as a healthy, crunchy topping for fruit compotes and fresh fruit salads.

Makes 12–20 x 30–50g servings (a 2-litre jar)

6 tbsp coconut oil, or olive or vegetable oil

2 level tbsp (about 30g) honey or soft brown sugar

300g rolled oats

200g other rolled grain flakes, such as rye, barley or quinoa

¼ tsp fine sea salt

150g mixed whole nuts, such as pecans, hazelnuts, almonds and cashews, roughly chopped

150g mixed dried fruit, such as raisins, sultanas, goji berries, chopped prunes and apricots

100g mixed seeds, including sunflower and pumpkin

To serve (per 30–50g serving)

A handful of berries or ½ apple or pear, skin on but chopped

A squeeze of fresh orange, lemon or lime juice

1 tsp ground flaxseed or hulled hemp seeds (optional)

1–2 tbsp natural yoghurt or kefir (page 246), optional

Preheat the oven to 160°C/Fan 140°C/Gas 3.

In a small saucepan, gently warm the oil and honey or sugar, stirring well, until warm. If you're using coconut oil, it should be completely liquid; don't worry if the honey or sugar doesn't dissolve completely.

Mix the oats, other rolled grain flakes and salt together in a large bowl. Trickle over the warm sweetened oil, mixing well so the oats and flakes are thoroughly coated.

Spread the oat mix in a shallow, even layer over 1 large or 2 smaller baking trays and place in the preheated oven. Bake for 20–30 minutes until golden brown, stirring halfway through (and swapping the trays around to ensure even baking if necessary). Leave to cool completely. Note the flakes won't be properly crunchy until cooled.

Once cooled, mix in the chopped nuts, dried fruit and seeds, then transfer the granola to an airtight container or jar. Use within 3–4 weeks.

Serve the granola with fresh berries or chopped apple or pear, and a squeeze of citrus juice. For extra omega-3s, you can sprinkle over 1 tsp ground flaxseed or hulled hemp seeds. A spoonful of yoghurt or kefir is very good with this too.

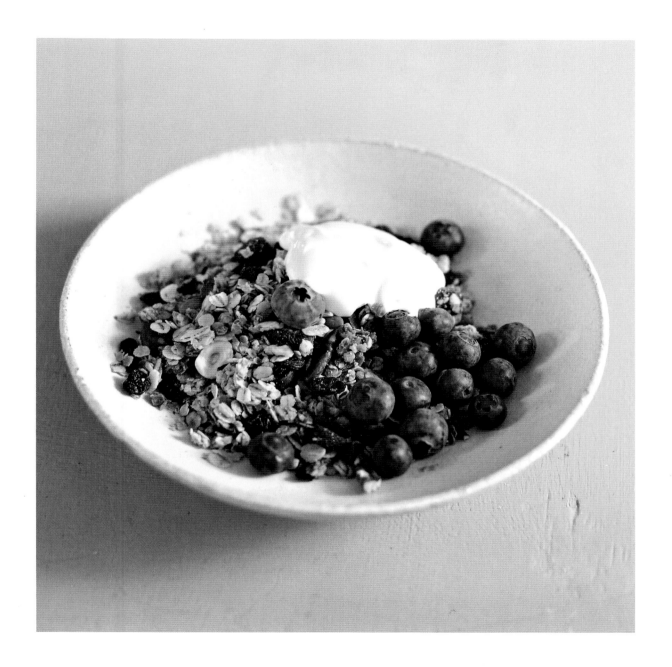

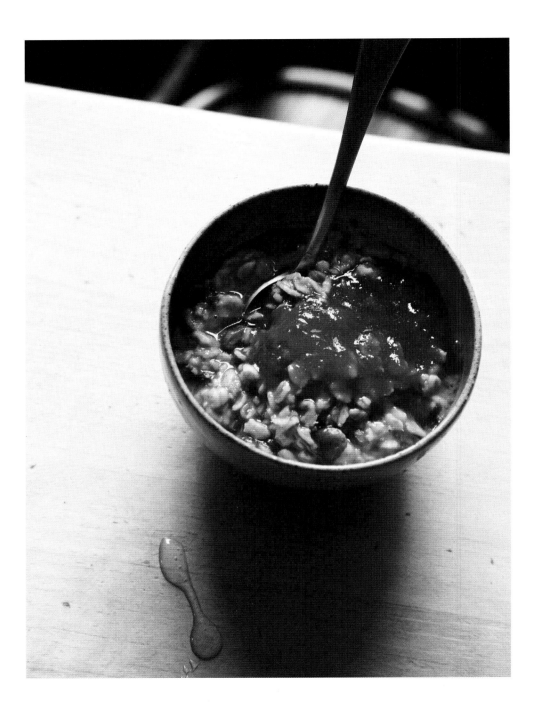

TEA PORRIDGE

A nice cup of tea and a hearty portion of porridge combined in one bowl – what could be better on a winter's morning? The tea not only brings some gut-friendly polyphenols (see page 84) but gently flavours the porridge, banishing any blandness. For even more of a kick, you can add some spice too. Raisins add sweetness, and if you want more of that you can finish with a little trickle of honey, too. You can serve this with a splash of milk, but I prefer it without. My favourite way to enjoy it is with a spoonful of roasted fruit compote.

Serves 4

2 heaped tsp loose-leaf tea (regular or decaff, rooibos is also good), or 2 tea bags

2 mugfuls (about 200g) of porridge oats or jumbo oats

50g raisins or sultanas

4 cardamom pods, bashed, and/or a good pinch of ground cinnamon or ground ginger (optional)

To serve (optional)

A little milk

Roasted fruit compote (pages 224–5)

A little honey or sugar

Brew the tea in a couple of mugs (or a jug) with 500ml boiling water for a good 3 minutes.

Put the oats, raisins or sultanas and the spices if using, into a saucepan and pour over the hot tea and another 500ml boiling water. Cook gently, stirring often, for about 7–10 minutes, until the oats are soft and the porridge is creamy and tender. Add a dash more hot water if needed.

Spoon the hot tea porridge into warm bowls (discarding the cardamom pods if used). Add a splash of milk if you wish. Spoon on some fruit compote if you like, and if you think it's needed, a restrained trickle of honey or a pinch of sugar.

Any leftover porridge can be refrigerated, then reheated later (or the next day), with a few tablespoonfuls of water added to loosen it.

TOAST FOR BREAKFAST

I try not to rely on bread so much these days (see page 109) and I no longer automatically 'toast up' at breakfast time. But I still like a toasty start to the day now and again. I favour a higher-fibre bread, made with at least 50% wholegrain flour – maybe a Scandi-style seeded rye loaf or a half-wholemeal sourdough. I love spelt-based breads too. And toast doesn't have to be smothered with jam or marmalade – I top my toast with as much goodness as I can, using combinations like these:

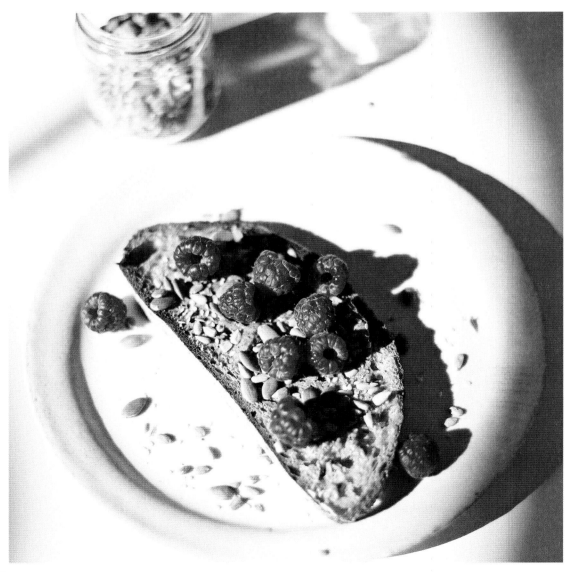

...with nut butter and berries

Per person

1 large or 2 small slices of wholegrain bread, such as spelt or rye

1 generous tbsp unsweetened nut butter, such as almond, cashew or peanut

A handful of raspberries or blueberries

A lemon wedge (optional)

2 tsp mixed seeds (optional)

Toast the bread. Allow it to cool for a minute or two then spread with your chosen nut butter. Add the berries, pushing them down lightly into the nut butter. Finish, if you like, with a squeeze of lemon and/or a sprinkling of seeds.

...with olive oil, honey and seeds

Per person

1 large or 2 small slices of wholegrain bread, such as spelt or rye

1 tbsp olive oil (or a bit of butter)

1 tsp honey

2 tsp mixed seeds or dukka (page 281)

Toast the bread. Allow it to cool slightly then trickle with olive oil (the combination of olive oil, honey and seeds is particularly good), or butter lightly. Trickle with the honey (or spread it if it's a thick honey) then finish with a good sprinkling of seeds or dukka.

...with avocado and seeds

Per person

1 large or 2 small slices of wholegrain bread, such as spelt or rye

½–1 medium avocado

1 tsp extra virgin olive oil, for trickling

A lemon wedge (optional)

½–1 tbsp mixed seeds or dukka (page 281), optional

A pinch of dried chilli flakes (optional)

Sea salt and black pepper

Toast the bread. Halve, peel and stone the avocado and either slice it or mash it roughly. Top the toast with the avocado and season with a pinch of salt and a twist of pepper. Trickle with the extra virgin olive oil and add a little spritz of lemon if you like. Finish with a sprinkling of seeds or dukka, and/or a pinch of chilli flakes for a touch of heat.

WHOLEGRAIN PANCAKES

These hearty, high-fibre vegan pancakes are delicious topped with a trickle of maple syrup (or honey, if you're not vegan) and/or fruit. Two large (or 3 slightly smaller) pancakes is enough for one serving. The whole seeds are optional – not everyone likes to crunch seeds in their pancakes – and the wholemeal flour and ground almonds/seeds already give plenty of fibre. Any leftover pancakes can be kept in an airtight container for up to 24 hours and gently reheated if you want them warm – popping them in the toaster is the easiest way, or you can place them in a low oven for a few minutes.

Serves 4 (makes 8–12 pancakes)

200g wholegrain spelt flour, or wholemeal 'cake' flour

50g ground almonds, ground flaxseed, or hulled hemp seeds

2–3 tbsp mixed whole seeds, such as sesame and sunflower (optional)

About 15g (1 tbsp) soft brown sugar

2 rounded tsp baking powder

A pinch of salt

2 tbsp vegetable or olive oil, or melted coconut oil

250ml almond, oat or soy milk (or cow's milk, if not vegan)

Vegetable oil, for cooking

To serve

Fresh berries or roasted fruit compote (pages 224–5)

Natural yoghurt (optional)

A little maple syrup or honey

Put the flour, ground almonds (or flax/hemp), whole seeds if using, sugar, baking powder and salt into a large bowl and use a whisk to combine them thoroughly. Make a well in the centre of the flour mix and add the 2 tbsp oil. Gradually pour in the milk, whisking all the time, to form a thick batter.

Heat a non-stick frying pan or a crêpe pan over a medium heat. Add a trickle of oil and use a silicone brush to brush it over the base of the pan in a thin layer. When the pan is hot, use a serving spoon to drop a large dollop of batter into the pan. Repeat so you have 3 or 4 pancakes in the pan.

Cook for about 2 minutes, until several bubbles form on the surface of each pancake. Using a broad spatula, flip the pancakes over and cook for a further 2 minutes or until golden brown on both sides. You can break one pancake open to check it is cooked through. If you find the pan getting too hot at any point, just take it off the heat for a moment or two. Transfer the cooked pancakes to a dish (you can keep them warm in a low oven at around 100°C/Fan 80°C/lowest Gas, if you like). Add a little more oil to the pan and cook the remaining batter in the same way.

Serve the pancakes warm with berries or roasted fruit compote, a dollop of yoghurt if you like, and a trickle of maple syrup or honey.

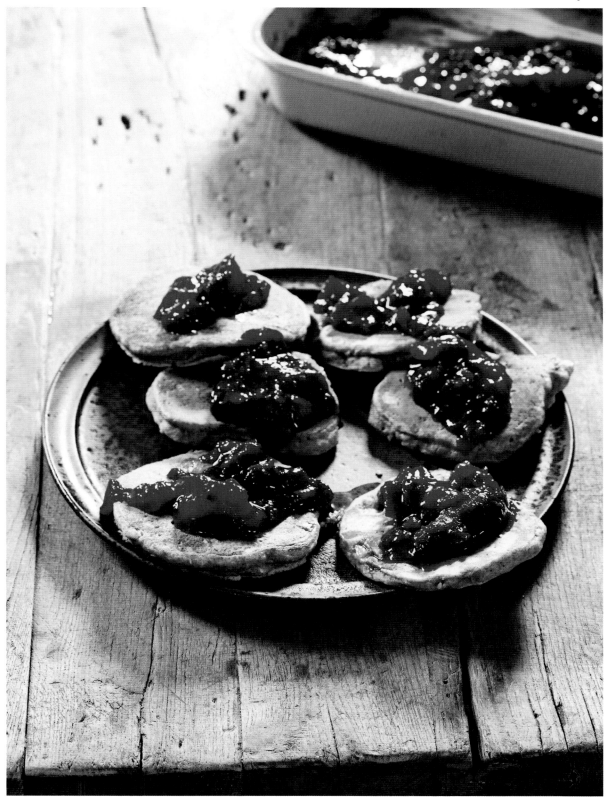

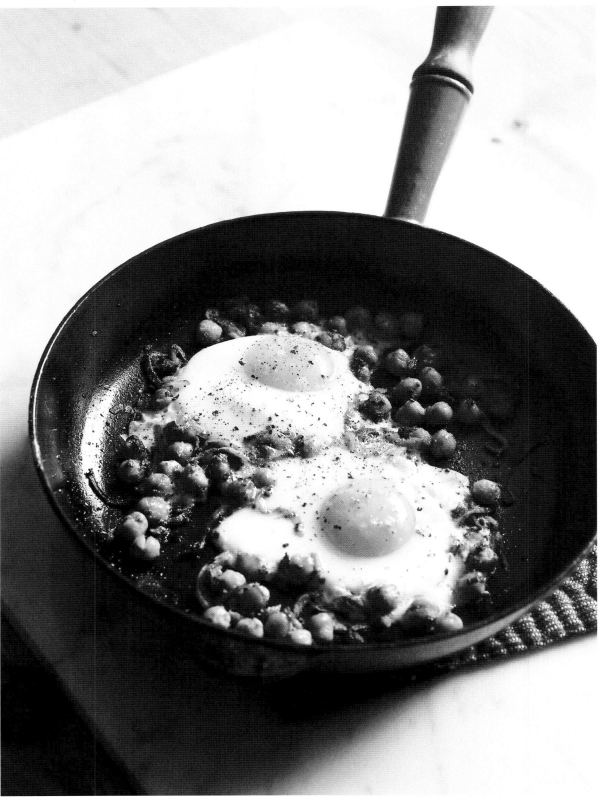

THE FRIED EGG OMELETTE

Easier than an omelette, more fun than egg on toast, this quick, filling dish can be customised in different ways (see below). Have your ingredients prepared and a warm plate ready because this cooks in minutes.

Per person

½ tbsp olive or vegetable oil

½ small or ¼ medium onion, finely sliced

60–120g cooked chickpeas or beans (¼–½ of a 400g tin), drained and rinsed

1 tsp of your favourite curry paste or powder

1–2 medium eggs

Sea salt and black pepper

Put a medium or large non-stick frying over a medium heat. Add the oil and, when it's hot, add the onion. Fry, stirring often, for about 3 minutes. It's fine if the onion colours a bit, but you don't want it to burn.

Add the chickpeas and curry paste or powder and stir through the onion. Cook for another minute.

Crack the egg(s) into the pan, letting the egg fall wherever it wants to – the white(s) will overlap and trap some of the onion and chickpeas, which is all good! Season with a pinch of salt and a twist of pepper and cook for a couple of minutes until the white is set. If, like me, you like your eggs flipped ('over easy' as they say in the US), you may find it easier to separate them with a spatula, then flip them one at a time, and cook for another 30 seconds, or to your liking.

Grind over some black pepper, then transfer the eggs, chickpeas or beans and all the tasty bits to a warm plate, and tuck in without delay.

AVOCADO, PUMPKIN SEED & CHILLI VARIATION
Peel ½ avocado and cut into 1cm thick slices. Thinly slice some fresh red chilli. Heat ½ tbsp oil in a non-stick pan. Add 2–3 tbsp (30–45g) pumpkin seeds and fry for about 3 minutes until toasted and popping. Add the avocado and chilli and fry for 30–60 seconds. Break in 2 eggs, season and cook as above.

TOMATO & CHILLI VARIATION
Halve about 100g cherry tomatoes and slice a couple of spring onions. Heat ½ tbsp oil in a non-stick pan and add the tomatoes and spring onions. Cook briskly for a few minutes, shaking or stirring now and then, until the tomatoes start to release their juices. Add a sprinkle of dried chilli flakes (or chopped fresh red or green chilli, or a dash of Tabasco). Break in 1–2 eggs, season and cook as above. You can also splice this with the main recipe by adding a couple of handfuls of chickpeas with the onions and tomatoes at the start.

POACHED EGG ON TOAST WITH KIMCHI

Rich with garlic and chilli, kimchi (page 286) is Korean-style fermented cabbage, and unpasteurised versions are full of beneficial live bacteria. Here, the spicy, salty sharpness of kimchi is offset nicely by the richness of the egg. If you prefer something milder, then any live kraut (see pages 282–4) works well. If your kimchi/kraut is in the fridge, ideally spoon out what you need and let it come up to room temperature before you put it on the toast, so it doesn't cool the egg down too much.

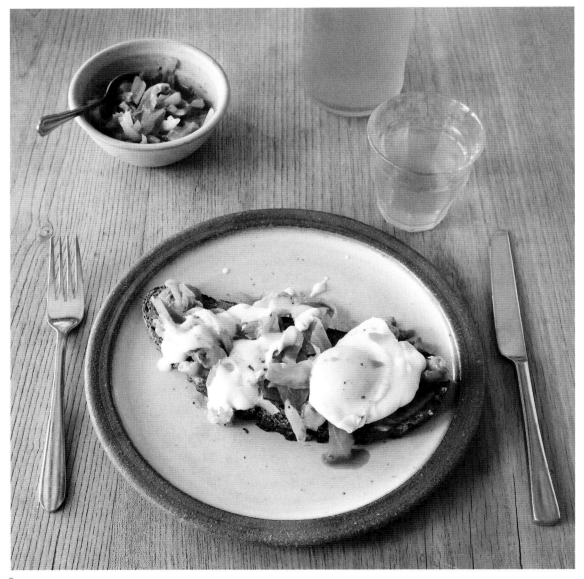

Per person

1–2 slices of wholegrain bread

1–2 medium eggs

1 tsp extra virgin olive or rapeseed oil

2 tbsp live kimchi (page 286) or a spicy kraut, ideally homemade (page 282), at room temperature

1 generous tbsp natural yoghurt (optional)

Black pepper

Boil the kettle, pour a 3–4cm depth of hot water into a medium saucepan (with a lid) and add a pinch of salt. Return to the boil then turn the heat down to its lowest setting. The water should be barely even simmering.

Meanwhile, get the bread in the toaster.

Have ready a slotted spoon. Break each egg into a ramekin or small cup. Carefully slip into the hot water, put the lid on the pan and immediately start timing 2 minutes.

Transfer the toast to a plate and trickle over the 1 tsp extra virgin oil. Spoon the kimchi or kraut on top.

After the 2 minutes' cooking time, carefully scoop up the poached egg(s) using the slotted spoon. Check that the white is set and not still jelly-ish (if necessary, return it to the water briefly). Allow as much water as possible to drain off the egg(s) through the spoon (you can dab away any excess water from the poached egg with the corner of a clean cloth).

Place the poached egg(s) on top of the kimchi or kraut, spoon on the yoghurt, if using, and season with pepper. You can also trickle over any kimchi juice left in the bowl. Eat straight away.

HUMMUS/AVOCADO VARIATION

If you're after a vegan breakfast, jettison the egg and yoghurt. Trickle half the oil directly onto the hot toast, then dollop on 2 tbsp of your favourite hummus or a beany pâté (see pages 277 and 274), and/or ½ avocado, sliced. Put the kimchi/kraut on top of this and trickle on a little more oil and kimchi juice, before tucking in.

EASY EGGS

If poaching eggs seems a bit of a faff, soft-boil them instead. Bring a pan of water to a rolling boil then lower 1 or 2 eggs (at room temperature) into the water, using a spoon. Time 4 minutes, then scoop the eggs out with a slotted spoon. Leave until just cool enough to handle, tap with a spoon to crack the shells and peel the eggs. (You can speed things up by peeling them under a trickling cold water tap, but be careful not to break the white!) Serve the eggs on top of the kimchi on toast, breaking them open with a fork so the yolk runs out.

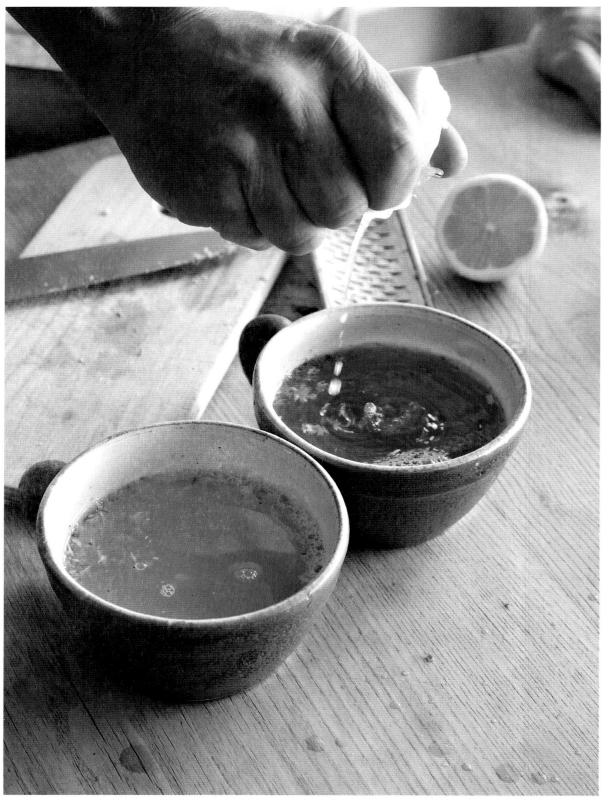

MORNING GINGER KICKER

This freshly brewed drink, which is a version of one I first encountered in the Filmore Café in York Station, is a fantastic way to start the day. The cider vinegar added at the end is optional but contributes a 'live' element.

Per person

A hazelnut-sized piece of fresh ginger, finely grated

A hazelnut-sized piece of fresh turmeric, finely grated (optional)

Black pepper or a pinch of dried chilli flakes

½ lemon

A dash of raw cider vinegar (optional)

Boil the kettle. Put the ginger and turmeric into a mug with a twist of black pepper or a pinch of chilli flakes. Pour in enough boiling water to half-fill the mug and leave to infuse for 4–5 minutes.

Squeeze in the lemon juice, at which point the brew will (if you've used turmeric) impressively change colour (as the acidic citrus reacts with the spice). Add a dash of cold water, and a dash of cider vinegar if using. Drink warm. You can actually eat the bits of ginger and turmeric left at the bottom of the mug – my wife likes to stir them into her overnight oats (see page 227).

MINT & LEMON VERBENA INFUSION

The two herbs we grow the most and use the most at home are probably mint (I grow both Moroccan mint and spearmint) and lemon verbena. They do find their way into recipes – especially the mint – but the way we use them most often is in this simple infusion, sometimes with one or the other, often with both. *(Pictured on page 161)*

Per person

A sprig of lemon verbena leaves

A sprig of mint

A small strip of lemon zest – one light stroke of the peeler, no pith (optional)

Boil the kettle and leave for a couple of minutes – or pour the boiling water into the cup you're using and leave for a minute. With the water at 80–90°C, you'll get a fresher taste from the herbs.

Add the herbs and lemon zest to the water (or vice-versa), cover with a small saucer to increase the aromatic hit and leave to infuse for a minimum of 3 minutes, ideally 5 or 10, before drinking. You can, of course, brew in a small teapot or infusion flask if you prefer.

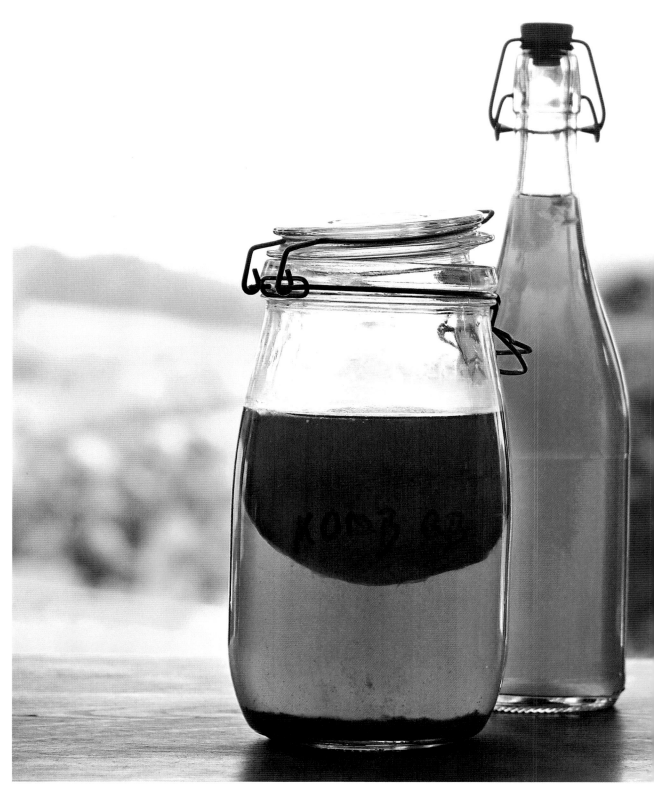

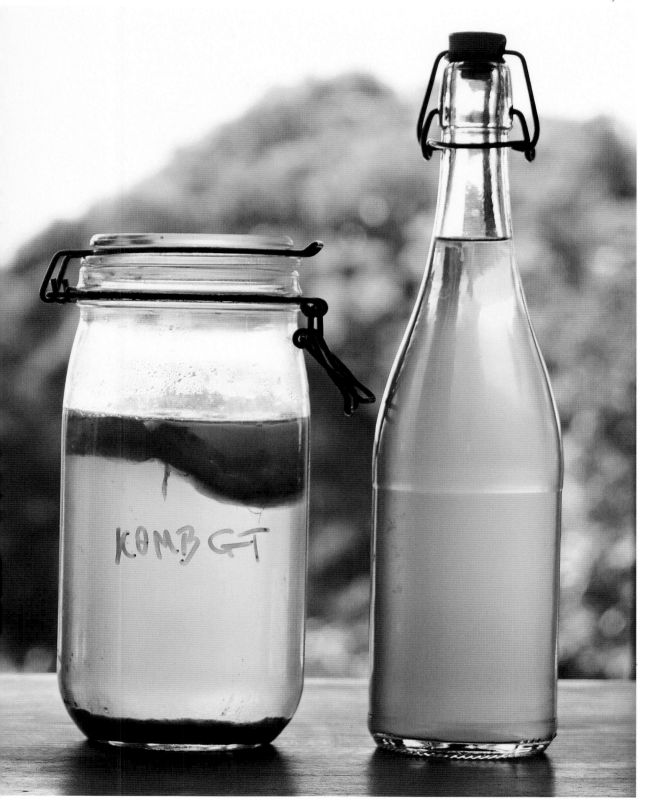

KOMBGT

My kombuchas

I have two kombuchas on the go, which I brew in 2-litre Kilner jars. One is based on organic green tea and the other on (caffeine-free) organic rooibos tea. What makes a kombucha happen is the 'SCOBY', which stands for symbiotic culture of bacteria and yeast, and it's the live bacteria which can benefit your gut (see page 82). You can buy a SCOBY starter online – or wangle one from a kombucha-brewing friend.

I feed my green tea kombucha with unrefined sugar. The received wisdom is to feed 8.5% sugar, i.e. 85g per litre of tea. I have gradually reduced this to 60g and my kombuchas are chugging along quite happily. You end up with less sugar than you put in and (unlike fermenting alcohol) less calories too. It's a complex process but to simplify, as the yeast consumes the sugar, ethanol is produced, which is then converted by the bacteria into acetic acid (similar to that in a live vinegar), consuming calories in the process. A typical finished kombucha has less than 4g of sugar (16 calories) per 100ml.

On that basis I think a couple of (175ml) wine glasses of chilled kombucha are a very reasonable replacement for an evening's moderate drinking. I also use kombucha to soak dried fruit and splash in my overnight oats (page 227). Here's the procedure...

GREEN TEA KOMBUCHA

I sometimes flavour this with half a dozen picked young nettle tops in spring, or a few sprigs of lemon verbena. And sometimes I make it 'straight up'.

Makes about 1 litre

4 level tbsp green tea leaves (or 4 green tea bags)

1 litre boiling water, ideally filtered

60g (4 level tbsp) unrefined sugar or rapadura sugar

A kombucha SCOBY starter

In a jug or teapot, combine the green tea (and the nettle tops or verbena if using) with the boiling water. Leave for a few minutes before stirring in the sugar, then leave to brew, stirring once or twice, until cooled completely. Strain through a muslin-lined sieve into a very clean kilner jar (at least 1.5 litre) and add your live SCOBY and its liquid. If the jar has a rubber seal, remove it, so the kombucha can 'breathe' (i.e. gas can escape). You can also brew kombucha in an open jar or jug, with a square of muslin over it. Leave to ferment at room temperature (18–22°C).

As it brews, kombucha becomes increasingly acidic. Taste it after 5 or 6 days. If you like the flavour, bottle it now. If you want it more tart, leave it for a couple more days. In a cool place, it may take 10 days or more to reach a pleasant level of acidity.

I strain my kombucha through a muslin-lined non-metal sieve into a plastic or glass jug, then pour it through a plastic funnel into a clean 750ml bottle with a rubber stopper. That leaves me a modest glassful for instant gratification, and enough live kombucha (at least 100ml) for my next brew.

If you are happy to drink flat kombucha (I am), bottle it and put it straight into the fridge. Chilling slows the fermentation right down and makes it nice and cold for drinking.

If you want a bit of sparkle in your kombucha, add another 1 tsp (5g) sugar to the kombucha at the bottling stage. Seal the bottle and leave it at room temperature for 2–3 days, while a secondary fermentation occurs, then transfer to the fridge.

Even in the fridge kombucha will continue to ferment slowly and become more acidic. If you find it too tart, you can rebalance it by diluting it with water or cold tea. Very acidic kombucha can be used like a live vinegar, in dressings and pickles.

ROOIBOS KOMBUCHA VARIATION
Instead of green tea, use rooibos tea leaves (4 level tbsp, or 4 tea bags). I feed mine with half honey, half sugar, and it goes well.

Maintaining your SCOBY

A good 100–200ml of leftover kombucha contains plenty of SCOBY (including the jelly-like plug often referred to as the SCOBY, although in fact the SCOBY is dissolved in both the liquid and the jelly). You can either crack on with your next brew immediately, or leave the remnant in the jar for a day or two. This will 'concentrate' it – i.e. up the levels of yeast and bacteria – and get the next brew off to a flying start. But don't leave it for more than a week without feeding it.

You can keep a constant brew on the go (with or without the pause for concentration), harvesting around 750ml every 6–10 days. And you can scale up the brew size according to your (and your family's) enthusiasm for kombucha! If you want to take a break, you can store your SCOBY (the plug and at least 100ml of liquid) in the fridge for up to 2 weeks. Any longer than that and you'll have to give it a 'maintenance feed' – a mugful (about 250ml) tea with about 20g sugar. Add the (cooled) sweetened tea to the SCOBY and leave at room temperature for a day or two to concentrate before returning to the fridge (or starting a new brew).

After a while, the jar will be getting a bit grubby, a residue will be gathering in the bottom and the jelly-like plug will have grown. To 'clean' the starter, pour the contents of the jar into a non-metallic container, thoroughly wash and rinse the jar, then return at least 50ml of liquid to it. Peel off a layer of the jelly and add that too. The rest of the liquid and jelly can be used to start a new brew or given to a friend to start one of their own.

KEFIR

Kefir is a fermented yoghurt-like drink, rich with beneficial bacteria and yeasts. You can buy ready-made kefir, in all sorts of flavours, but making your own is very satisfying – not to mention far more sustainable. To make kefir, fresh milk is fermented with kefir 'grains' – rather strange-looking clusters that harbour lots of active beneficial micro-organisms.

You can use a freeze-dried culture (available from health food stores) to make your kefir, in which case you simply need to follow the instructions on the pack. Alternatively, order some live kefir grains online – they are firm little curds, a bit like the lumps in cottage cheese but harder. Or get some from a friend – that's what I did, nabbing both a little cluster of kefir grains and a heap of good advice from my friend Rachel de Thample, a talented food writer (and resident River Cottage fermentation expert). This method is based closely on hers.

Makes 500ml

500ml unhomogenised whole milk
(ideally organic)

1 tbsp kefir grains (not measured with
a metal spoon)

Pour the milk into a large, clean jar or jug, making sure it is not filled to the brim. Add the kefir grains and stir with a non-metal spoon (the grains are damaged by contact with metal). Cover and leave to ferment at room temperature for 12–24 hours.

Tilt the jar a little and you will see the milk has slightly thickened or curdled. Strain through a non-metallic sieve into a clean non-metallic container and reserve the grains in the sieve, returning them to a clean jar for your next 'brew'. Your strained kefir is a slightly thickened, tangy, yoghurt-like liquid – ready to drink, or store in the fridge for a few days. It may well separate, but can be gently stirred back together again.

Drink your kefir chilled, either neat or whizzed up in a blender with fresh fruit, such as berries or bananas. Many people like to take their kefir in this way, particularly at first, as the sharp flavour can take a little getting used to. Strained kefir will continue to gently ferment in the fridge so is best drunk within a week. I am very happy to drink 'neat' kefir – sipping, not glugging. And it's delicious poured over granola or muesli, or used instead of yoghurt in Bircher/overnight oats.

Between brews, you can store the kefir grains in a clean jar in the fridge with just enough liquid kefir to cover them. You don't have to keep a constant brew on the go but you should feed them with fresh milk or kefir at least every 2 weeks and rinse them occasionally with fresh milk or water in a non-metal sieve.

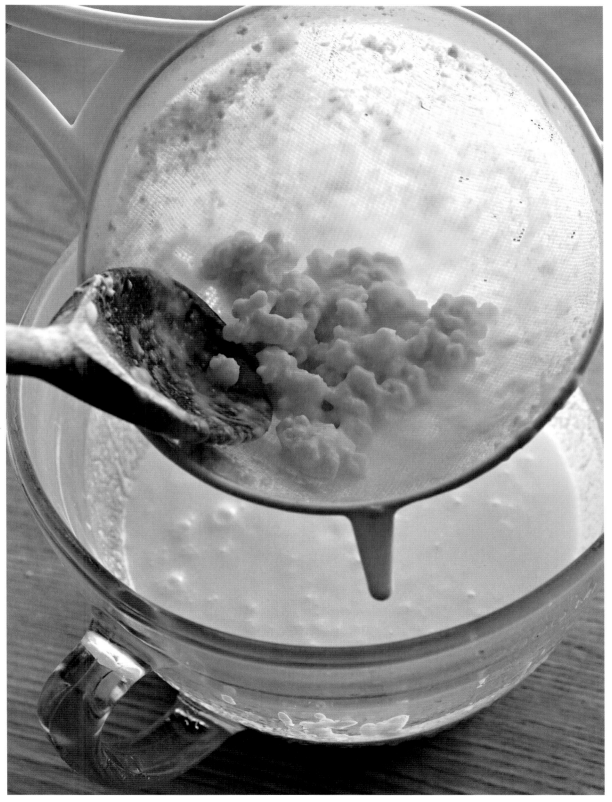

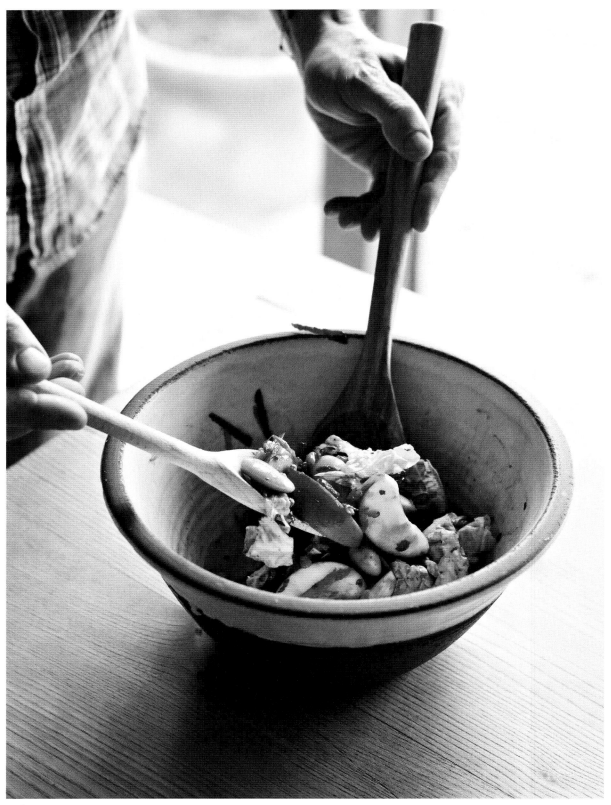

QUICK LUNCH(BOX)ES

As with breakfasts, weekday lunchtimes are a fantastic opportunity to massively up your game with diverse and delicious whole foods. The trick is to put together these quick lunches as simple assemblies of good things. They don't need to involve 'making' much, certainly not cooking much – more just throwing together a selection of lovely, fresh ingredients that will please the senses and nourish you well. The building blocks are simple: fresh vegetables and fruits (often raw), nuts and seeds, whole grains, cooked or tinned pulses, tinned fish, eggs. Bursting with wholeness and fibre, these ingredients can easily be made tangy and tasty with punchy dressings and crunchy sprinkles.

There are a few things that require some prep: 'hard-boiled' eggs, plain-cooked whole grains (see below), flavoursome pestos, hummuses and 'blitzes'. But the work required is minimal and, once made, they can happily sit in the fridge for several days, to be dipped into whenever you choose. It is useful to have some kind of food processor to help you produce these. But beyond that, the most advanced equipment you require is a decent knife, a sturdy box grater and, of course, a reusable lunchbox...

As you'll see, most of the recipes in this chapter give quantities 'per person', with a degree of flexibility to allow for your appetite, or where you are for portion size on my weight-loss meal plan (on pages 196–7) if you are following it.

GRAINS AT THE READY

Several of these simple combos include some kind of whole grain – usually spelt, barley or brown rice. I like to have at least one tub of grain pre-cooked, cooled and sitting in the fridge ready to use. In all cases, it helps to soak the whole grain first for anything up to 4 hours in cold water. It plumps up the grains, and speeds up the cooking a bit too. Rinse well, then put into a pan, cover with cold water and bring to the boil. Lower the heat and simmer, covered, until the grain is tender. For wholegrain spelt and rice, this will probably be 25–30 minutes; for pearl barley, perhaps 35–40. Once cooked, drain and, if you're not eating the grains straight away, spread out on a cold plate to cool completely then transfer to the fridge.

It's important that cooked grains, particularly rice, are not left sitting around at room temperature for ages, as occasionally a harmful bacteria can grow on them. So, keep the grains in the fridge until you come to mix up your lunchbox and keep the combo cool, ideally in the fridge at work, until you come to eat.

This first run of 'recipes' showcases the kind of fast-and-loose mix-and-match of great ingredients that go together well. To emphasise the principle of creative combining and the interchangeability of the elements, I've called the dishes simply by their main ingredients, and subtitled them with the generic family that each ingredient comes from. This will help you see your way to an almost infinite variety of improvised delicious combinations that you can play with.

BEETROOT, CARROT, SPELT, BEANS, APPLE

roots / grain / pulse / fruit / leaf

Per person

1 small raw beetroot, scrubbed or peeled

½ raw carrot, scrubbed or peeled

A handful of cooked whole spelt or barley grains (see page 249)

2 handfuls of cooked butter beans (⅓–½ of a 400g tin), drained and rinsed

1 crisp apple, cored and cut into wedges

½ little gem lettuce, roughly torn

For the dressing

1 tsp freshly grated ginger

1 tbsp vegetable oil

1 tbsp olive oil

1 tbsp raw cider vinegar

A pinch of sea salt

A twist of black pepper

Whisk the dressing ingredients together. Coarsely grate the beetroot and carrot and combine with the other ingredients in another bowl. Pour on the dressing and tumble everything gently together. Eat straight away or pack into a lunchbox for later.

LENTILS, PEAR, CELERIAC, PARSLEY

pulse / fruit / root / herb / seeds

Per person

A handful of cooked Puy lentils (freshly cooked or from a tin)

1 just-ripe pear, cored and cut into slices

2 tbsp raisins, ideally pre-soaked in apple or orange juice, or kombucha (page 244) or water

1 tbsp pumpkin seeds

A handful of grated raw celeriac

A handful of parsley leaves

A squeeze of lemon juice

Extra virgin olive or rapeseed oil

Sea salt and black pepper

Combine the lentils, pear slices, raisins, pumpkin seeds, grated celeriac and parsley in a bowl. Squeeze on a little lemon juice, and add a trickle of extra virgin oil, a pinch of salt and a twist of pepper. Tumble it all together and serve or pack into a lunchbox.

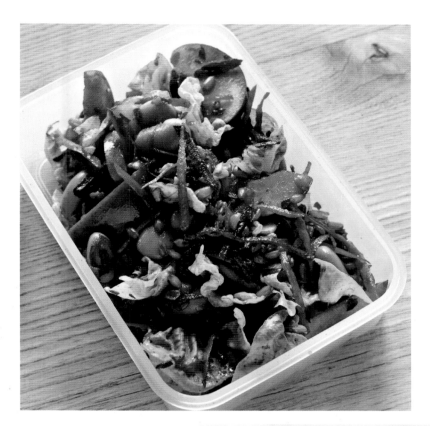

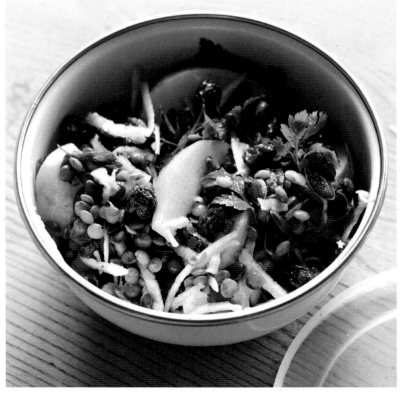

FENNEL, BEANS, SPELT, APPLE, ORANGE

crunchy veg / pulse / grain / fruit / herb

Per person

1 tbsp virgin rapeseed or olive oil

A squeeze of lemon juice

½–1 fennel bulb (or 1–2 celery stems), sliced

A couple of handfuls of cooked white beans, such as haricot or cannellini (⅓–½ of a 400g tin), drained and rinsed

A handful of cooked whole spelt or barley grains (see page 249)

1 crisp apple, cored and cut into chunks or wedges

1 orange, peeled, segmented and cut into chunks

A few mint leaves, shredded

Sea salt and black pepper

Combine the oil and lemon juice in a bowl with a pinch of salt and a twist of pepper. Add all the other ingredients and tumble them gently together. Eat straight away or pack into a lunchbox for later.

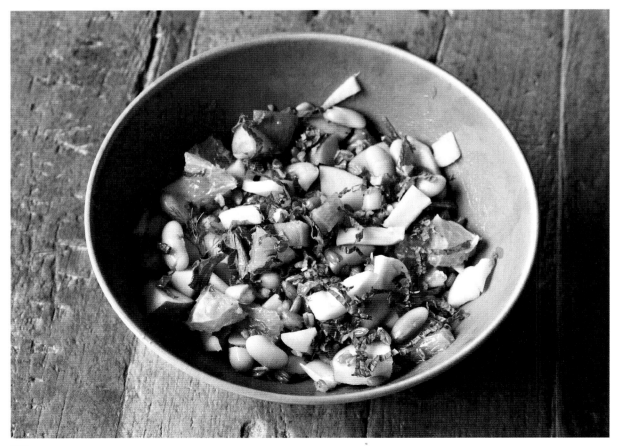

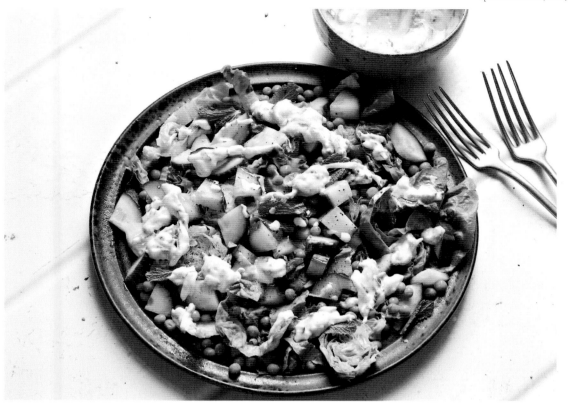

LITTLE GEMS, CUCUMBER, PEAS, MINT

leaf / crunchy veg / pulse / herb

<u>Serves 2</u>

100g frozen peas or petits pois

2 little gem lettuce

1 medium cucumber

A handful of mint leaves

6 tbsp natural yoghurt

1 tbsp extra virgin olive oil

A scrap of garlic (about ¼ clove), crushed or finely grated

Juice of ½ lime

Sea salt and black pepper

Put the peas or petits pois into a pan, cover with boiling water and return to the boil. Drain in a sieve, run briefly under cold water and set aside.

Slice the little gems across into 1–2 cm rounds. Arrange on a serving plate. Cut the cucumber in half. Quarter one half lengthways and slice it into 1–2cm chunks. Add these to the lettuce on the plate. Scatter over the peas and mint.

Grate the remaining cucumber into a bowl and add the yoghurt, olive oil, garlic, lime juice, a pinch of salt and a twist of pepper. Stir to combine and make a dressing. Spoon over the salad and add an extra grinding of pepper to serve.

BEETROOT, RADICCHIO, PLUMS, BEANS

root / leaf / fruit / pulse

Per person

About 1 tbsp extra virgin olive oil

About 1 tbsp raw cider vinegar

A pinch of dried chilli flakes

1–2 small-medium raw beetroot, scrubbed or peeled and coarsely grated

A handful of radicchio or chicory leaves, shredded

2–3 small-medium plums, halved, stoned and cut into thin wedges

A handful of cherry tomatoes, halved

A handful or two of cooked kidney beans (¼–½ of a 400g tin), drained and rinsed

Sea salt and black pepper

1 large radicchio leaf or ½–1 wholegrain flatbread, to serve

Combine the olive oil, cider vinegar and chilli flakes with a pinch of salt and a twist of pepper in a bowl. Add the grated beetroot, shredded radicchio or chicory, plum wedges, cherry tomatoes and beans and tumble gently together. Serve wrapped in the extra radicchio leaf or flatbread. Or pack in a lunchbox to eat later.

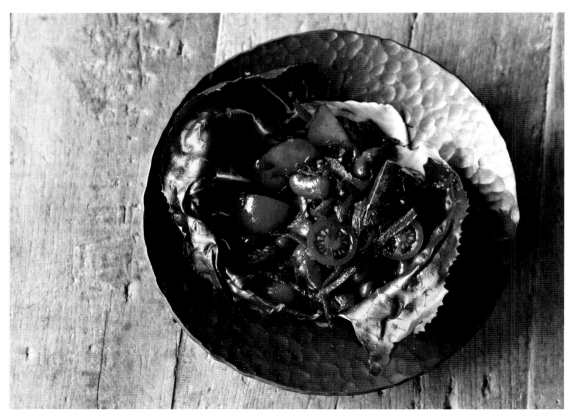

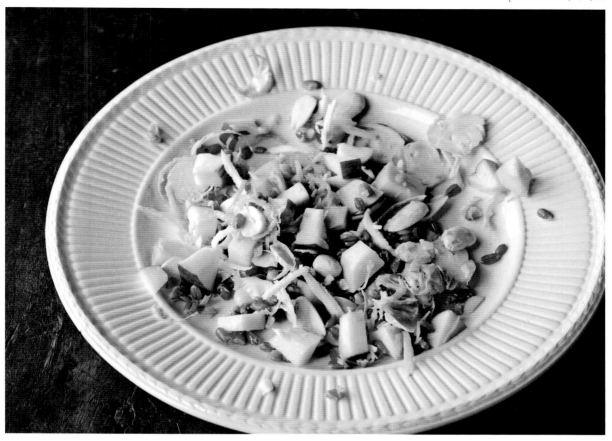

PARSNIP, BRUSSELS, APPLE, SPELT, ALMONDS

root / brassica / fruit / grain / nut

Per person

1 small parsnip, scrubbed or peeled and coarsely grated

4 Brussels sprouts, shredded

1 crisp apple, cored and roughly chopped

A handful of cooked whole spelt or barley grains (see page 249)

8–10 whole, skin-on almonds, soaked and skinned, split in half

For the dressing

1 tbsp extra virgin olive oil, or vegetable or rapeseed oil

1 tsp honey

1 tsp English mustard

A pinch of sea salt

A twist of black pepper

Whisk the dressing ingredients together in a bowl. Combine the other ingredients in another bowl. Pour on the dressing and tumble everything gently together. Eat straight away or pack into a lunchbox.

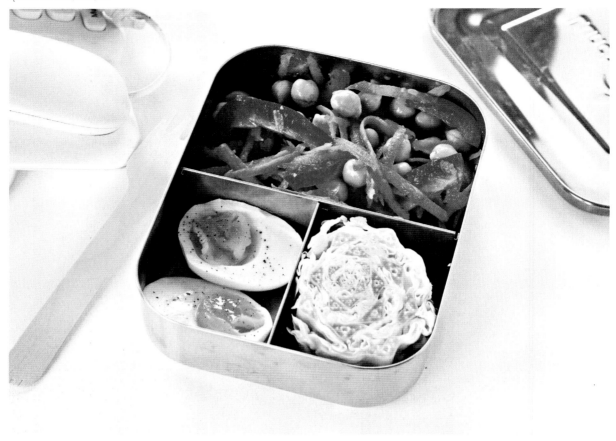

RED PEPPER, CARROT, CHICKPEAS, EGG

crunchy veg / root / pulse / egg

Per person

2 tsp harissa paste

Juice of ½ orange

1 red pepper, cored, deseeded and thinly sliced

1 medium carrot, coarsely grated

A couple of handfuls of cooked chickpeas (⅓–½ of a 400g tin), drained and rinsed

Sea salt and black pepper

To serve

1 'hard-boiled' egg (see page 268), halved

½ little gem lettuce

Stir the harissa and orange juice together in a bowl. Add the sliced pepper, grated carrot and chickpeas and turn gently to coat. Season the halved boiled egg and lettuce with a pinch of salt and a twist of pepper. Assemble on a plate to eat straight away or pack into a lunchbox.

EGG, CAULIFLOWER, KRAUT, PARSLEY

egg / crunchy veg / fermented veg / herb

Per person

1–2 tbsp natural yoghurt

1 tbsp extra virgin olive oil

1–2 tbsp kraut, ideally homemade (page 282)

1–2 'hard-boiled' eggs (see page 268), peeled and roughly chopped

A handful of thinly sliced raw cauliflower

A handful of parsley leaves, chopped

Sea salt and black pepper

3–5 seeded oatcakes, to serve

Put the yoghurt, olive oil and kraut into a bowl with a pinch of salt and a twist of pepper and stir to combine. Add the chopped boiled egg(s), sliced cauliflower and chopped parsley and stir gently. Transfer to a plate or a lunchbox and eat with oatcakes.

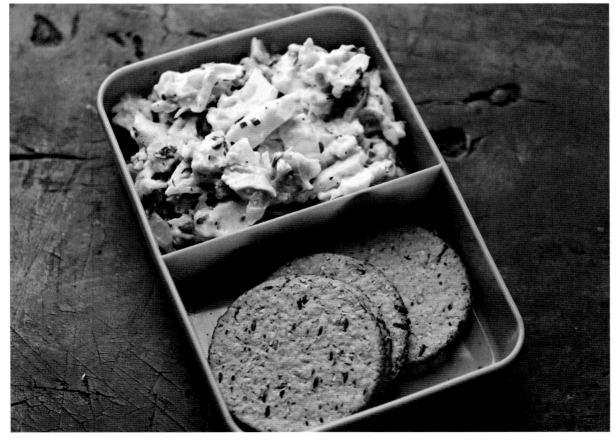

KIMCH-EREE

Grain / nut or pulse / fruit / fermented veg / egg

<u>Per person</u>

A couple of handfuls of cooked brown rice

A few whole, skin-on almonds, soaked and skinned, or a handful of cooked chickpeas (about ⅓ of a 400g tin), drained and rinsed

1–2 tbsp raisins, ideally pre-soaked in apple or orange juice, or kombucha (page 244) or water

A handful of cherry tomatoes, cut into wedges

1 tbsp kimchi, ideally homemade (page 286)

1–2 'hard-boiled' eggs (see page 268), peeled and cut into wedges

A trickle of olive oil

Sea salt and black pepper

Put the rice, almonds or chickpeas, raisins, tomato wedges and kimchi into a bowl, add a pinch of salt and a twist of pepper and stir gently. Add the boiled egg wedges, trickle over a little olive oil and turn gently again. Eat straight away or pack into a lunchbox.

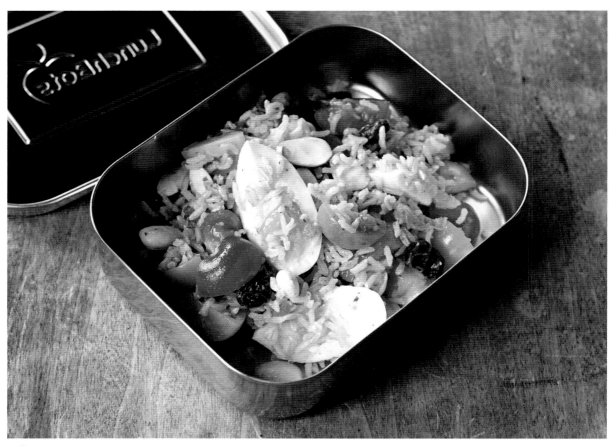

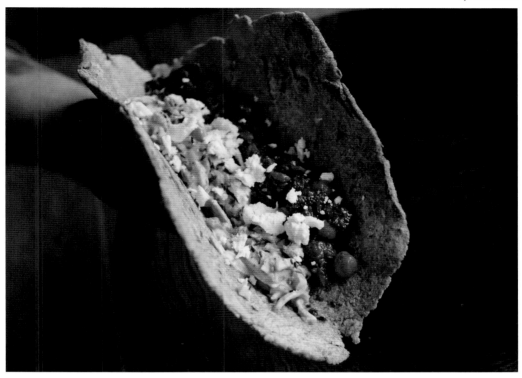

BASHED BEETROOT & CHICKPEA (WRAP)

Root / pulse / nut / fermented veg

Per person

1 large or 2 medium cooked beetroot

A handful of cooked chickpeas (about ¼ of a 400g tin), drained and rinsed

A handful of walnuts, roughly bashed

2 tbsp extra virgin olive oil

2 heaped tsp tahini

Juice of ½ lemon

1 tbsp natural yoghurt

1 tbsp kraut, ideally homemade (page 282)

1 tsp toasted cumin seeds

½ wholegrain wrap or a small pitta or flatbread (warmed if you like), or a few oatcakes to serve (optional)

A little feta cheese (optional)

Sea salt and black pepper

Roughly chop the beetroot, put into a bowl and mash roughly. Add the chickpeas, walnuts, olive oil, tahini, lemon juice, a pinch of salt and a twist of pepper and stir together. In a separate bowl, combine the yoghurt, kraut and cumin seeds.

Spread the beetroot mix down the middle of the wrap (or in a split pitta or flatbread). Spread the yoghurt mix next to it. Crumble over the feta, if using, and eat straight away. Or box up the beetroot mix and take with the wrap/pitta for later, lunchtime assembly. It is also delicious as a salad, without the wrap. Or you can shovel it onto a few oatcakes.

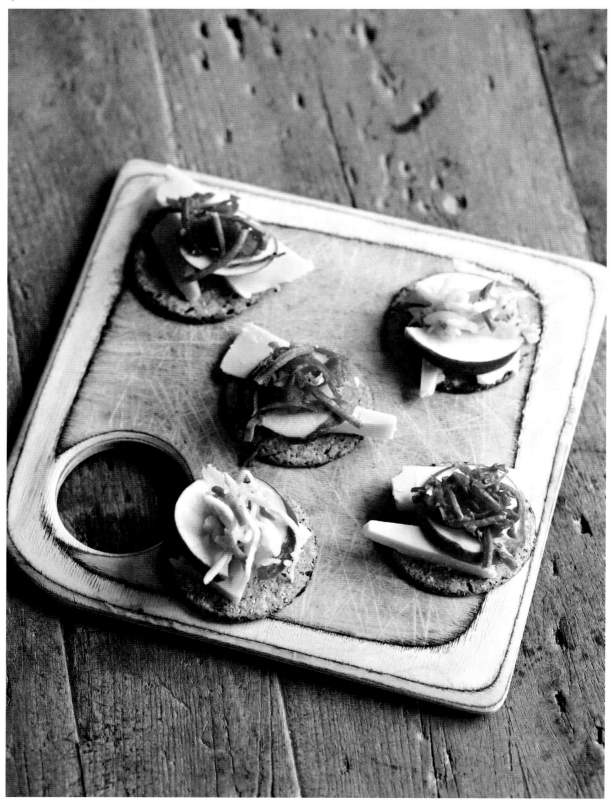

OATCAKES WITH CHEESE, APPLE & KRAUT

Cheese and oatcakes make a perfectly legitimate lunch. An apple and a spoonful of live kraut make them healthier, tastier and even more satisfying. You can top oatcakes in all kinds of fun, tempting and healthy ways, and I often do! See my variations below.

Per person

3–5 oatcakes

A piece of Cheddar or other cheese (40–60g), sliced

1 crisp apple, cored and sliced

1–2 tbsp kraut, ideally homemade (page 282)

Pack up the ingredients separately in a lunchbox, ready to assemble just before eating: top each oatcake with one or two slices of Cheddar, a couple of pieces of apple and a spoonful of kraut.

BERRY & RICOTTA VARIATION

Take the cheese/fruit theme in a different direction, with ricotta, or fresh goat's curd, and sliced strawberries or whole raspberries or blueberries and, if you have it, a little chopped mint. You can layer the ricotta, strawberries and mint, or mix them lightly together and pile onto the oatcakes. Finish with a tiny splash of balsamic vinegar, if handy.

EGG VARIATION

For a more savoury snack lunch, roughly chop a 'hard-boiled' egg or two (see page 268), bind with a little mayonnaise or yoghurt, and pile onto oatcakes. Top with kraut or kimchi (pages 282–6), or slices of cucumber or spring onion.

FISH VARIATION

Tinned fish, especially sardines, is great mixed with a dollop of yoghurt and a chopped spring onion or a sprinkle of capers. Pile onto oatcakes and finish with a slice of cucumber or fennel.

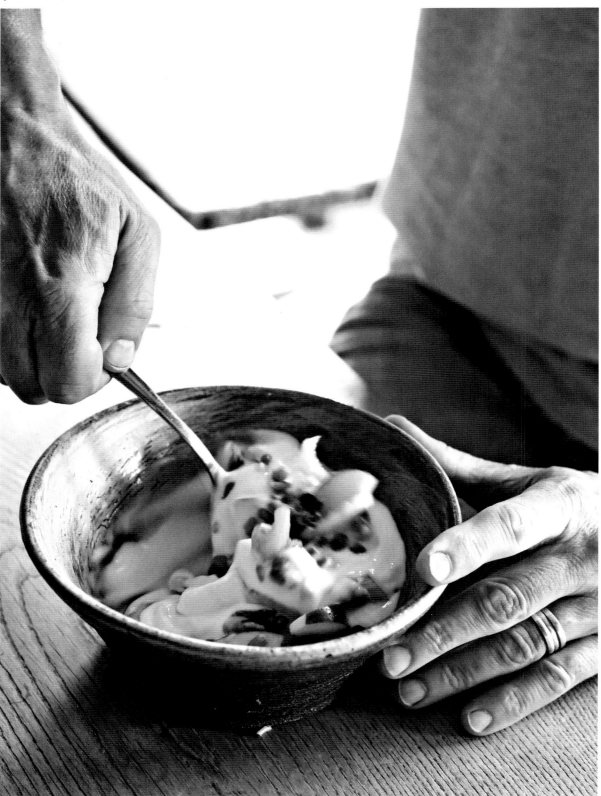

WALDORF YOGHURT

This takes a breakfast approach to yoghurt and makes it a satisfying lunch. It's quirky but delicious, and ripe for customisation.

Per person

1 tender inner celery stem, sliced

½ crisp apple, cut into thin wedges

1–2 tbsp raisins, ideally pre-soaked in apple or orange juice, or kombucha (page 244) or water, or a handful of grapes, halved

6–8 walnut halves

1 or 2 handfuls of cooked whole spelt or barley grains (see page 249)

150g natural yoghurt

Sea salt and black pepper

In a bowl, combine the celery, apple, raisins, walnuts, grains, a pinch of salt and a twist of pepper and tumble together.

Either put the yoghurt into a serving bowl, tip the celery mix on top and gently combine, or pack the fruit/veg mix and the yoghurt separately in a lunchbox and combine just before eating.

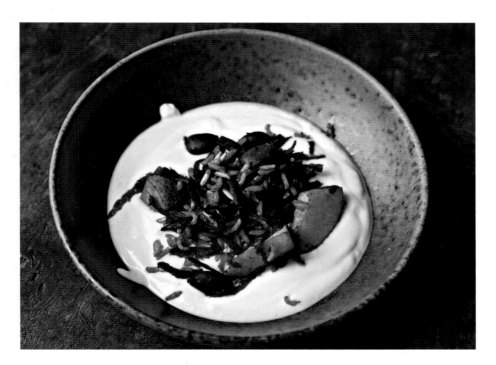

BEETROOT & PEAR VARIATION
Replace the Waldorf mix with 1 small grated raw beetroot, 1 pear cut into chunks, a handful of cooked brown rice and a dozen or so peeled, soaked whole almonds.

SARDINE MAYO WITH CAPERS & RED ONION

I love tinned fish for a quick, easy and healthy snack lunch, and sardines (sustainably sourced) top the list. More often than not I do something like this with them.

Serves 4

1 tbsp natural yoghurt

1 tbsp mayonnaise

2 tins sardines or mackerel in oil or water, drained (about 80g each drained weight)

1 tbsp capers, drained

½ small red onion, finely chopped

Sea salt and black pepper

To serve (per person)

A small chicory bulb, or little gem lettuce, separated into leaves

1 heaped tbsp kraut or kimchi, ideally homemade (pages 282–6), optional

Oatcakes or wholegrain bread/toast (optional)

Combine the yoghurt and mayo in a bowl with a pinch of salt and a twist of pepper. Add the tinned fish and mash to combine, then stir in the capers and onion. Transfer to a serving dish or pack into lunchboxes. Eat with chicory or little gem leaves, and kimchi or kraut if you like. To make it more filling, serve on oatcakes, or wholegrain bread or toast.

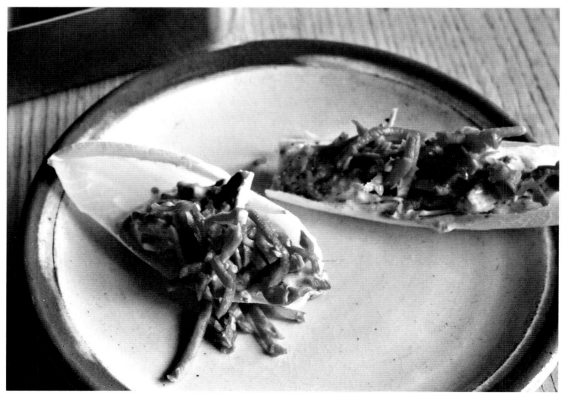

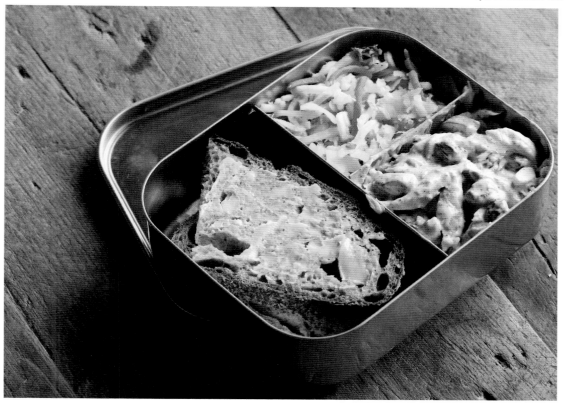

CORONATION CHICKEN

A lovely lunchbox version of the picnic classic, this also works with leftover roast pork, or even sausages.

Per person

1–2 tbsp natural yoghurt

1–2 tsp mayonnaise

A handful or two (80–120g) of roughly shredded cold cooked chicken

1 tbsp raisins, ideally pre-soaked in apple or orange juice, or kombucha (page 244) or water

8–12 whole, skin-on almonds, soaked and skinned

Sea salt and black pepper

To serve

A spoonful of kraut or kimchi, ideally homemade (pages 282–6)

1–2 slices of wholegrain bread/toast, (optional)

Combine the yoghurt and mayo in a bowl with a pinch of salt and a twist of pepper. Add the chicken, raisins and almonds and stir in. Transfer to a plate or a lunchbox and eat with the kimchi or kraut. To make it more substantial, you can serve a slice or two of wholegrain bread or toast on the side.

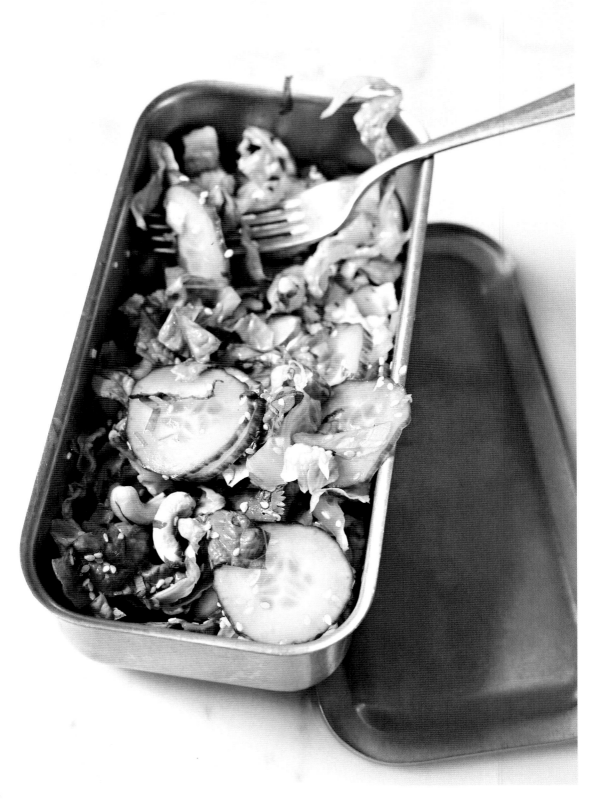

CUCUMBER, LETTUCE & CASHEWS

Fresh herbs, lime juice and soy sauce give this lively green salad plenty of flavour, while cashews and sesame seeds add protein and texture. I like to finish the dish with slices of avocado.

Per person

½ cucumber (about 200g), sliced

½ romaine/cos lettuce, roughly shredded

2–3 tbsp cashew nuts

1–2 tbsp sesame seeds

A few mint or coriander leaves, or both, chopped

Juice of 1 large lime

1 tbsp tamari or soy sauce

Black pepper

To serve (optional)

½–1 avocado

A few dried chilli flakes

Tumble the cucumber, lettuce, cashews, sesame seeds and herbs together in a bowl. Trickle over the lime juice and tamari or soy, add a twist of pepper and toss lightly.

Transfer the salad to a bowl, or a lunchbox for later. If using avocado, halve, stone and peel it then slice thickly and add to the salad, with a pinch of chilli flakes if you like.

FENNEL/APPLE VARIATION

Replace the cucumber with slices of raw fennel or apple, or both.

NUT/SEED VARIATION

Raw or lightly toasted peanuts can stand in for the cashews. Or you can sprinkle with the tamari-roasted seeds/nuts described on page 281.

SARDINES & BEANS

Tinned sardine and mackerel fillets are such an easy way to get some delicious, healthy oily fish into my day and make a very tasty addition to protein-rich salads like this one. Look for sustainable tinned fish – I like the Fish 4 Ever brand.

Per person

1–2 eggs

A couple of handfuls of cooked white beans, such as cannellini or haricot (⅓–½ of a 400g tin), drained and rinsed

½–1 tin sardines or mackerel in oil or water, drained (40–80g drained weight), plus 1 tbsp oil from the tin or 1 tbsp extra virgin olive oil

2 tbsp small capers

1 tsp English mustard

Juice of ½ lemon

2–3 tbsp chopped parsley

Sea salt and black pepper

To 'hard-boil' the eggs, fill a pan with enough water to cover the eggs and bring to the boil. Gently lower the eggs into the pan on a spoon, then immediately start timing 7 minutes, keeping the water at a simmer. When the time is up, drain off the water, place the pan in the sink and run cold water over the eggs to stop the cooking. Leave them to cool before peeling.

Put the beans into a large bowl. If the fish is tinned in oil, add 1 tbsp of it to the bowl with the beans. Drain off the rest of the oil, then add the fish to the bowl too. (If the fish is tinned in water, drain that off, and add the fish to the bowl along with 1 tbsp olive oil.)

Add the capers, mustard, lemon juice, chopped parsley, a pinch of salt and a twist of pepper. Tumble everything together, breaking up the fillets of fish as you go.

Transfer to a serving plate or lunchbox. Halve the boiled eggs or slice them thickly and add to the salad. Serve or pack up to eat later.

'SAUER-DINE' VARIATION
Replace the capers, mustard, lemon juice and parsley with 1 heaped tbsp kraut or kimchi, ideally homemade (pages 282–6).

SMOKED MACKEREL & LENTIL VARIATION
Swap the tinned fish for a fat fillet of smoked mackerel, flaked off the skin. Toss this with a couple of handfuls of pre-cooked or drained and rinsed tinned Puy or brown lentils (⅓–½ of a 400g tin), 1 tbsp olive oil, the capers, mustard, lemon juice, chopped parsley, a pinch of salt and a twist of pepper. Transfer to plates or lunchboxes and finish with slices of crisp apple rather than boiled eggs.

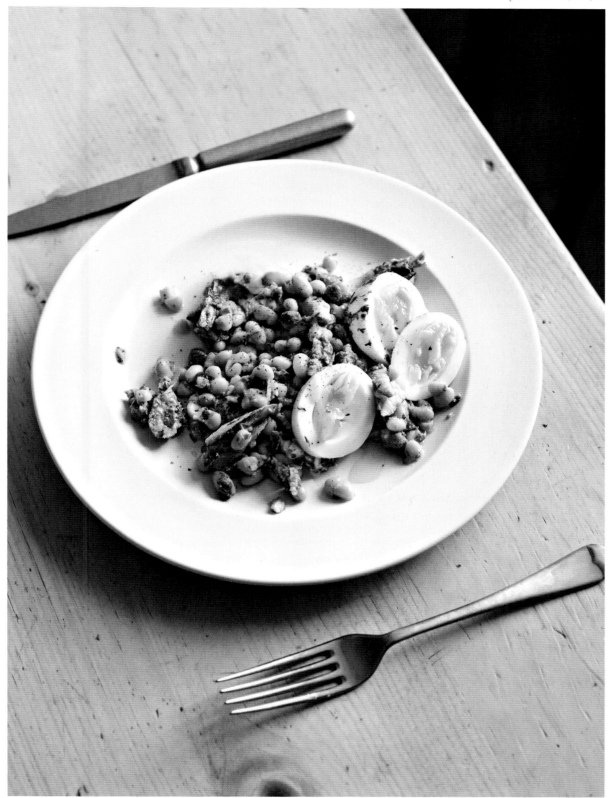

CURRIED CARROT BLITZ

This raw 'blitz' – a sort of chunky carrot hummus, flavoured with curry spices – takes moments to throw together in a food processor. To simplify it further, you can replace the spice seeds and chilli with 2 tsp of your favourite curry powder. Tasty and filling, the blitz makes a great lunchbox standby. Eat it with cucumber sticks (or other raw veg crudités) and oatcakes, or a slice of wholegrain bread or toast, or some slices of avocado and a dollop of natural yoghurt.

Serves 4

500g carrots, trimmed

2 x 400g tins chickpeas, drained and rinsed

Juice of ½ lemon, or to taste

50g raisins

1 tsp cumin seeds

1 tsp coriander seeds

A pinch of dried chilli flakes or ½ medium-hot fresh chilli, deseeded and chopped (optional)

A scrap of garlic (about ¼ clove), finely grated

1 tsp freshly grated ginger

4 tbsp olive oil

Sea salt and black pepper

To serve (per person)

A handful of raw veg crudités, such as cucumber, carrot, peppers, cut into fingers or wedges

A few oatcakes, or 1 or 2 slices of wholegrain bread or toast

Cut the carrots into small chunks and place in a food processor with all the other ingredients, adding a pinch of salt and a twist of pepper. Blitz to a thick, chunky, chopped-up mixture. Stop to scrape down the sides of the processor a couple of times. Make sure everything is well combined but don't reduce the ingredients to a paste – you want a bit of chunky texture.

Taste the mix and add more salt, pepper and/or lemon juice if you think it is needed. Transfer to a bowl if you're serving it straight away, or pack into a plastic tub and keep in the fridge.

CASHEW & CORIANDER VARIATION
Replace the chickpeas with 200g cashew nuts, soaked for a few hours, and the lemon juice with lime juice. Leave out the raisins and cumin seeds, but include the coriander seeds, chilli, garlic, ginger, oil, a pinch of salt and a twist of pepper. Blitz as above. Serve scattered with coriander leaves. To eat, try scooping it up with a few slices of avocado wrapped up in little gem lettuce leaves.

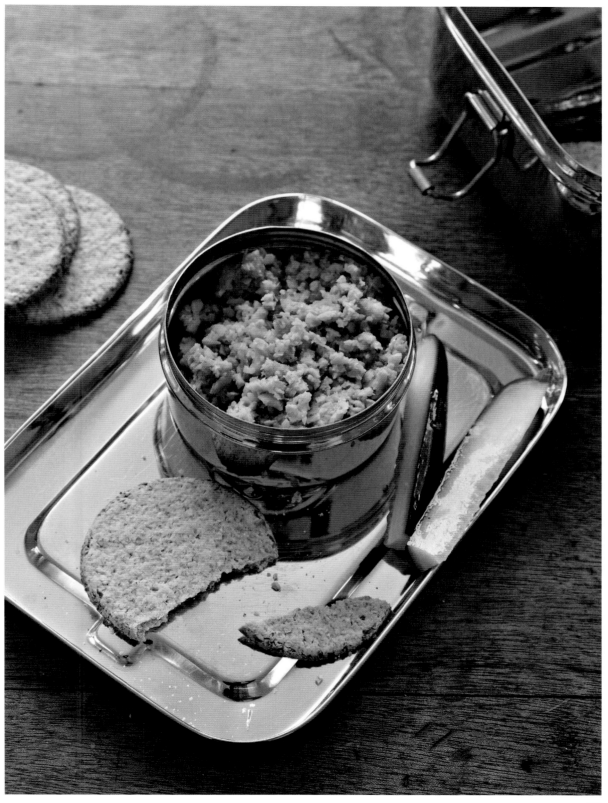

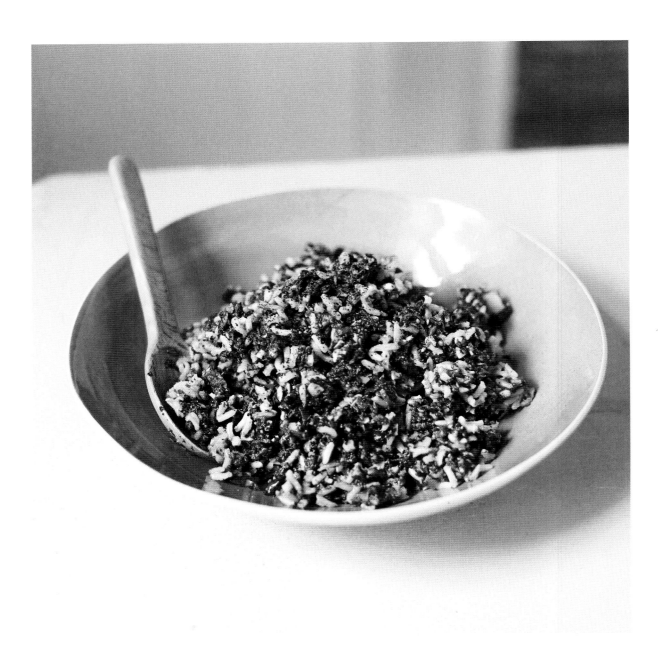

MUSHROOM, ALMOND & OLIVE BLITZ

I do love a 'blitz' – a chunky, whizzed-up mix of raw, healthy ingredients, somewhere between a salad and a dip. This mushroom and olive example is really tasty.

Serves 4

300g chestnut or portobello mushrooms, broken into pieces, stalks and all

100g whole, skin-on almonds, soaked for a couple of hours if time

100g pitted black olives, such as kalamata

A scrap of garlic (about ¼ clove), finely grated

¼ medium-hot red chilli, deseeded and finely chopped (optional)

A handful of parsley leaves

2 tbsp extra virgin olive oil

A squeeze of lemon juice

Sea salt and black pepper

To serve (per person)

A handful of raw veg crudités, such as carrot, celery, fennel, cut into fingers or wedges, and/or salad leaves

OR

A handful or two of cooked brown rice (50–100g), or cooked chickpeas or lentils (⅓–½ of a 400g tin), drained and rinsed

Put all the ingredients, except salt and pepper, into a food processor and blitz until the mixture is coarsely chopped. Taste the mixture and add a pinch of salt and a twist of pepper if needed.

You can eat the blitz straight away but it's particularly good if it's left to stand in a cool place for a few hours to allow the flavours time to develop.

Give it a stir before serving, then serve as a dip with raw veg, or turn it into a salad (as pictured) by stirring in some cold, cooked brown rice (but note that cooked rice shouldn't be kept out of the fridge for any length of time, see page 249).

Alternatively, pack a portion of blitz in a lunchbox with some raw vegetables or salad leaves and some cooked lentils or chickpeas. You can also serve it in a wrap, with a bit of shredded cabbage and/or grated carrot.

BASHED BEAN PÂTÉ WITH CRUDITÉS

This white bean pâté – flavoured with mustard, parsley, capers and a hint of garlic – couldn't be easier. It's a lovely, flavoursome way to turn a heap of raw veg into lunch and doesn't even require a food processor: you can knock it together with a fork in a few minutes. I like to serve it with carrot, celery and/or fennel, with maybe a few slices of apple too.

Serves 4

2 x 400g tins white beans, such as butter beans, cannellini or haricot, drained and rinsed

A scrap of garlic (about ¼ clove), finely grated

2 tbsp small capers

1 tsp English mustard

A handful of parsley leaves, chopped

Juice of ½ large lemon, or to taste

6–8 salted anchovy fillets in oil, roughly torn up (optional)

3 tbsp extra virgin olive oil

Sea salt and black pepper

To serve

Lots of raw veg crudités and/or fruit, such as carrot, celery, fennel and apple, cut into fingers or wedges

Place the beans on a large plate or in a wide, shallow dish (it's easier to mash them on a flat surface than in a bowl). Use a fork to roughly mash them up.

Add the garlic, capers, mustard, parsley, lemon juice, anchovies and olive oil. Using two forks this time, mash and stir everything together. Taste and adjust the seasoning with a pinch of salt and a twist of pepper and a little more lemon juice if required. Transfer to a bowl or pack portions into tubs. Serve with lots of raw veg and/or fruit.

KRAUT/KIMCHI VARIATION
For a vegan version of this dip, leave out the anchovies. You can also replace the capers, mustard, lemon and anchovies with 1 heaped tbsp kraut or kimchi, ideally homemade (pages 282–6); if you buy the kimchi, make sure it's a vegan version, without fish sauce or dried shrimp.

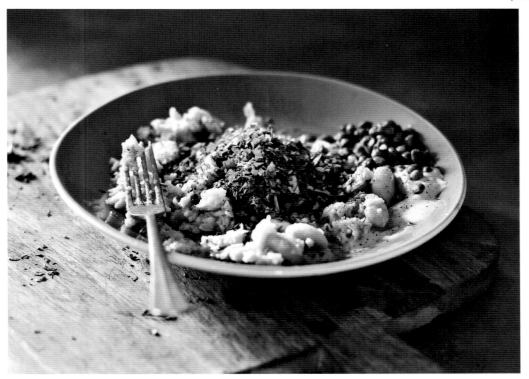

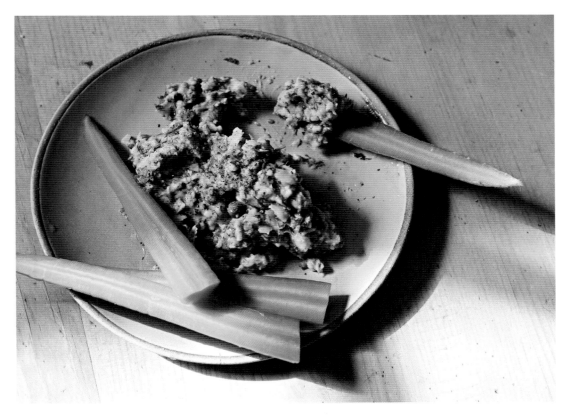

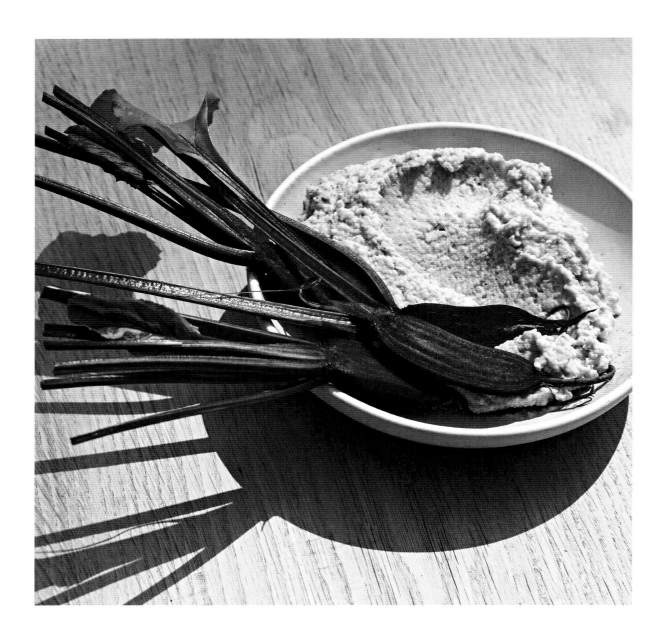

NUTTY CITRUS HUMMUS

This fresh, zesty take on a classic hummus is great for those who are not keen on the flavour of tahini (though if you are a tahini fan, you can swap it in for the nut butter). You can serve it with any crunchy, raw veg – carrot, celery and cucumber being the most obvious – but don't overlook the possibilities of crisp lettuce hearts, thin wedges of cabbage, cauliflower florets and, as here, young, sweet beetroot.

Serves 4

2 x 400g tins chickpeas (or white beans, or one of each), drained and rinsed

2 tbsp (about 50g) nut butter, such as peanut or almond

Finely grated zest and juice of 1 lemon

Finely grated zest and juice of 1 orange

A scrap of garlic (about ¼ clove), grated

2 tbsp extra virgin olive oil

Sea salt and black pepper

To serve

Raw veg crudités, such as carrot, peppers, cucumber, baby beetroot, cut into fingers or wedges

Put the drained chickpeas into a food processor with the nut butter, citrus zest and juice, garlic, a pinch of salt and a twist of pepper. Blitz to a coarse purée, then keep blending, trickling in the olive oil. If necessary, trickle in a little water too, to achieve a loose, spoon-able texture. Taste to check the seasoning and adjust if you need to, then it's ready to eat.

CURRIED ROAST VEG VARIATION

Add leftover roasted root veg, such as carrots, parsnips or beetroot, and a spoonful of curry paste or powder to the processor as you blitz the hummus to make a tasty, textured veg-packed dip. If you like this variation (and you will!), you can even roast some roots especially. Leftovers of almost any veg curry work well too.

PESTOMEGA

This is a blitzed-up, flavour-packed, cheese-free powerhouse of a pesto, rich in plant-based omega-3 fats – a delicious vegan way to get more of these crucial nutrients into your life. It is mega-versatile too: stir it into salads, swirl on soups, slather in a wrap, use as a dip or toss through hot wholegrain pasta. The seaweed is optional – it gives a nice umami hit in the absence of cheese but it does make the pesto darker.

Serves 4 with wholegrain pasta,
6–8 as a swirl or dressing

50g walnuts or pumpkin seeds, or a mix

50g hulled hemp seeds or sunflower seeds

1 small garlic clove, roughly chopped

50g flat-leaf parsley and/or basil leaves

About 10g dried seaweed flakes, rehydrated in water (optional)

Juice of ½ lemon, or to taste

Up to 150ml walnut oil, hemp oil or virgin rapeseed oil, or a mix

Sea salt and black pepper

Lightly toast the nuts and seeds in a dry pan for a few minutes. This will release their fragrance and oils.

Transfer the toasted mix to a food processor, add the garlic and process until finely chopped but still with some texture. Add the herb leaves, and seaweed if using, and blitz again to chop the leaves.

Add the lemon juice, then begin trickling in the oil, with the food processor running. Stop blending when you have a loose but still pleasingly granular texture (not a green mayonnaise!). Taste, and add salt, pepper and more lemon juice if you like.

Store in the fridge – if you completely cover the surface with oil, so all air is excluded, it will keep for at least a couple of weeks.

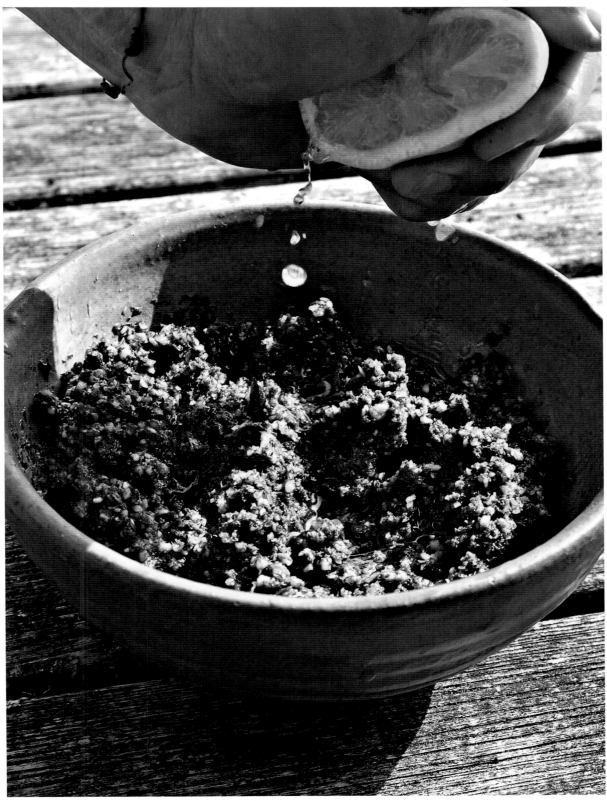

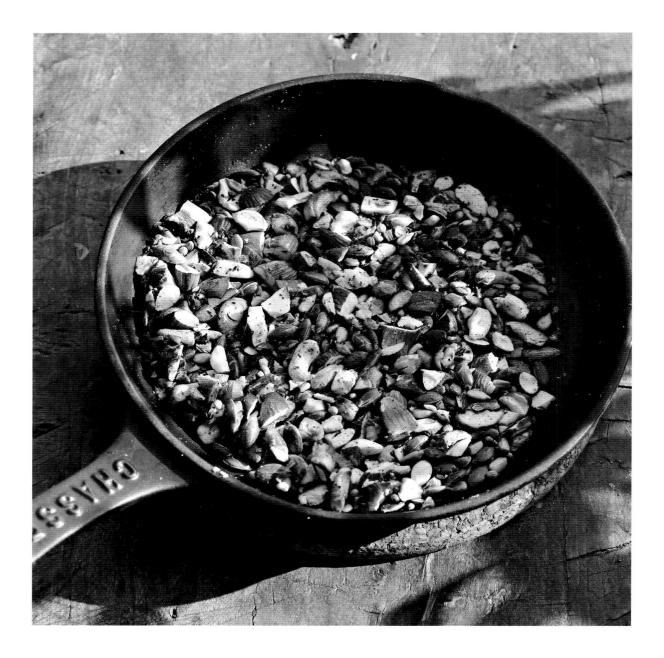

DUKKA

I keep sticking recipes for this nutty, seedy sprinkle in my books because it's just so darned delicious, and is a great way to give some super-healthy dishes an extra boost. Scatter it over salads, seared or roasted veg, soups and dips to add flavour, texture, goodness, and an irresistible hit of spice. You'll find lots of suggestions in other recipes in the book for the deployment of this lovely stuff. And once you see how transformative it can be, I'm sure you'll think of many more.

Makes 10–12 generous sprinkles

30g whole, skin-on almonds or hazelnuts, roughly chopped or bashed

30g cashew nuts or peanuts, roughly chopped or bashed

30g pumpkin seeds or sunflower seeds, or a mix

2 tsp cumin or caraway seeds

2 tsp coriander seeds

1 tsp fennel seeds (optional)

A good pinch of flaky salt

A few twists of black pepper

A small pinch of dried chilli flakes

A few sprigs of mint, coriander or rosemary, leaves only, chopped (optional)

Set a small, heavy pan over a medium-high heat. Add the nuts and pumpkin or sunflower seeds to the pan and toast them for 2–3 minutes, shaking the pan regularly so they take on some even colour.

While the seeds and nuts are toasting, lightly crush all the spice seeds using a pestle and mortar – breaking rather than grinding the spices; leaving a few whole seeds is fine. Add these to the pan of nuts and seeds, along with the salt, pepper and chilli flakes. Continue to heat for 2–3 minutes, moving or turning the mix now and then – you're toasting the nuts and spices, almost-but-not-quite burning them (and beware, the small seeds/spices burn quite easily). When done, tip onto a plate and set aside to cool.

You can use the dukka immediately, or store it in an airtight container for a week or so.

If you want to add a lovely fragrant note, stir in some of the suggested chopped fresh herbs just before serving. Once you've added the herbs you'll need to use the dukka within the day, or it will lose its crunch.

TAMARI-ROASTED SEED VARIATION
Another lovely seedy sprinkle with an Asian note can be achieved by tossing 150g pumpkin seeds – or a mix of pumpkin seeds, sunflower seeds and broken cashew nuts – with 2 tbsp tamari (or soy sauce). Spread out on a large, non-stick baking tray and toast in the oven at 180°C/Fan 160°C/Gas 4 for 10–12 minutes, stirring once or twice, until dark and there is no more liquid tamari visible. As you take the tray from the oven, give the seeds a final stir, then leave to cool and dry. Store and use as above. (Makes enough for 6–8 generous sprinkles.)

SPICY CABBAGE & CARROT KRAUT

Eating live, fermented veg – like this tangy, tasty sauerkraut – is one of the simplest ways to boost your gut health, delivering not only beneficial bacteria but also fibre and phytonutrients to your tum (see page 32). If this is your first bit of home-fermenting, you'll soon see how simple, cheap and satisfying it is, and I bet it won't be your last.

This is a gateway recipe: the brine method here, using a 4% brine to ferment 1kg veg (mainly cabbage), is very easy and adaptable, as you can see from the variations overleaf. The traditional method (massaging 2% salt – i.e. 20g per 1kg veg – directly into your shredded white cabbage/veg) also works well, but is a bit more risky, as air pockets can form and the wrong microbes can get involved.

Serve your kraut with salads or roasted veg, cram some into a pitta with falafel and hummus, or spoon it on top of soups or beside hearty stews. You can even eat it for breakfast with eggs or avocado (see page 238). And don't discard the salty-spicy-savoury brine – try using a splash in dressings and sauces to add oomph and probiotic goodness, too.

Makes at least 10 servings

40g fine sea salt

½ large white cabbage (about 750g)

2 large or 3 medium carrots (about 250g in total)

2 tsp ground turmeric or 1 tbsp finely grated fresh turmeric

A thumb-sized knob of fresh ginger (about 25g), finely grated

A good pinch of dried chilli flakes (optional)

Thoroughly wash and dry a 2-litre preserving jar, such as a Kilner jar. Remove the rubber seal from the lid of the jar – this will allow gas to escape as your kraut ferments. Add the salt to 1 litre cold water and stir until completely dissolved to form a brine.

Remove any dirty outer leaves from the cabbage and rinse the outside of the cabbage well. Take one good large leaf and set aside. Cut the cabbage half into 2 or 3 wedges and, using a box grater or a food processor, coarsely grate or shred the whole lot, barring perhaps the fibrous base of the stem. Thinly slice any larger bits of leaf that fall off while you're grating, with a knife. Put all the shredded cabbage into a large bowl.

Coarsely grate, shred or julienne the carrots and add to the cabbage. Add the turmeric, ginger and chilli flakes, if using. Mix well – the turmeric will stain the mix golden-yellow.

Pack the mixture into the prepared clean preserving jar, pressing the veg down and leaving at least 5cm head-space at the top. Pour the brine slowly into the jar, allowing it to filter down through the veg. Keep going until there is enough brine in the jar to come about 3cm above the veg when you press the veg down with your (very clean) hand (the veg will want to float). Keep any leftover brine for now.

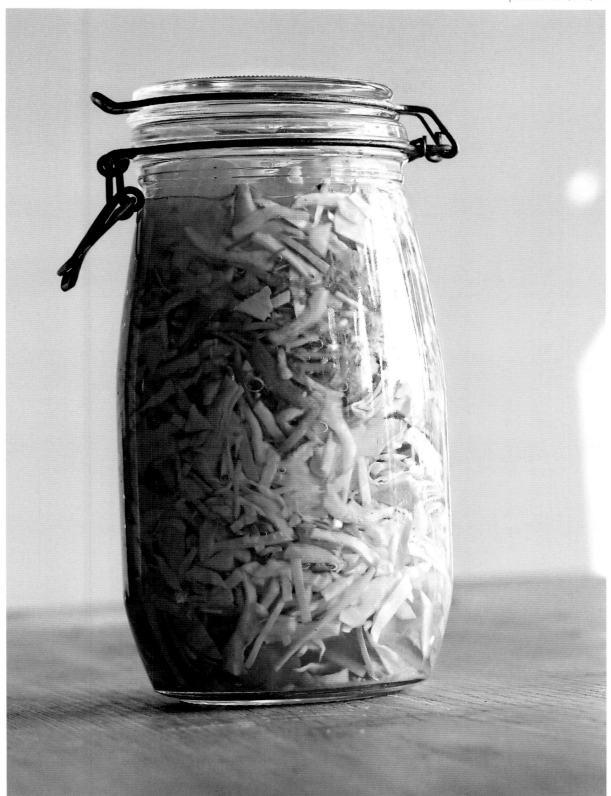

Tip the jar this way and that a few times to help release any air bubbles. Put the reserved cabbage leaf over the top of the shredded veg. You now need to weigh down the veg in the jar so that it stays submerged under the brine. Veg that is exposed to air above the brine tends to go mouldy and this can spoil the whole jar. Begin by putting the reserved whole cabbage leaf on top of the brined veg and pressing it down so the brine rises above it. This might be enough but you can further weight the veg with a very clean beach pebble, a glass paperweight or a specially designed glass fermentation weight (available from online suppliers), or even a small glass or china cup – but nothing metallic. Close the jar.

Stand the jar on a cloth to catch any escaping brine and leave to ferment at cool room temperature for 1 week. Have a look at it every day – you should be able to see bubbles of carbon dioxide forming inside. Every couple of days, open the lid to let any excess gas escape, then close it again.

After a week, taste the kraut. It should be pleasantly sour and tangy, which means it is ready to eat. If it doesn't have that tang yet, leave it another day or two. Otherwise, transfer it to the fridge.

Your kraut will keep for weeks, as long as the veg in the jar stays submerged in brine. If it does go mouldy on the top, you might get away with removing and discarding the top layer and recovering with brine, but if it develops a bad or really 'off' smell or taste (as opposed to the natural pungency of fermented cabbage!) them I'm afraid you'll have to discard the whole lot.

CLASSIC KRAUT VARIATION
Omit the carrots and use an extra 250g white cabbage (i.e. 1kg in total). Leave out the ginger and turmeric, replacing them with 1–2 tsp caraway or fennel seeds. You can also add 1–2 tsp juniper berries if you have some to hand.

PURPLE KRAUT VARIATION
Use red rather than white cabbage and replace the carrots with about 250g peeled raw beetroot, coarsely grated or shredded. As for the classic kraut, omit the ginger and turmeric, replacing them with 1–2 tsp caraway or cumin seeds and a generous grinding of black pepper.

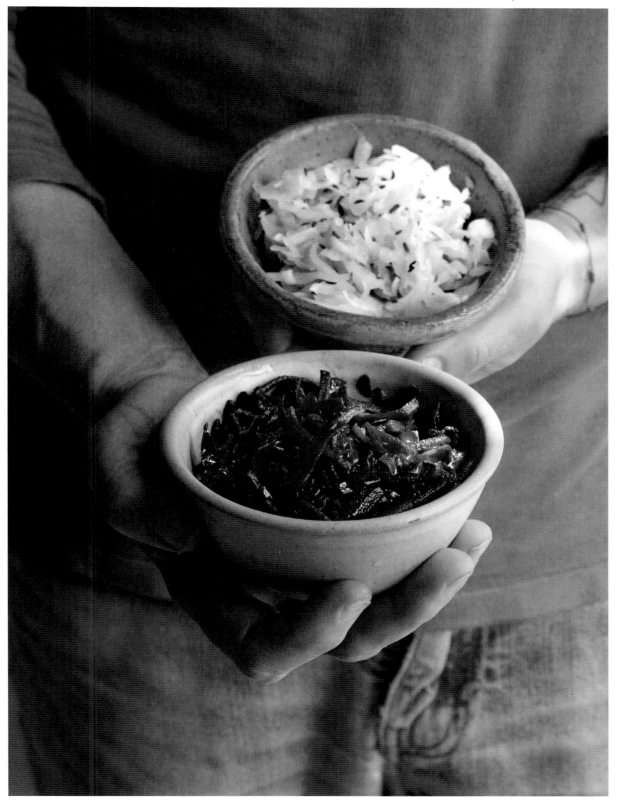

GILL'S VEGAN KIMCHI

Former River Cottage head chef and long-time collaborator, Gill Meller still helps me brainstorm recipes and cooks with me on photoshoots. He turned up to one with this lovely homemade kimchi, and I asked him if I could put it in the book. I'm so glad he obliged; it's pleasingly simple and very versatile.

The radishes and turnips/kohlrabi add a lovely extra crunch, but If you're struggling to get hold of them, you can leave out one (or both) and just add another half (or whole) cabbage instead. The seaweed is also optional – and not all vegans eat it – but it does add to the umami hit.

Makes a 2-litre jar

2 medium summer cabbages, such as hispi/sweetheart (about 1.2kg in total)

About 6 small turnips (200–250g in total) or the same weight of kohlrabi (optional)

A bunch of radishes (200–250g), optional

150ml boiled water, cooled to room temperature

40g fine sea salt

½ thumb-sized piece of fresh ginger, finely grated

2 garlic cloves, finely crushed or grated

4 tbsp Korean dried chilli flakes (or use a scant tsp standard dried chilli flakes with seeds, which are much more fiery, plus 2 tbsp sweet paprika)

1 tsp coriander seeds, lightly toasted and crushed

1 tbsp dried seaweed flakes, ideally kombu/kelp or dulse (optional)

Wash and sterilise a 2-litre preserving jar. Remove the base of the stem from each cabbage and peel away any damaged or tired leaves. Slice the cabbage in half from top to bottom, then slice each half into quarters or fifths, giving you 8–10 thin wedges held together by a fragment of stem. Any leaves that come loose can go in the jar too.

Peel the turnips or kohlrabi, if using, and cut in half only if they are large. Slice into thin rounds, or half-rounds, 2–3mm thick. If using radishes and they have tops that are fresh and green cut these off, rinse and set aside. Halve the radishes from top to bottom.

Place all the vegetables, including the radish tops if using, in a large bowl. Combine the cooled water with the salt, ginger and garlic and pour this over the veg. Sprinkle over the chilli flakes (or chilli and paprika), toasted coriander seeds and seaweed if using. With very clean hands, tumble and squeeze all the ingredients together for 2–3 minutes. Let the veg stand in the bowl for 30 minutes, then repeat this squeezing and tumbling process again. You're working the salt into the vegetables and the veg juices out into the bowl, which will give you the spicy aromatic brine, essential for fermentation.

Pack the veg into the sterilised 2-litre jar, packing them down tightly with clean hands as you go. Pour over the brine from the bowl: it needs to come up over the top of the veg; if it doesn't, push the veg down firmly to drive more brine upwards.

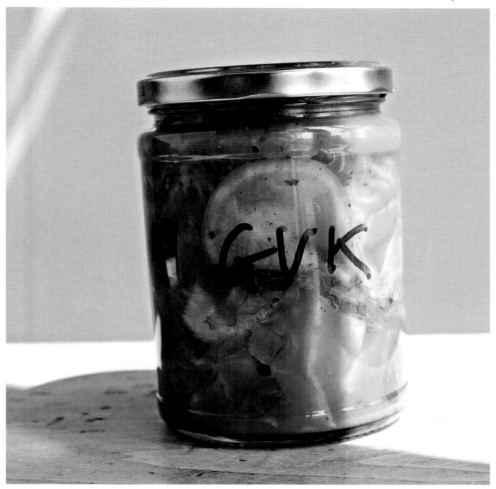

To keep the vegetables submerged in the brine, cover the surface with a circle of clean cabbage leaf then pop a scrupulously clean beach pebble, glass paperweight or bespoke fermentation weight, or even a small glass or cup (but nothing metallic), on top of that. It needs to be heavy enough to keep the veg submerged (but not so big that it doesn't fit in the jar).

Cover the jar with a loose-fitting lid or a piece of cotton cloth and leave it to ferment at room temperature (but no more than 22°C) and out of direct sunlight.

After 8–10 days your kimchi should be ready to eat. You can keep it in the fridge in the same jar, or decanted into a few small jars. Remember it is a living product and even in the fridge it may continue to ferment very slowly. It's a good idea to loosen the tops of jars to 'burb' the kimchi once a week or so.

You can eat your kimchi as a condiment with almost any meal – and there are lots of suggestions for using it in other recipes in this book.

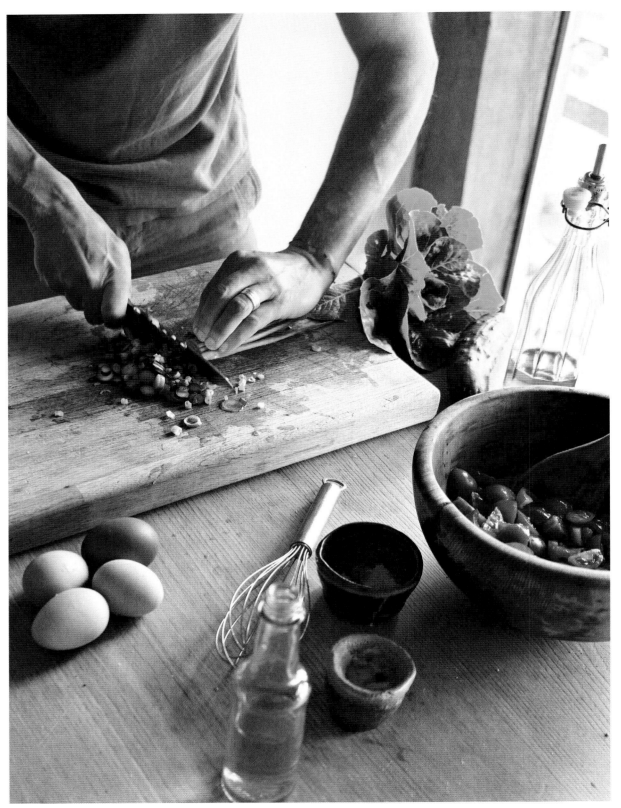

SATISFYING SALADS

A 'salad' needn't mean 'skinny', or 'light'. It can be appealing and generous, signifying all kinds of good things. It's about much more than just leaves (lovely components as these can be), and it certainly mustn't mean boring or unsatisfying. For me, a salad simply suggests an eclectic mix of flavourful ingredients (mostly plants), tumbled together usually with some kind of dressing. Beyond that, there are no rules!

Here, I've focused on salads that are really satisfying, which means some of them use cooked veg and often include some kind of protein – pulses, nuts, seeds, egg, fish or a yoghurt dressing. They can all perform brilliantly as a filling lunch, or a light evening meal – and, as with the offerings in the previous chapter, most will also pack up well in a lunchbox (and may even taste better after mingling for a while at close quarters!). They will work particularly well served (in combinations of two, three or more) as dishes to mix, match and share, mezze-style. This, more and more, is the way I like to feed my family and friends.

Like so many of my recipes, these are not intended as final words, rather as springboards. Feel free to swap in different veg, pulses or nuts, and to tweak the dressings to your taste. I have a few suggestions for such variations, as ever, but I heartily encourage you to plough your own furrows...

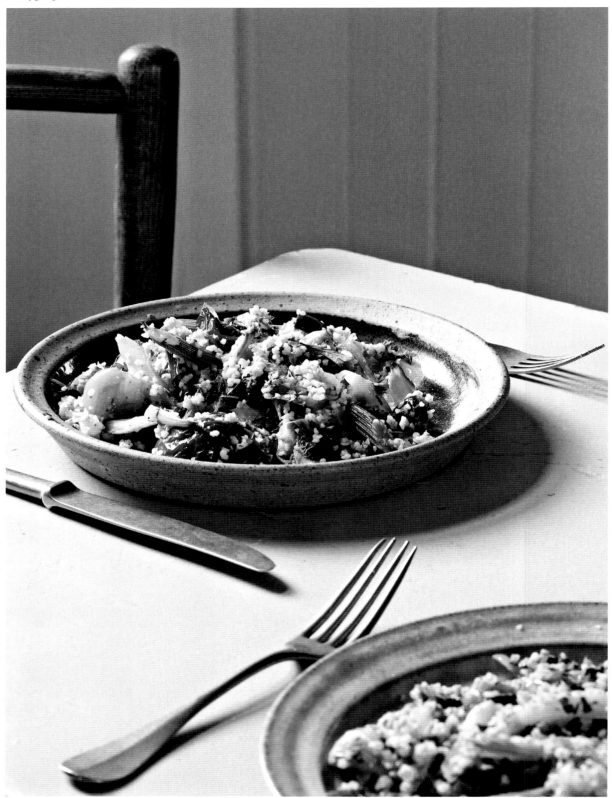

ROAST FENNEL & TOMATO TABBOULEH

An authentic tabbouleh has loads of green herbs and not much bulgar wheat at all (see page 369 for a lovely version with lamb). This salad is a little more generous with the whole grain and also uses delicious, sweet, roasted veg, spices and lots of lemon.

Serves 3–4

3 medium fennel bulbs (500–600g in total)

2 medium red or brown onions, roughly chopped

2 garlic cloves, thickly sliced

300g cherry tomatoes

2 tbsp olive or rapeseed oil

150g bulgar wheat

1 tsp ground cumin

1 tsp ground coriander

A good pinch of hot smoked paprika or cayenne

Finely grated zest and juice of 1 lemon

A bunch of flat-leaf parsley (25g), leaves picked and roughly chopped

A bunch of mint, basil or coriander (25g), leaves picked and roughly chopped

Sea salt and black pepper

To serve

Green salad leaves

Extra virgin olive oil

Lemon juice

Preheat the oven to 200°C/Fan 180°C/Gas 6.

Roughly chop the fennel bulbs, including the core. Put the fennel, onions, garlic and cherry tomatoes into a very large roasting tray (or divide between two roasting trays, to avoid crowding the veg). Trickle over the oil, add a pinch of salt and a twist of pepper and toss together. Roast for 30–35 minutes, stirring halfway through, or until tender and lightly caramelised.

Meanwhile, pour 250ml water into a medium saucepan. Add the bulgar wheat, spices and a pinch of salt. Stir well. Bring to the boil, reduce the heat and simmer for 3 minutes. Turn off the heat, cover the pan tightly and leave to stand for 10 minutes.

Use a fork to fluff up the bulgar wheat, replace the lid and leave to stand until the roasted veg are done. Once cooked, add the contents of the roasting tray(s) to the bulgar. Add the lemon zest and juice and turn everything together gently using a fork.

The tabbouleh is best served warm or at room temperature so give it some time to cool down if you can. Just before serving, fold in the chopped herbs and add more salt and pepper if needed. Eat with green leaves, dressed with a little olive oil and lemon juice.

VEG VARIATIONS

Try replacing the fennel and tomato with mushrooms and cubed squash for an autumn version, or with roots, such as swede, parsnip and carrot in the winter.

POTATO, BEANS & SMOKED MACKEREL

Smoked mackerel is rich, intense and delicious – you don't need a great deal of it to add real character to a dish. In this hearty salad, the mackerel is mixed with a little yoghurt, mustard and seasoning then folded together with freshly cooked young veg. As well as being a lovely at-home lunch, this one packs up well as a portable meal.

Serves 4

700g new potatoes or salad potatoes (unpeeled)

200g green beans, trimmed

2 medium fillets (about 200g) smoked mackerel

3 tbsp natural yoghurt

2–3 tsp wholegrain mustard

A squeeze of lemon juice

A good handful of flat-leaf parsley, roughly chopped (optional)

Sea salt and black pepper

Cut the potatoes into large bite-sized pieces, place them in a pan and pour on enough water to cover. Bring to a simmer and cook for about 7–8 minutes, until almost tender. Throw in the beans, and cook for a further 3 minutes. Drain the veg well in a colander and leave to cool.

Meanwhile, peel away the skin from the mackerel fillets and roughly break up the flesh, dropping it into a bowl. Add the yoghurt, mustard, lemon juice and a twist of pepper and combine with a fork to create a coarse-textured mixture – still with flakes of fish visible, not a pâté.

Add the mackerel mixture to the cooled potatoes and beans, with the chopped parsley if using, and toss together. Taste and add a little pinch of salt if needed (the fish may provide enough) and more pepper or lemon juice if you like. Transfer to a serving platter or individual dishes and serve.

VEG VARIATIONS
You can replace the green beans with another tender green vegetable such as asparagus or broccoli (standard, Tenderstem or purple sprouting).

FISH VARIATIONS
A couple of tins of mackerel or sardine fillets, drained and broken up, can be used instead of the smoked fish.

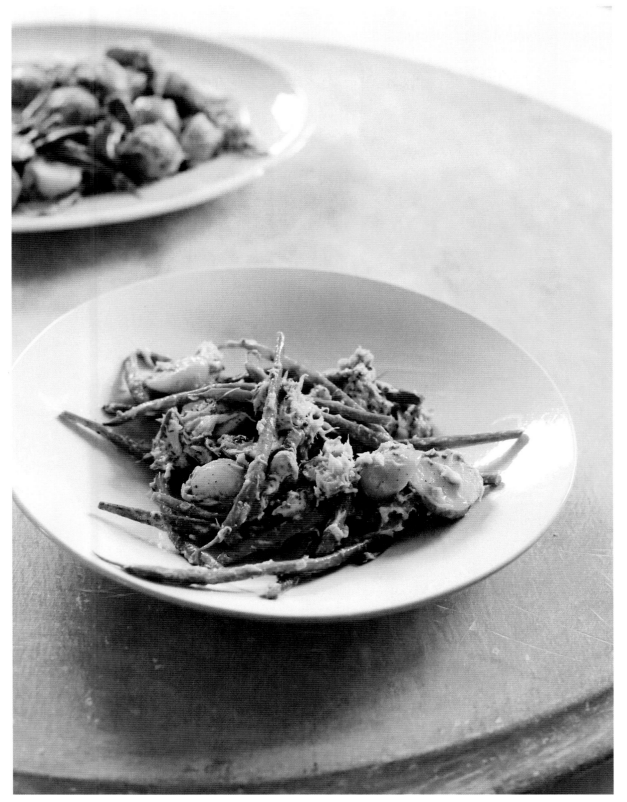

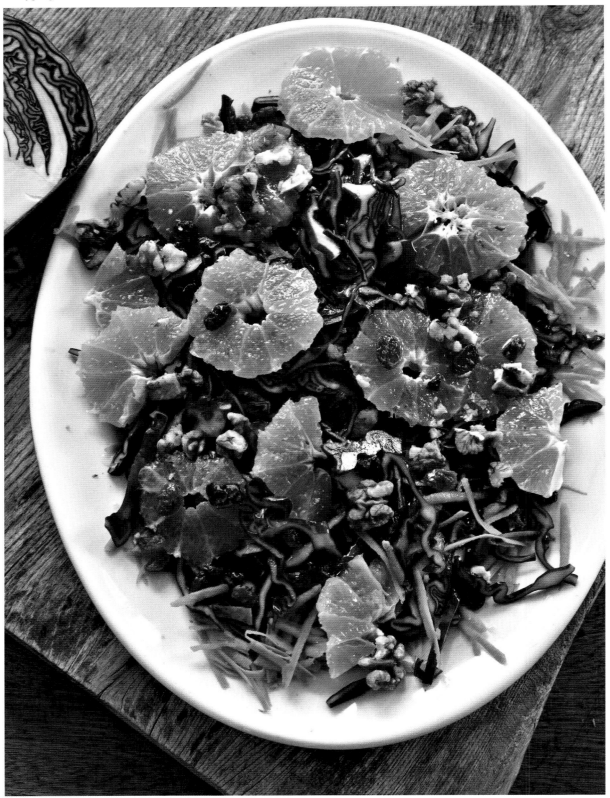

RED CABBAGE, CARROT & CLEMENTINES
with raisins & walnuts

With its amazing colours, this is a stunning dish: a lovely mingling of crisp raw veg, juicy citrus, sweet raisins and slightly bitter walnuts. It's a perfect choice for winter days – a light, refreshing alternative to heavy, stodgy fare.

Serves 4

250–300g red cabbage (½ small cabbage, or ¼ large one)

75g raisins

2 tbsp raw cider vinegar

4 clementines (or 'easy-peelers')

3 medium carrots (200–250g in total)

100g walnuts, broken into pieces or very roughly chopped

Sea salt and black pepper

Extra virgin olive oil, to finish (optional)

Remove the core from the piece of cabbage, then use a very sharp knife or a food processor to shred the cabbage as thinly as possible. Place it in a large bowl.

Add the raisins and cider vinegar to the cabbage. Squeeze in the juice of one of the clementines and add a pinch of salt and a twist of pepper. Tumble everything together and leave to stand for 15–20 minutes. This will slightly soften the cabbage and plump up the raisins.

Grate the carrots coarsely and scatter them over a large serving platter. Give the cabbage and raisins a good stir, pile on top of the carrots, and pour over any juice left in the bowl.

Peel the remaining 3 clementines and use a very sharp knife to slice them into 1cm thick rounds (don't worry if some of the rounds fall apart). Lay the fruit over the top of the cabbage. Scatter over the chopped walnuts. Finish, if you like, with a trickle of extra virgin olive oil, and serve.

VEG/SEED/NUT VARIATIONS
Some obvious and easy swaps here would be white cabbage for red, celeriac or beetroot for carrots, and pumpkin seeds or almonds for the walnuts.

BRASSICAS, LENTILS & LIVE DRESSING

Simply cooked veg need never be dull – a good dressing is all you need to ensure that it's tasty and satisfying. This particular dressing uses a richly savoury miso paste, made from fermented soya beans, which adds to the 'live' element, along with the yoghurt and kefir (but you can use a dash of good soy sauce instead).

Serves 4

150g dried Puy lentils or 300g cooked (1⅓–1½ x 400g tins, rinsed and drained)

400g purple sprouting broccoli, calabrese or Tenderstem

1 small or ½ large spring (pointed) or savoy cabbage

A little extra virgin olive oil

Sea salt and black pepper

For the dressing

1 tbsp raw cider vinegar

1 tbsp unpasteurised white/shiro miso paste, or a dash of soy sauce

2 tbsp natural yoghurt or kefir (page 246)

1 tbsp virgin olive or rapeseed oil

A scrap of garlic (about ¼ clove), crushed or finely grated

To finish (optional)

Sesame seeds

Black onion seeds

If you are cooking the Puy lentils from scratch, put them into a pan, cover with cold water and bring to the boil. Turn down the heat and simmer for about 15 minutes, until just tender. Drain in a colander, then run under the cold tap to cool them down. Leave to drain thoroughly.

Halve any larger broccoli spears, retaining all the leaves and stalk, except for any fibrous bits (slim spears can be left whole). Cut the cabbage into 4 or 8 wedges, keeping the core intact.

Boil the kettle. Put the broccoli and cabbage into a large pan, cover with boiling water and bring to the boil. Reduce the heat and simmer for 3–5 minutes, until the core of the cabbage pieces is just tender. Drain, then run under the cold tap to cool down. Leave to drain thoroughly.

To make the dressing, mix all the ingredients together in a small bowl. Don't worry if the oil doesn't amalgamate completely – it looks nice like this!

When all the elements are ready, arrange the cooked cabbage and broccoli on a serving plate. Scatter over about half of the lentils, trickle with a little extra virgin olive oil and season with a pinch of salt and a twist of pepper. Spoon the dressing over the veg, then scatter the remaining lentils over the top. If you like, you can finish with a generous sprinkle of sesame and/or black onion seeds.

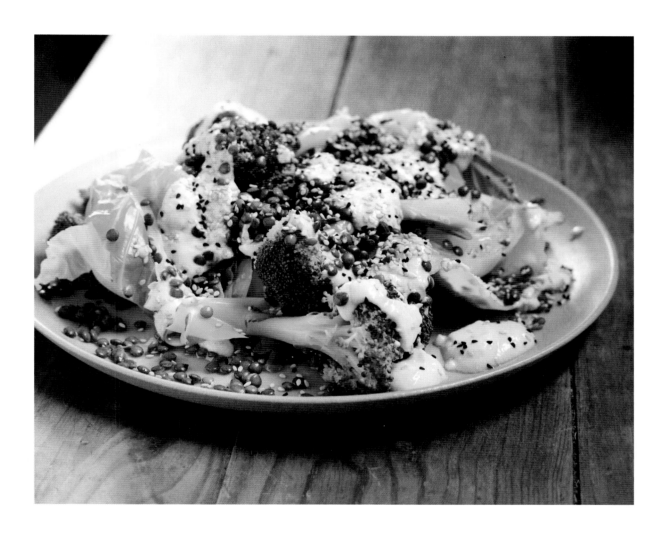

SPICY ROAST PARSNIPS
with barley, raisins & walnuts

Parsnips are delicious with curry spices, particularly when roasted so that their thin, tapering ends turn delectably sweet and caramelised. Here, spicy roasted parsnips are tumbled with nutty whole grains, raisins and a scattering of walnuts to create a dish with lots of satisfying textures. I like to add some crisp leaves for contrast, too.

Serves 4

150g pearl barley, pearled spelt or whole spelt grain

500g parsnips

2 tbsp curry paste

3 tbsp olive or rapeseed oil

50g walnuts, roughly chopped

75g raisins

A bunch of leaves, such as watercress, rocket or flat-leaf parsley

Juice of ½ orange or lemon

Sea salt and black pepper

Soak the pearl barley or spelt in cold water for anything from 20 minutes to a couple of hours then drain and rinse well. Put the grain into a saucepan, cover with plenty of cold water and bring to the boil. Reduce the heat and simmer until tender. This will take about 20–25 minutes for spelt, more like 35–40 minutes for barley. Drain.

Meanwhile, preheat the oven to 190°C/Fan 170°C/Gas 5. Peel the parsnips and trim the base and tip from each. Cut each parsnip in half lengthways then cut each half from top to bottom into long batons, no more than 2cm at the thick end. Don't worry if they are a bit wobbly and uneven – this all adds to their charm!

Put the curry paste and 2 tbsp of the oil into a large bowl and mix together. Add the parsnips with a pinch of salt and a twist of pepper and toss the parsnips in the curry spice so they are all coated – you may find a pastry brush helpful for this.

Scatter the parsnips in a large, shallow roasting tray. Roast for about 40 minutes, stirring once, until starting to caramelise. Add the chopped walnuts, raisins and cooked spelt or barley to the roasting tray, stir everything together and return to the oven for 5 minutes.

Remove from the oven and let cool slightly for 5 minutes then toss with the leaves and transfer to a platter or individual plates. Squeeze over a little citrus juice and trickle over a touch more olive oil before serving.

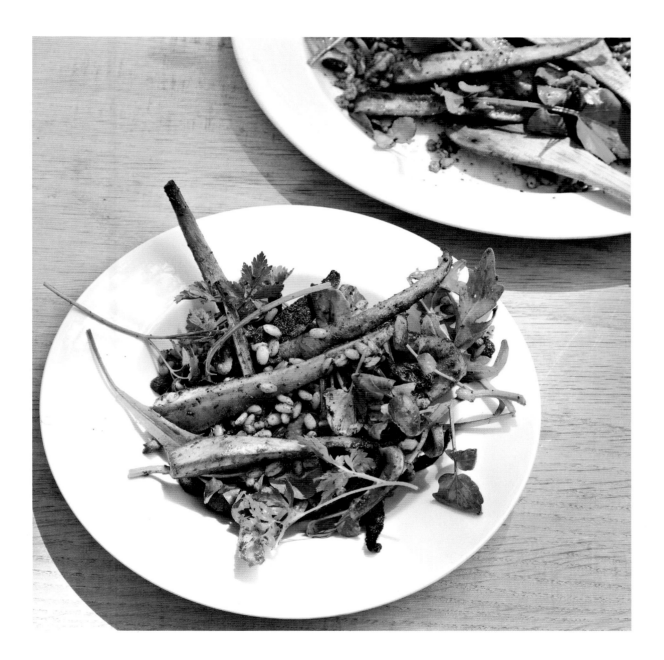

SIMPLE SUMMER SALAD
with egg (& niçoise variations)

This recipe takes the most obvious and easy-to-find 'salad veg' and combines them in a slightly unexpected and rather lovely way. The secret is to cut everything quite small, so that each forkful has quite a lot going on, without any two bites being quite the same. It might not be the most exciting ingredients list in the book – but it is delicious!

Serves 4

500g cherry and/or other ripe tomatoes

A small crisp-hearted lettuce

3–4 spring onions, trimmed

1 small or ½ regular cucumber

4 'hard-boiled' eggs (see page 268)

For the dressing

1 tsp English mustard

1 tbsp raw cider vinegar or lemon juice

2 tbsp olive oil

A scrap of garlic (about ¼ clove), crushed or finely grated

Sea salt and black pepper

To make the dressing, simply whisk all the ingredients together in your salad bowl, adding a pinch of salt and a twist of pepper.

Now prepare the salad veg, adding them to your salad bowl as you go. Quarter cherry tomatoes or cut them even smaller if you like; roughly chop bigger ones. Finely shred the lettuce. Thinly slice the spring onions on an angle. Peel the cucumber if you like (or 'semi-peel' it, so it's still streaked with green), cut lengthways into quarters then into eighths, then cut across into 1cm chunks. Roughly chop the 'hard-boiled' eggs.

Toss everything well to combine. Leave for a few minutes to allow everything to marry and mingle, then toss once more, gently, before serving.

NIÇOISE VARIATIONS
You can easily build on this salad by adding some or all of the following, which take it increasingly in the direction of a classic niçoise salad: sliced cooked new potatoes; sliced cooked French (green) beans; a handful of olives, chopped; a small tin of sardines, mackerel or (pole-and-line-caught) tuna, flaked; a few chopped anchovies.

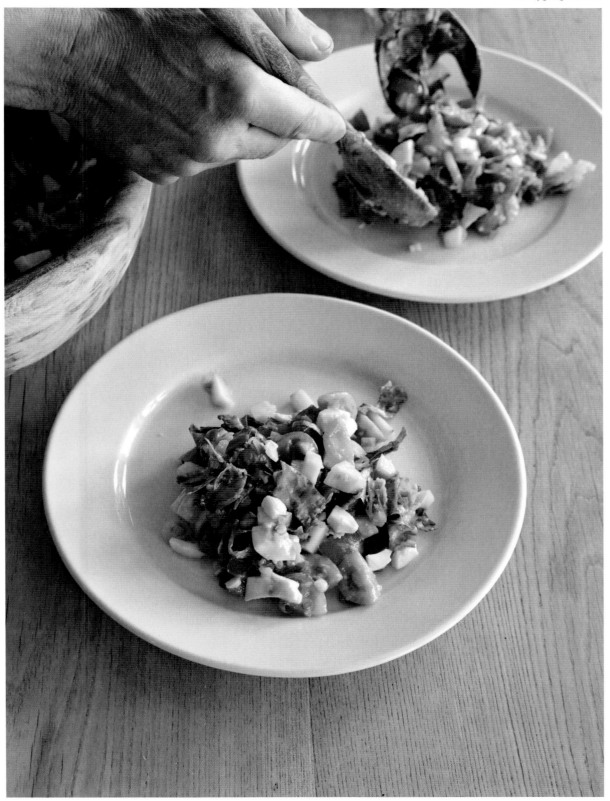

OMELETTE SLAW

Dressed with soy, sesame oil and a little ginger, this combination is a neat East Asian riff on a simple raw cabbage and carrot slaw. Strips of freshly cooked omelette go on top, adding contrasting texture and a protein punch that makes the salad really satisfying.

Serves 2

A wedge of white or red cabbage (about 150g)

1 large or 2 medium carrots (about 150g)

1 tbsp tamari or soy sauce

1 tbsp toasted sesame oil

Juice of ½ lime or small lemon

1 tsp finely grated fresh ginger

A scrap of garlic (about ¼ clove), finely grated

2 tsp sesame seeds, toasted if you like (optional)

2–3 medium eggs

A pinch of dried chilli flakes (optional)

A few drops of vegetable oil, for frying

1–2 tbsp tamari-roasted seeds (page 281)

Sea salt and black pepper

Remove the hard core from the cabbage wedge, then use a large, sharp knife or food processor to shred the cabbage as finely as possible. Put into a large bowl.

Coarsely grate the carrot(s), using a box grater or a food processor; add to the cabbage. Add the tamari or soy, sesame oil, lime or lemon juice, ginger, garlic and sesame seeds, if using, and mix thoroughly. Leave to stand, covered, while you make the omelette.

Whisk the eggs together with a pinch of salt and a twist of pepper, and a few chilli flakes if you fancy. Set a non-stick frying pan over a medium heat and add a few drops of oil. When hot, add the whisked eggs and tilt the pan until the egg covers the base. Cook for a minute or two until the surface of the egg is just barely set, then take the pan off the heat and leave to cool. (You can speed the cooling by transferring the omelette to a plate.) Roll up the cooled omelette and slice it into 1cm strips.

Give the slaw another stir. Taste it and add a twist of pepper and a squeeze more lime or lemon if needed (the soy should give enough salt). Toss half the omelette strips through the slaw and leave for a few minutes to absorb the dressing.

Divide the slaw between two dishes and scatter the remaining omelette slices over the top. Finish with a sprinkle of the tamari-roasted seeds, if you like, and serve.

VEG VARIATIONS
Replace the carrot with coarsely grated celeriac or beetroot – both are delicious.

AVOCADO/TOFU VARIATIONS
For a vegan slaw, replace the egg with slices of avocado and toasted cashew nuts, or strips of fried tofu.

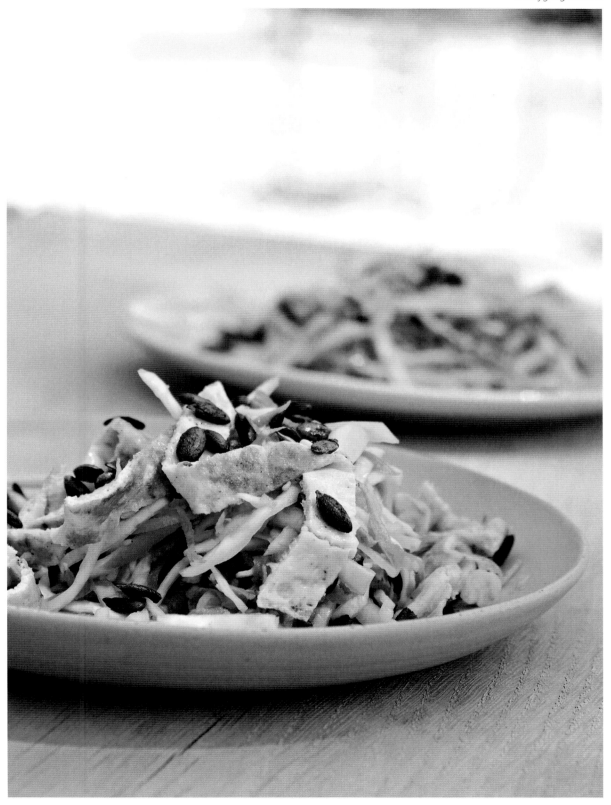

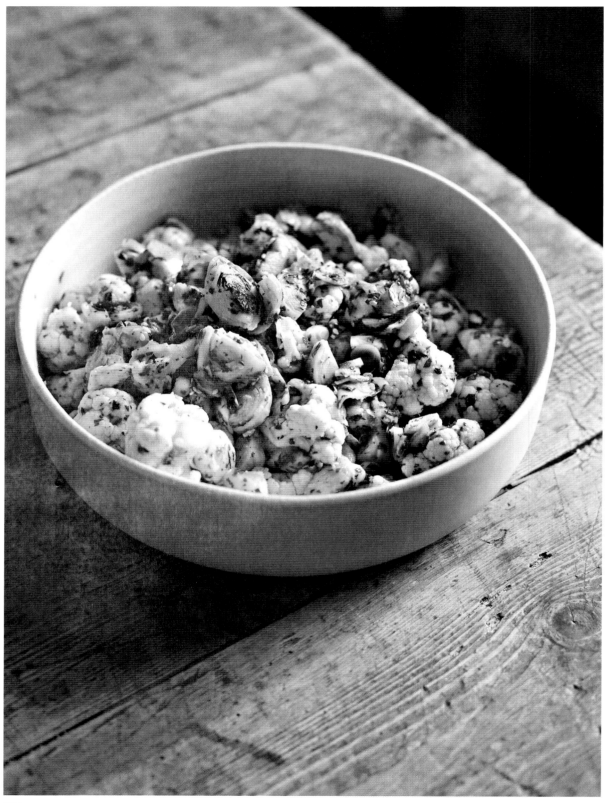

SEARED CAULI & SPROUTS
with soy dressing

This surprisingly filling dish is made by blasting cauliflower and Brussels sprouts in a very hot wok for just a few minutes, before tossing them in a vibrant, Asian-inspired dressing. It's great as part of a mix-and-match mezze. To make more of a meal of it, toss a handful of cooked brown rice or other whole grains into the pan with the veg as it cooks. Or you can serve the seared veg alongside brown rice cooked to order.

Serves 3–4

1 small–medium cauliflower (about 800g)

200g Brussels sprouts

A little vegetable oil, for frying

Sea salt

For the dressing

2 tbsp tamari or soy sauce

Juice of ½ lime or small lemon

A scrap of garlic (about ¼ clove), finely grated

1 medium-hot red chilli, chopped (and deseeded if you prefer less heat), or a pinch of dried chilli flakes

1 tsp honey

4 spring onions, thinly sliced

1 tsp finely grated fresh ginger

1 tbsp toasted sesame oil

1 tbsp sesame seeds

2 tbsp chopped coriander leaves (optional)

Trim the cauliflower, then cut it into small pieces, about 2cm. As well as the florets, include most of the stalk and the small, tender inner leaves. Trim and quarter the Brussels sprouts. Set the veg aside for a moment. Combine all the ingredients for the dressing in a large bowl.

Set a wok or a large frying pan over a high heat. When it is hot, add a splash of oil, then throw in half of the veg with a pinch of salt. Fry, without moving, for a good 30 seconds then give it a shake or stir and leave again; let the veg get some patches of rich, brown colour – this will enhance the flavour. Keep cooking the veg in this way for between 2 and 4 minutes until it is nicely patched with brown all over (it will be just cooked, but still *al dente*). Tip the hot veg into the bowl of dressing.

Pour a little more oil into the pan and cook the second batch of veg in the same way, keeping the pan really hot and letting the colour develop, then add to the rest of the veg.

Once all the veg is in the dressing, give it a good stir. You can eat the salad straight away, or allow it to sit for 15–20 minutes, macerating in the dressing, before serving.

VEG VARIATIONS
Replace the Brussels sprouts with some red or white cabbage, core removed and cut into 1cm wide strips; or broccoli, cut into chunks and florets like the cauli.

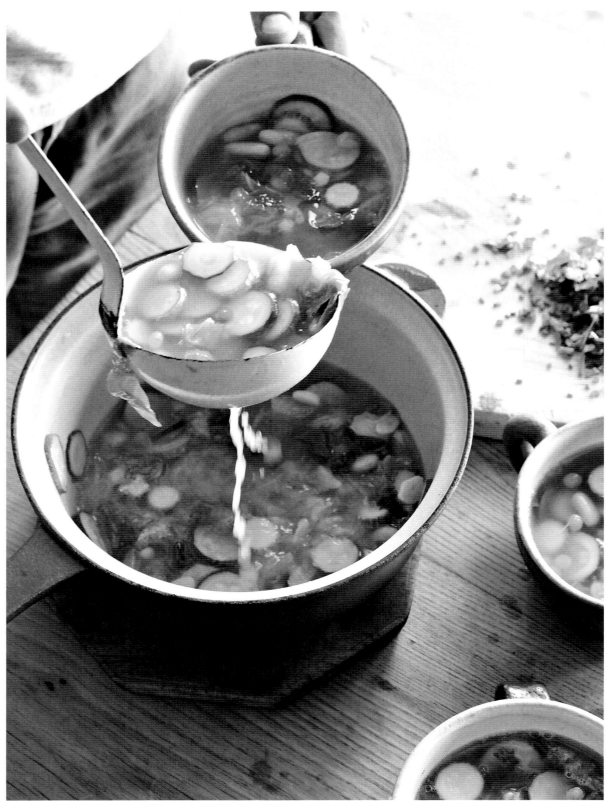

SUSTAINING SOUPS

If you harbour suspicions that a bowl of soup can never quite cut it as a main meal, this chapter has been devised to gently insist that you revise that view! The recipes that follow – steaming aromatic broths full of vegetables and herbs, hearty bowls of blitzed-up veg-and-pulse goodness, and some gorgeous twists on fish and shellfish classics – are tasty, hearty and soothing in equal measure.

I've also built these recipes to be brilliant ways to push your whole food count to the max – one serving can easily contain three, four or more lovely fresh vegetables, before we even get to the pulses and proteins that guarantee your hunger is sated, and the herbs and spices that take you eagerly to the bottom of the bowl. It's not a crime to have some (good, wholegrain) bread with these soups. But it's definitely not needed to 'complete' them.

Soups are fantastic make-ahead dishes, too. Find a few you really like, cook them up (in double batches if you like), then freeze in portions and you've got an almost-instant healthy meal to hand. And that might just stop your fingers fumbling for the food-delivery phone app!

Many of these recipes use vegetable stock as a base. A stock cube or granules are fine (I sometimes use low-salt organic ones), but I've also included a recipe for a very quick and simple homemade veg stock (on page 325), which will take your soups to a whole new level (and give you an extra treat of a supper on the side).

ROAST MUSHROOM & ARTICHOKE SOUP

Jerusalem artichokes are an under-appreciated winter vegetable, with a unique, earthy, nutty-sweet flavour. They are also a fantastic source of inulin, a prebiotic fibre that is highly beneficial to our gut bacteria (see page 84). The veg are roasted and then blitzed with hot stock and some cashews or chickpeas for a slightly creamy texture – a few tasty bits left whole as a chunky garnish. A warning note here: Jerusalem artichokes (aka 'fartichokes') are notorious for their gas-producing effect, which is linked to their prebiotic power! If your gut is on the sensitive side, stick to a small portion the first time you try this.

Serves 4

300g Jerusalem artichokes

300g chestnut mushrooms

1 medium onion, chopped

2 garlic cloves, sliced

100g cashew nuts or cooked chickpeas (about ½ a 400g tin, rinsed and drained)

1 tbsp olive or vegetable oil

700ml hot veg stock (page 325)

Sea salt and black pepper

1 tbsp chopped parsley, to finish (optional)

Preheat the oven to 180°C/Fan 160°C/Gas 4. Scrub the artichokes and chop into chunky pieces, about 2cm. Roughly chop the mushrooms (stalks and all).

Put the artichokes, mushrooms, onion, garlic and cashews or chickpeas into a large roasting tray. Trickle over the oil and toss the veg together. Roast for 35–40 minutes, stirring once or twice, until tender and golden. Put about a quarter of the roasted veg mix to one side; keep warm.

Transfer the remaining veg mix to a blender with the hot stock and blitz until smooth, adding a splash of hot water if the soup seems excessively thick. Taste the soup and add a little salt and pepper if needed.

Reheat the soup if necessary and ladle into warm bowls. Scatter the reserved veg over the top, along with the chopped parsley if using. Add a grinding of pepper and serve.

CELERIAC VARIATION
Celeriac is delicious with mushrooms and makes a very good swap for the Jerusalem artichokes (it will need peeling and cutting into chunks before roasting).

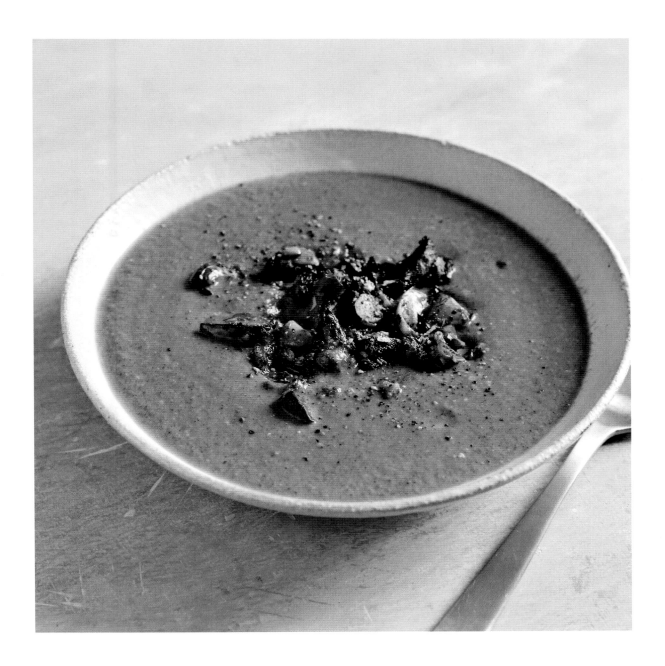

CURRIED CAULI, LETTUCE & PEA SOUP

Light but filling and full of flavour, this vegan soup is warming and delicious. It's very good when made with individual spices, but you can also cheat and use a ready-made curry powder or paste (using 1 tbsp to replace the ground coriander, cumin, turmeric and dried chilli).

Serves 4

1 small–medium cauliflower (about 800g)

2 tbsp olive or vegetable oil

1 medium onion, chopped

3–4 large garlic cloves, finely grated

A thumb-sized knob of fresh ginger, finely grated

1 tsp ground coriander

1 tsp ground cumin

1 tsp ground turmeric

¼ tsp dried chilli flakes

200ml coconut milk

500ml hot veg stock (page 325)

100g frozen peas or petits pois

2 little gem lettuce, thickly sliced or cut into thin wedges

8 spring onions, sliced

1 rounded tsp tamarind paste or juice of ½ lime or lemon

Sea salt and black pepper

A small bunch of coriander, leaves picked and chopped, to finish (optional)

Cut the cauliflower into small florets, including the tender parts of the stalk and small, tender leaves.

Put a large saucepan over a medium heat and add the oil. When hot, add the onion and sweat gently, stirring often, for 5–6 minutes until softened.

Add the garlic and ginger, then the individual spices (or the curry powder/paste). Fry gently with the onion for a couple of minutes, stirring frequently so the spices don't burn. Add the cauliflower florets and stir them into the spicy mixture.

Pour in the coconut milk, veg stock and 200ml boiling water and bring to a simmer. Cook for 3 minutes, then stir in the peas, lettuce and spring onions (don't worry, the lettuce will wilt down). Let the soup return to a simmer, then cook for another minute.

Remove from the heat and stir in the tamarind paste or citrus juice. Taste and add a little salt and pepper if needed. Ladle the soup into warm bowls and finish with chopped coriander if you like.

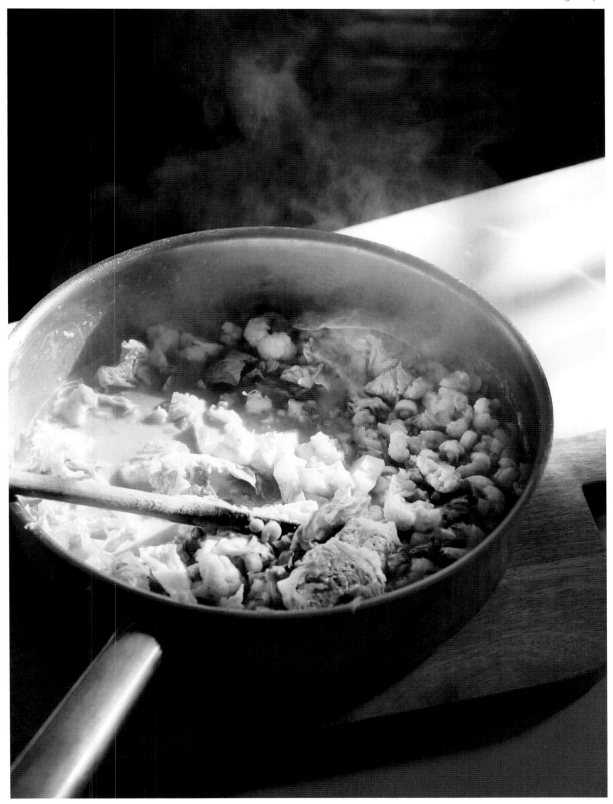

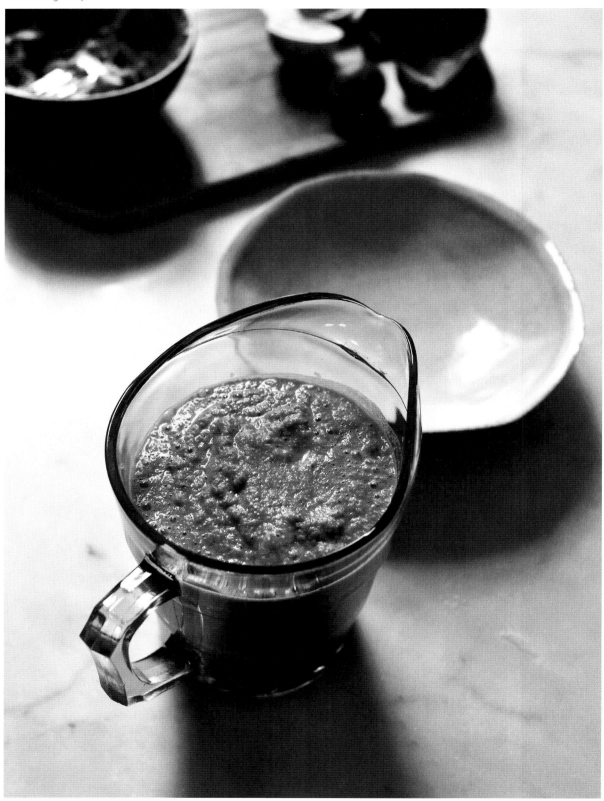

SPICED GAZPACHO
with bashed avocado

This tempting gazpacho – a soup made with raw veg – is probably more of a light lunch than a hearty supper, but it's so delicious, I had to include it. This version, like many, is based on tomatoes – and they need to be flavoursome. Cherry tomatoes on-the-vine are usually a pretty safe bet, taste-wise, but big tomatoes are great too if you can find properly ripe ones. Depending on the power of your blender, you might get little flecks of tomato skin left in the finished soup – all good fibre – but if they bother you, sieve them out. For a contrasting crunch, you could serve the gazpacho with wholegrain croûtons or some good-quality corn chips.

Serves 4 as a light lunch

50g cashew nuts, soaked in 100ml cold water for at least 1 hour (up to 4 hours)

400g ripe, tasty tomatoes, cut up if big

1 red pepper, cored, deseeded and chopped

½ medium cucumber (200g), chopped

1 garlic clove, finely grated

2 tbsp extra virgin olive oil, plus a little extra to finish

1 tbsp red wine vinegar or sherry vinegar

½ tsp cumin seeds, crushed (or ½ tsp ground cumin)

¼ tsp smoked paprika

Sea salt and black pepper

For the bashed avocado

1 large, ripe avocado

Juice of ½ lime

1–2 tbsp chopped coriander (optional)

1 tbsp extra virgin olive oil

Tip the cashews and their soaking water into a blender. Add the tomatoes, red pepper, cucumber, garlic, olive oil, vinegar, spices, a pinch of salt and a twist of pepper. Blitz until smooth – but don't worry if a few flecks of skin remain. You might need to stop the blender a few times and tamp everything down to get it all blending. It's intended to be quite a thick soup, but if it seems too thick, add more cold water (up to a small glass).

Taste the soup and adjust the seasoning (including the vinegar) if needed, then transfer to a large jug and chill well in the fridge (for at least an hour). It's a good idea to chill your soup bowls at the same time.

Prepare the avocado just before serving: halve, stone and peel the avocado then roughly mash the flesh (keeping some chunks for texture) with the lime juice, coriander if using, olive oil, a pinch of salt and a twist of pepper.

Give the gazpacho a good stir then divide it between cold bowls. Top with a spoonful of the bashed avocado and finish with a trickle of your best olive oil.

BEANS & GREENS SUMMER SOUP

This is a lovely chunky green bowlful. The generous garlic and beans robustly underpin the whole thing, and the summer veg and herbs add lovely fresh flavours and goodness.

Serves 2

1 tbsp olive or rapeseed oil

½–1 whole garlic bulb (at least 6 cloves), separated, peeled and thinly sliced

2 small courgettes (or 3–4 baby ones), sliced

100g freshly podded peas or frozen petits pois

400g tin white beans, such as cannellini or haricot, drained and rinsed

1 litre hot veg stock (page 325)

1 little gem, cos or butterhead lettuce, coarsely shredded

Sea salt and black pepper

To finish

A small bunch of parsley, leaves picked and roughly chopped

AND

A small bunch of chives, snipped, or a few spring onions, sliced (optional)

OR

4 tsp pestomega (page 278)

Heat the oil in a large saucepan over a medium heat. Add the sliced garlic and allow to sizzle for 1 minute. Add the courgettes and sweat for another couple of minutes.

Add the peas and beans and pour on the hot stock. Bring to a simmer and cook for 2 minutes or until the peas are tender. Add the lettuce with a pinch of salt and a twist of pepper, stir in and cook for just another minute. Taste and check the seasoning.

Spoon the soup into warm bowls and finish with a generous sprinkling of chopped herbs or add 1 tsp pestomega to each.

SUMMER VEG VARIATIONS
Instead of (or as well as) the lettuce, thinly slice a small fennel bulb and add with the courgettes at the start. Another good addition is a few finely shredded summer cabbage leaves; or you can include a small bunch of chard (add the chopped stalks at the start, the shredded leaves at the end). Green (French) beans or runner beans can certainly go in. And if you're lucky enough to have sweet, fresh broad beans to hand, swap those for the tinned white beans.

AUTUMN/WINTER VEG VARIATIONS
Replace the courgettes with 2 sliced medium carrots and/or ½ medium celeriac, or parsnip, cut into small batons, and sweat for a few minutes longer to soften. Use shredded kale or spinach instead of lettuce.

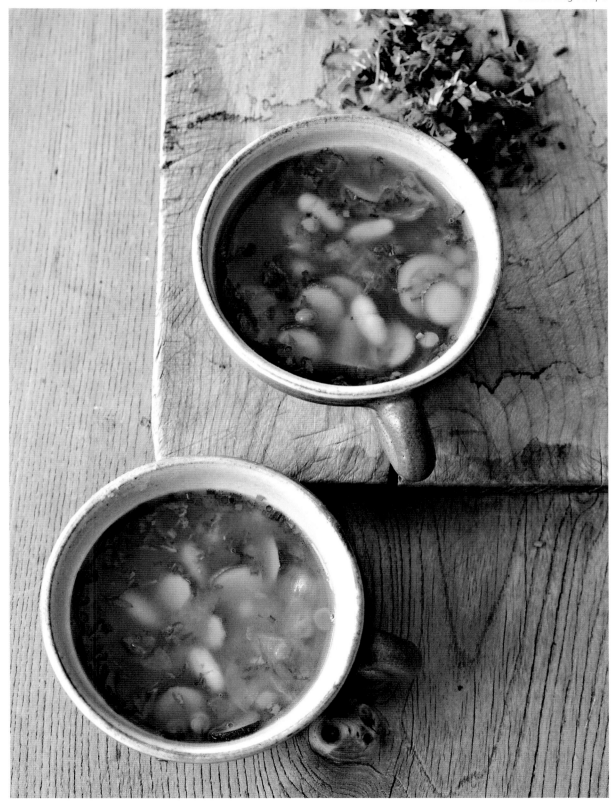

STORECUPBOARD TOMATO & BEAN SOUP

At its most basic, this super-easy soup requires only an onion and a couple of storecupboard staples – tinned tomatoes and beans – and it's well worth making if that's all you put into it (perhaps with a dash of chilli). But you have the option of building in some fresh veg too, depending on what you have to hand. Either way, it's a lovely, thick soup. If you want to loosen it and make it more soupy, add some hot veg stock with the tomatoes; you won't need more than a mugful (250–300ml).

Serves 4

1 tbsp olive or vegetable oil

1 large onion, chopped

2 x 400g tins whole tomatoes

250–300ml hot veg stock (page 325), optional

1 red chilli, deseeded and chopped, or 1 tsp smoked sweet paprika, or a good dash of chilli sauce (optional)

2 x 400g tins white, black or kidney beans, or chickpeas, drained and rinsed

Sea salt and black pepper

Optional extra veg

1 carrot, chopped

1 celery stem, thinly sliced

1 red pepper, cored, deseeded and thinly sliced

1 fennel bulb, thinly sliced

To finish (optional)

Extra virgin olive oil or pestomega (page 278)

Place a large saucepan or a small stockpot over a medium heat. Add the oil and, when hot, add the onion with a pinch each of salt and pepper. This is also the time to add any or all of the optional extra veg – carrot, celery, pepper and/or fennel. Turn the heat down a little and sweat the veg for about 5 minutes to soften a little.

Add the tomatoes with their juice, crushing them with your hands as you drop them in, and picking out the little white stalky ends if they bother you. Add the stock, if you like, and the chilli, paprika or chilli sauce, if using. Stir well and bring to a gentle simmer. Cook, uncovered, for about 15 minutes to reduce, stirring a few times and mashing the tomato down a little with a fork or spoon as it cooks.

Before adding the beans, you can part-blitz the soup with a hand blender if you like – either roughly, or until smooth. Or just leave it chunky and unblitzed (my preference).

With the back of a spoon (or your fingers) break up the beans slightly, before stirring them into the soup. Simmer gently for another 5 minutes or so. Season with salt and pepper and ladle into warm bowls. Finish with a trickle of good olive oil or a spoonful of pestomega and a grinding of pepper.

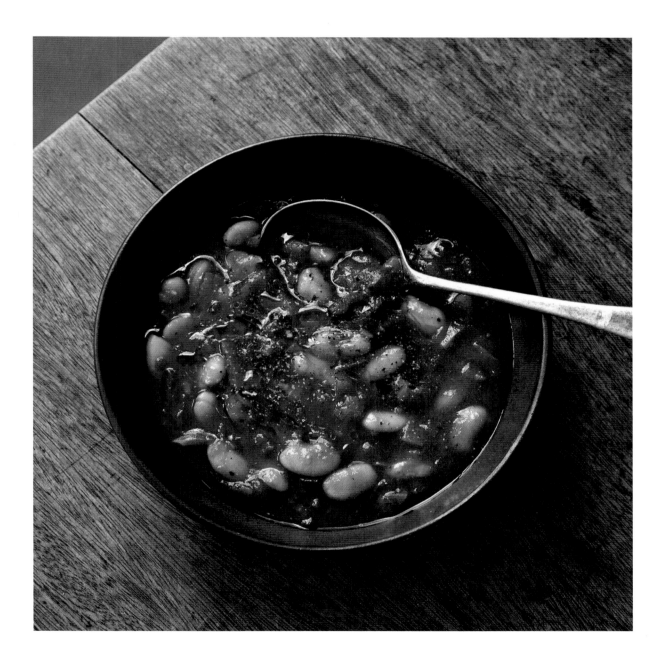

YELLOW SPLIT PEA SOUP
with harissa & almonds

Made with basic storecupboard ingredients, this soup is healthy, filling, and an absolute doddle. Ideally, I soak the split peas for a few hours before cooking, but it's not essential, so this can still be a fairly spur-of-the-moment soup! I like to top it off with a garnish that provides a contrast of colour, texture and flavour – so it looks and tastes pretty special. Here I have used toasted nuts seasoned with a good dollop of spicy harissa paste.

Serves 4

3 tbsp olive or vegetable oil

2 leeks, trimmed, quartered lengthways and thinly sliced, or 2 onions, chopped

2–3 garlic cloves, sliced

250g yellow split peas, soaked if possible (for up to 4 hours), rinsed well

1 litre veg stock (page 325)

Sea salt and black pepper

To finish

50g whole almonds

2 tsp harissa paste, or to taste

Set a large, heavy-based pan over a medium heat. Add half the oil, followed by the leeks or onions and garlic. Sweat, stirring often, for about 5 minutes until softened.

Add the split peas and stock, bring to a simmer then turn the heat down. Cook gently, uncovered, for around 30 minutes, stirring from time to time, until the split peas are completely soft. It might take a little longer (45–50 minutes) if they haven't been soaked.

Use a stick blender to blend the soup thoroughly in the pan (or transfer to a jug blender to blitz). Add a dash of hot water if the soup seems excessively thick, then taste and add a pinch of salt and a twist of pepper as needed.

Heat the remaining oil in a small frying pan. Add the almonds and fry for a few minutes, stirring often, until lightly toasted. Remove from the heat and stir in the harissa. Ladle the soup into warm bowls, top with your harissa-spiked almonds and trickle over any spicy oil left in the pan. Finish with a grinding of pepper. Serve a slice or two of wholegrain bread on the side if you're having this for a main meal.

FINISHING OPTIONS
Instead of almonds, you can toast hazelnuts or use dukka (page 281). Or replace the nuts with about 100g cubed halloumi, frying it (with just a scrap of oil) for a few minutes until nicely coloured and crispy at the edges before tossing with the harissa. And you can do something similar with meaty leftovers – roast lamb or chicken for example – frying the scraps of meat until starting to become crispy, then tossing them with the harissa before scattering over the soup.

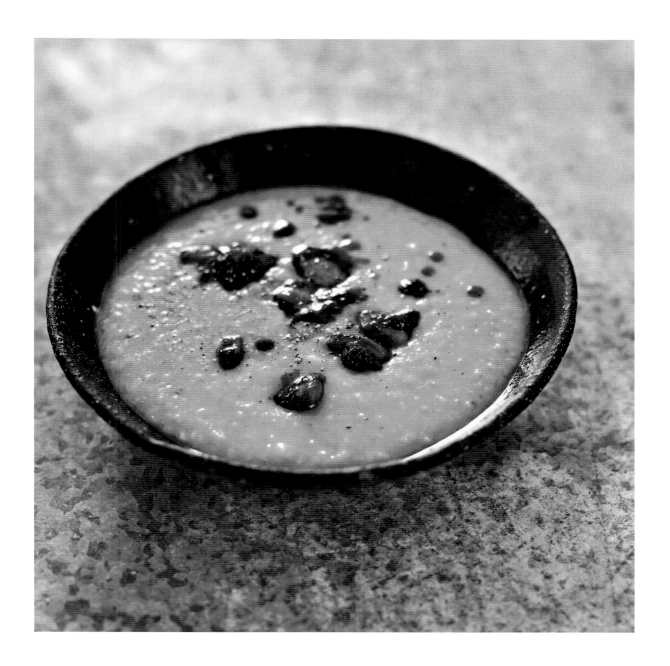

MUSSEL SOUP WITH LEEK & POTATO

Mussels are delicious, rich in nutrients (including omega-3 fats) and a great example of a sustainable seafood. They're also simple to cook, as this hearty soup demonstrates. I like to leave a few mussels in their shells, or 'in the half-shell'. They look great, and it's fun to pick them out of the soup to eat with your fingers as you go.

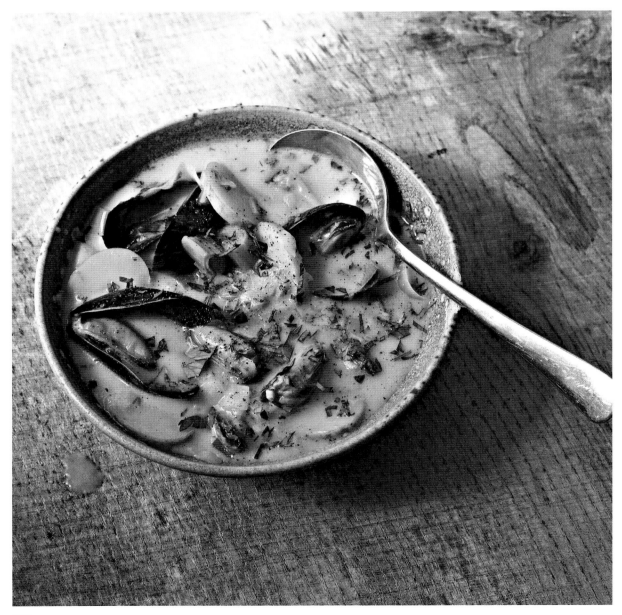

Serves 2

1kg live mussels

200g new or waxy potatoes

2 large or 3 medium leeks, trimmed

1 tbsp olive or vegetable oil, or butter

100ml dry white wine or dry cider

1–2 garlic cloves, sliced

400ml hot veg stock (page 325)

1 tsp English mustard

1 tbsp crème fraîche

Black pepper

Chopped parsley, to finish (optional)

Put the mussels into a colander and give them a good rinse, shaking them about a bit, under cold running water. If the shells have any 'beards' (little clumps of wiry fibres), pull them off. Discard any mussels with broken shells, and any that are open and do not close when you give them a sharp tap (these ones may be dead).

Cut the potatoes into slices, the thickness of a £1 coin. Cut the leeks into 5mm thick slices. Heat a large saucepan over a medium heat. Add the oil or butter, then the potatoes and leeks and a few twists of pepper. Turn the heat down, cover the pan and let the veg sweat for about 5 minutes, so it starts to soften, then take off the heat while you sort the mussels.

In a second large pan (with a tight-fitting lid), heat the wine or cider until boiling, then add the garlic and mussels. Put the lid on and cook for 2–3 minutes, shaking the pan once or twice. Lift the lid. Almost all of the mussels should be open; if not, cover the pan and give them another minute. Tip the mussels into a sieve over a bowl, to catch the juices. (Discard any mussels that still aren't open at this stage.)

Add the hot stock to the veg pan, return to the heat and let it come to a gentle simmer. Cook, uncovered, for about 5 minutes until the potatoes are tender. Meanwhile, start taking the cooked mussels out of their shells, dropping them back into the sieve and making sure any juices go into the bowl. Leave a dozen or so mussels in their shells, or 'in the half-shell' if you like.

When the veg is tender, tip all the mussels (shelled and in shell) into the soup. Carefully pour in the mussel-y, cidery juice from the bowl too, except for the last bit, which may be slightly gritty. Stir well and take off the heat. Taste the broth and add more pepper if needed. Stir in the mustard and crème fraîche. Ladle into warm bowls and sprinkle with chopped parsley if you like.

CURRIED VARIATION
Sweat the leeks and spuds with 2 tsp curry powder or paste. Finish the soup with 2 tbsp coconut milk and a squeeze of lemon or lime, instead of mustard and cream.

WHITE BEAN VARIATION
Swap the potatoes for a 400g tin cannellini or haricot beans, drained and rinsed; these only need to be heated through. (This works with the curried variation, too.)

CURRIED BEANY CULLEN SKINK

Cullen skink is an old Scottish friend that I keep welcoming back to my kitchen, in various guises. This time round the usual spuds are swapped for creamy beans, there's a healthy dose of greens in the form of spinach, and a dash of curry gives lovely warmth and extra comfort.

Serves 4

2 tbsp olive or vegetable oil

2 medium leeks or onions, trimmed, halved and sliced

3 garlic cloves, sliced

2 bay leaves (optional)

1 rounded tbsp medium-hot curry powder or paste

300ml whole milk

500ml veg stock (page 325)

About 300g smoked haddock or pollack fillet, skinned and cut into bite-sized pieces

400g tin cannellini or borlotti beans, drained and rinsed

About 200g baby spinach (or regular spinach, tough stalks removed, leaves roughly chopped)

2 tbsp chopped flat-leaf parsley or coriander (optional)

Black pepper

Place a large saucepan over a medium heat. Add the oil and then the leeks or onions, garlic, bay leaves if using, and curry powder or paste. Sweat, stirring regularly, for 3–4 minutes.

Pour in the milk and stock, bring to a simmer and cook for a further 2–3 minutes.

Add the smoked fish and beans followed by the spinach, adding it a handful at a time as it wilts down in the simmering soup. By the time the spinach is wilted (in just a few minutes), the fish will be cooked.

Add the chopped parsley or coriander if using, and season with a few twists of pepper (the smoked fish should make it salty enough). Ladle into warm bowls and serve.

KIPPER VARIATION
You can use kipper fillets instead of the smoked haddock or pollack.

VEG VARIATIONS
Add sweetcorn (frozen or even tinned) or peas, instead of, or as well as, the beans. And, of course, potatoes can replace the beans for a classic cullen skink – peel and roughly chop the spuds, add them to the simmering stock and cook until just tender before adding the smoked fish.

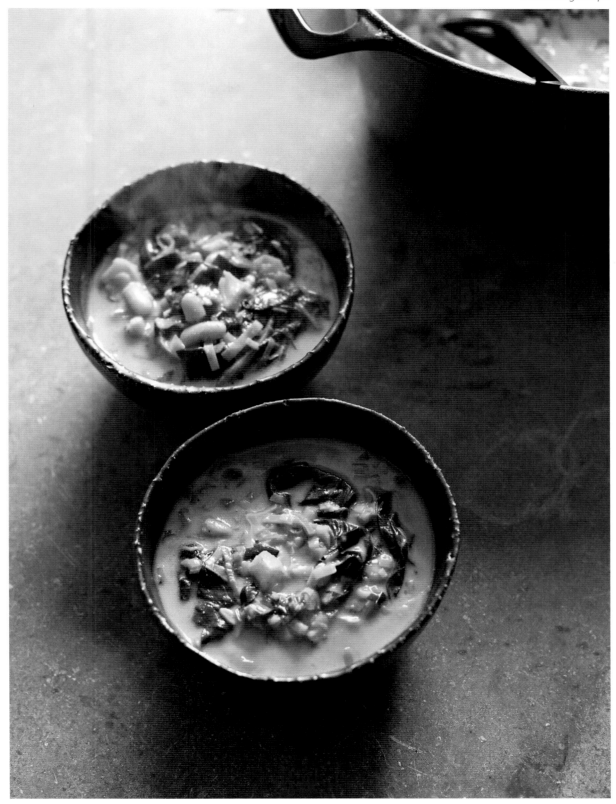

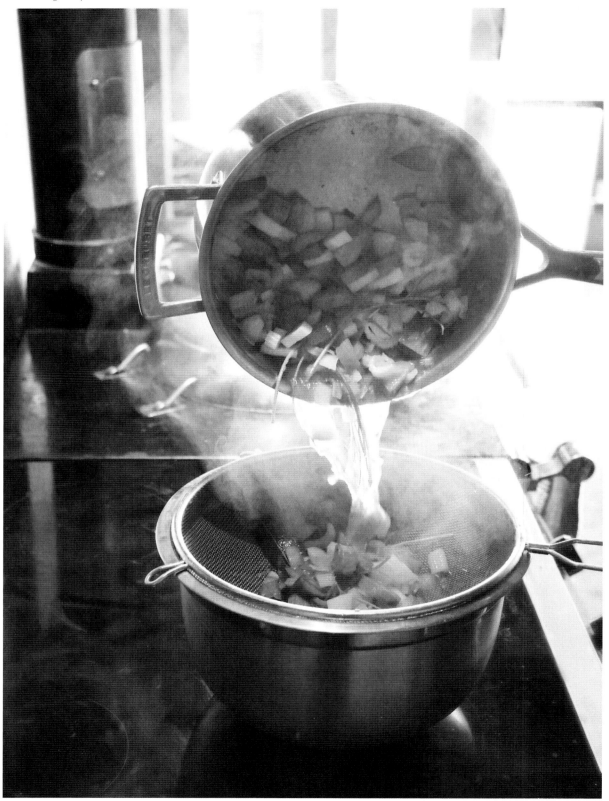

VEG STOCK

I use veg stock a lot – not just in soups but in stews and curries too. Sometimes I resort to a stock cube (the organic, low-salt kind) but a homemade vegetable stock is always nicer (not to mention less processed), and doesn't take long to make. Gently sweating the veg in a little oil before adding the water helps to develop the flavour, but if time is of the essence you can skip this stage and just add the water straight away.

Makes about 1.2 litres

A dash of olive or vegetable oil

1 large onion, roughly chopped

1 large leek, or a couple of green leek tops, roughly chopped

2 medium carrots, chopped

3–4 celery stems, coarsely chopped

1 parsnip or a chunk of celeriac, peeled and chopped (optional)

A bunch of parsley, stalks only (optional)

2–3 bay leaves

A good twist of black pepper

Put all the ingredients into a large saucepan or small stockpot and set over a medium-high heat. Sweat the veg, stirring regularly, for 4–5 minutes until lightly golden. Pour over 1.5 litres water and bring to the boil. Lower the heat and let simmer fairly gently, uncovered, for 15–20 minutes, or until the liquid tastes good. It should be tasty enough that you could use it, once seasoned with salt and pepper, as the base for a broth.

Pour through a sieve into a bowl to strain out the veg and the stock is ready to use, or to chill and freeze. Keep the cooked veg to make the hash below.

CHICKEN STOCK

If you've roasted a chicken, don't discard the bones or carcass – instead, use them to make a tasty stock for soups and stews. Follow the recipe above, adding the broken-up chicken carcass and bones after you've sweated the veg, and simmer very gently for at least 1½ hours – up to 3 hours – before straining.

STOCK VEG HASH AND EGG

Don't discard the strained veg from your veg stock – they make a good 'hash'. Let them steam off until cool, pick out the parsley stalks and bay leaves, and keep the veg in the fridge until you want to use them. Heat a little olive or veg oil in a pan, and fry 1 or 2 chopped garlic clove(s) for a minute until just starting to brown. Add the leftover stock veg (plus any other leftover veg you have, including cooked potatoes). Keep frying fairly fast, turning occasionally, until the veg is browning nicely and season well with salt and pepper as a nice golden crust starts to form. If spuds are included, you can usually squash the veg into a nice 'cake' and turn the whole thing, but it still works if broken up a bit. When well caramelised (and borderline burnt in parts!) pile onto a plate. Fry an egg or two in the same pan (or poach separately) and serve with, or on, the hash.

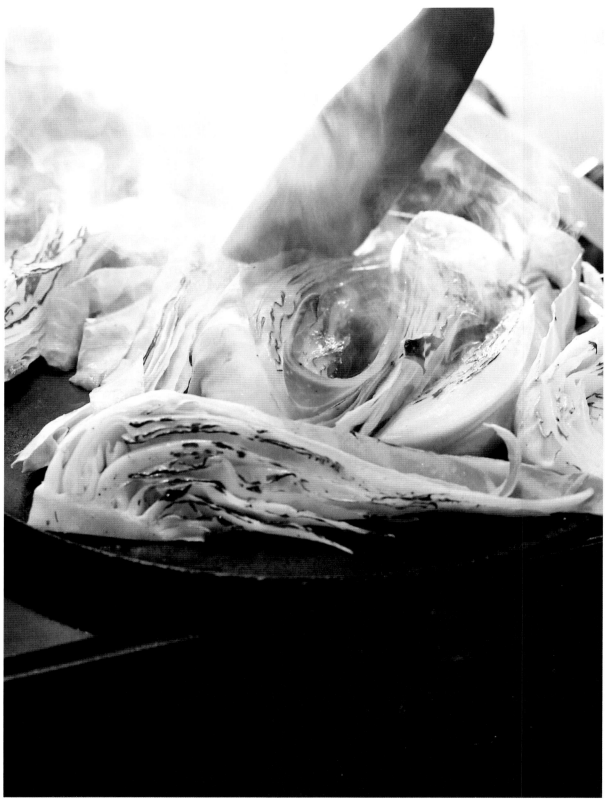

VITAL VEG MAINS

Hearty meals based around vibrant, diverse, tasty veg are my passion (borderline obsession) these days. Whole, varied and high in fibre, these dishes form the bedrock of my eating, and I hope they will do the same for you.

I've long since thrown out the old 'meat-and-two-veg' template for composing a meal. Rather I'm usually thinking 'veg-and-more-veg'. And veg means edible plants in the broadest sense, including proteinaceous pulses and beans, nuts, seeds, and indeed fruits. Because in my kitchen, fruits often share the plate with – and lend their tart and aromatic qualities and natural sweetness to – the plant groups we more conventionally call vegetables. With plenty of herbs, spices and aromatics to join the party, there is no limit to the tempting plant-centred main courses you can enjoy.

Put these dishes front and centre in your meal planning, and I can offer a slam-dunk guarantee that you will be eating better. If you are looking for a place to start, try my Family Veg Audit on pages 62–5; it'll remind you which veg you like (even if you've been neglecting them) and will point you in the direction of the dishes most likely to be a hit straight off. And don't forget to check out the recipe variations – there are alternative veg options in almost every case.

These recipes have been designed to be complete, without the need for a carby dose of bread, spuds or pasta on the side. If you do want them to go a little further (or you are feeding hungry mouths on active bodies!) then the best option would be to serve with a modest side of whole grains, or a sensible (maximum fist-sized, see pages 170–1) portion of spuds.

ROAST ASPARAGUS & LITTLE GEMS
with lentils & boiled eggs

I like the way that roasting vegetables intensifies their flavours and caramelises the cut edges. It's an easy win with roots and brassicas, but it also works surprisingly well here with spears of asparagus and wedges of tight-hearted little gem lettuces. The lentils and eggs make a fine fulfilling meal of it.

Serves 2

A bundle of asparagus (about 200g)

2 little gem lettuce, quartered lengthways

4–5 spring onions, trimmed

4 tbsp olive oil

2 'hard-boiled' eggs (see page 268), peeled and roughly chopped

2–3 tbsp cooked or tinned Puy lentils, drained and rinsed

1 tbsp white wine vinegar

1–2 tsp English mustard, to taste

A small handful of roughly chopped parsley (optional)

Sea salt and black pepper

Dukka or tamari-roasted seeds (page 281), to serve (optional)

Preheat the oven to 200°C/Fan 180°C/Gas 6. Trim off the base of the asparagus spears if they look at all woody or tough.

Put the asparagus spears, lettuce wedges and spring onions into a roasting tin or oven dish, trickle with 2 tbsp olive oil, season with a pinch of salt and a twist of pepper and turn to coat. Roast for about 15 minutes until the asparagus is tender and everything is nicely golden.

Meanwhile, combine the chopped boiled eggs and lentils with the remaining 2 tbsp oil, the wine vinegar, mustard and chopped parsley, if using. Season with salt and pepper.

When the veg are cooked, allow them to sit for 10 minutes or so, then spoon on the egg mixture. Before serving, sprinkle with a handful of dukka or tamari-roasted seeds if you like.

VEG/PULSE VARIATIONS
Try courgettes, cut into long batons, or fennel, cut into wedges, instead of asparagus. You can also swap in chunks of leek or regular onion wedges for the spring onions. And feel free to swap out the lentils with tinned chickpeas or beans.

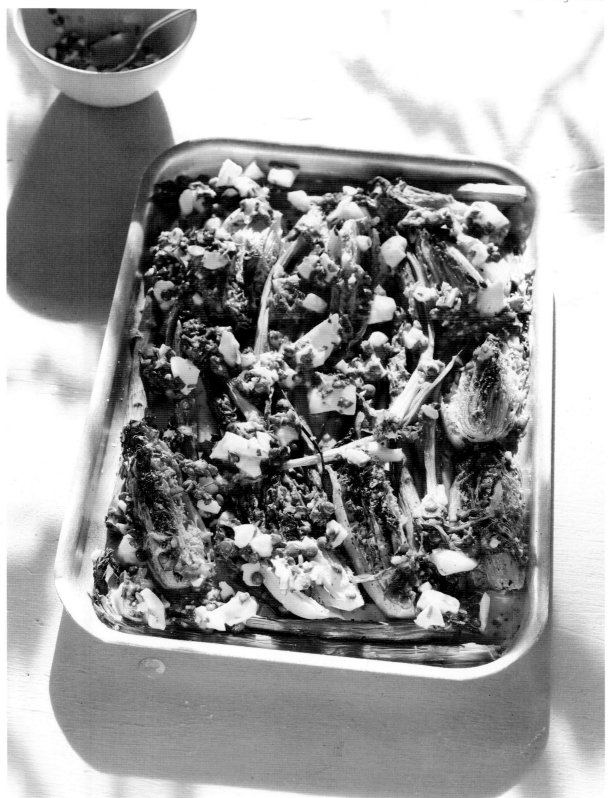

NUTTY BEANY BEETROOT CURRY

This is a fantastic way to eat beetroot – great for anyone who isn't normally a fan of this amazing vegetable! The carby beetroot, pulse-y beans and nutty cashews make it pretty substantial, so you don't really need rice or bread. A spoonful of plain, creamy yoghurt on the side is a nice addition, or bashed avocado works well for a vegan meal.

Serves 4

1–1.2kg beetroot (ideally with leaves, or you could use a few spinach leaves)

2 tbsp olive or vegetable oil

1 large onion, chopped

A thumb-sized piece of fresh ginger, grated

4 garlic cloves, grated

2 tbsp curry paste or powder

150g cashew nuts

500ml tomato passata

500ml hot veg stock (page 325)

400g tin kidney or cannellini beans, drained and rinsed

Sea salt and black pepper

Natural yoghurt, to serve

Peel the beetroot and cut into 2–3cm chunks; you can wash and reserve any leaves if they are in good nick.

Set a large saucepan or a small stockpot over a medium heat and add the oil. When it is hot, add the onion. Once the onion is sizzling, lower the heat a little and fry gently for 8–10 minutes. Add the ginger, garlic and curry paste or powder and fry, stirring, for another 2–3 minutes.

Add the beetroot and cashews and stir them into the spicy mix. Add the passata and stock and bring up to a brisk simmer. Lower the heat and simmer gently, uncovered, until the beetroot is tender, stirring now and again. It should be cooked in around 20 minutes, but can take a bit longer, depending on the beetroot. As the sauce simmers, it will reduce down and thicken. If you think it's reduced too much, add a splash of boiling water.

Stir the beans into the curry for the last 5–10 minutes of cooking. If using beetroot or spinach leaves, shred these into thick strips and stir them in at the same time.

Taste the curry and add salt or pepper if needed, then spoon into warm dishes. Top with a generous dollop of yoghurt and finish with a grinding of pepper.

VEG/PULSE VARIATIONS
Try replacing the beetroot with cubed squash, or a mix of squash and parsnips. And, in place of beet tops, stir in some shredded chard, kale, spring greens or spinach. Chickpeas can go in instead of the beans.

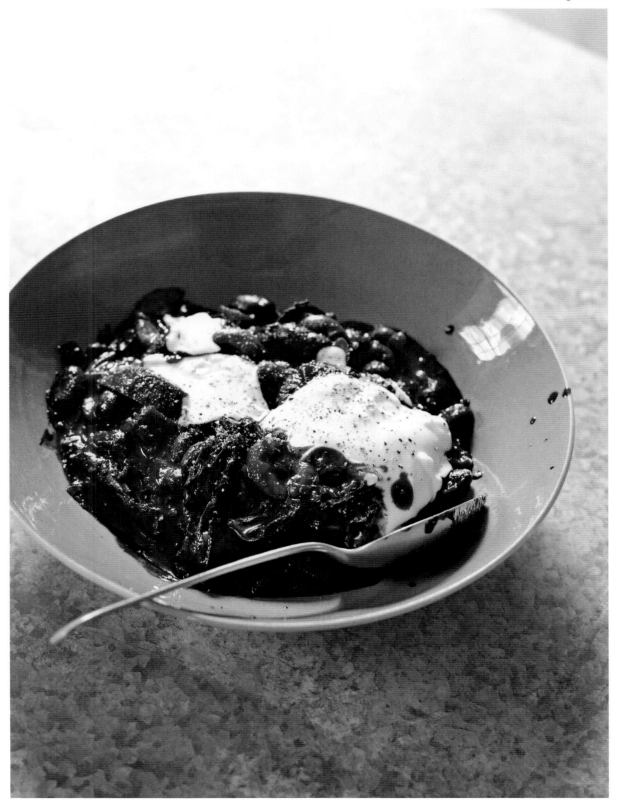

ROASTED VEG & BASHED CHICKPEAS

I've extolled the virtues of tray-roasting veg for a while now, and I'm not about to stop any time soon! This hearty outing makes the most of delicious winter veg, complementing them with a sort of deconstructed hummus made by roughly bashing up chickpeas and nuts with some tasty seasonings.

Serves 4

1 head of broccoli, calabrese or a bunch of purple sprouting broccoli (about 300g)

1 small–medium cauliflower, or spring (pointed) or savoy cabbage (about 800g)

2 tbsp olive oil

1 tsp cumin seeds

3–4 large banana shallots, or 2 onions

3–4 medium carrots

1 tsp coriander seeds

Sea salt and black pepper

For the smashed chickpeas

50g whole, skin-on almonds (soaked or dry)

2 x 400g tins chickpeas, drained and rinsed, or 450g freshly cooked chickpeas

¼–½ garlic clove, finely grated or crushed

3 tbsp olive oil

Grated zest and juice of ½–1 lemon

A good pinch of hot smoked paprika or a sprinkling of dried chilli flakes (optional)

Preheat the oven to 190°C/Fan 170°C/Gas 5.

Cut the broccoli into large pieces, including any green leaves and as much of the stalk as possible (just discard any bits that look fibrous). Put into a large roasting tray. Cut the cauliflower into similar sized pieces, again using most of the stalk, too. Or, if you're using cabbage, cut into 8–10 slim wedges, keeping the central stem intact. Add the cauli or cabbage to the broccoli with 1 tbsp olive oil, the cumin seeds and some salt and pepper. Toss together.

Cut the shallots or onions into slim wedges. Cut the carrots into chunky batons. Put the carrots and shallots or onions into a second roasting tray with 1 tbsp olive oil, the coriander seeds and some salt and pepper. Toss together.

Put both trays of veg in the oven (placing the carrots and shallots on the higher shelf) and roast for 40–45 minutes, taking them out halfway through to stir the veg.

Meanwhile, for the smashed chickpeas, bash the almonds using a large pestle and mortar until roughly ground, then tip into a bowl. Put the chickpeas into the mortar and bash these to a coarse mash, retaining some whole bits. Add to the almonds with the garlic, olive oil, most of the lemon zest and juice, and paprika or chilli. Season with a pinch of salt and a twist of pepper and mix well. If it looks a bit dry, you can add a splash of water. Taste and add more spice and/or lemon if needed.

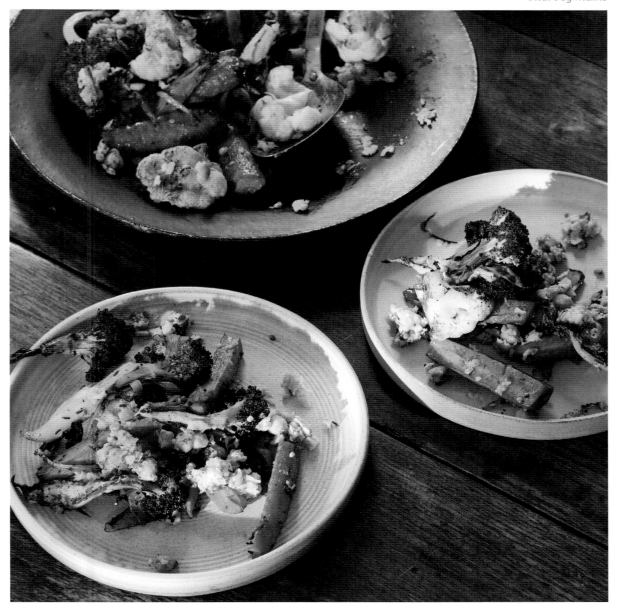

Once the veg is tender and caramelised in places, tip it all into one tray and toss lightly together. Transfer to a large serving dish. Spoon the chickpea mix on top of the roasted veg and serve.

VEG/NUT/PULSE VARIATIONS

You can use halved Brussels sprouts in place of the cauli or cabbage, and other root vegetables can join, or be swapped for the carrots – parsnips and swede are particularly good here. Walnuts work just as well as the almonds, giving a slightly more bitter-sweet flavour – and of course other tinned pulses, like cannellini or kidney beans, can be bashed up instead of chickpeas.

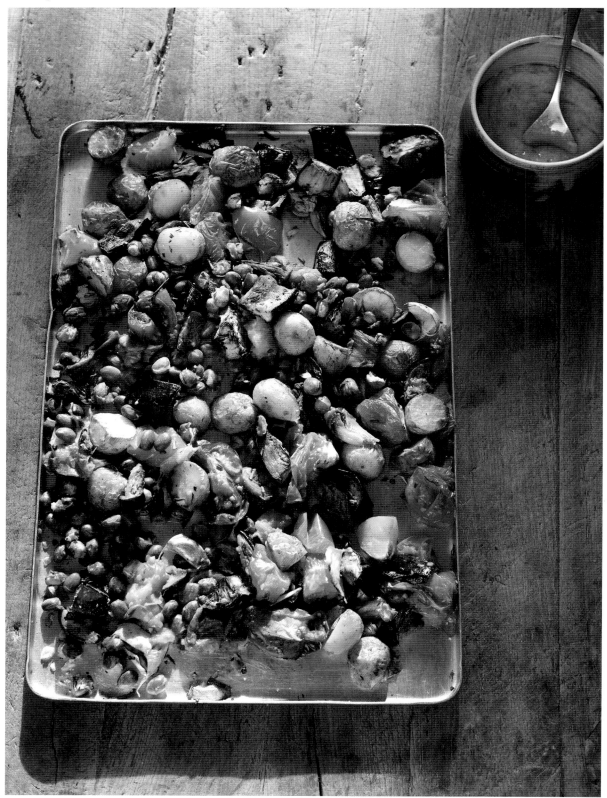

AUBERGINE, POTATO & TOMATO TRAY ROAST
with miso dressing

It surprises some to hear that these three wonderful vegetables are related, so different are their forms and flavours. But they are all members of the deadly nightshade family! Here they couldn't be more alive, coming together in perfect harmony with a knock-out dressing. If you don't need this dish to be vegan, a more old-school dressing with a crumbling of good cheese is another lovely way to finish it (see the variation below).

Serves 3–4

1 medium aubergine (about 300g)

About 300g new potatoes

4–6 garlic cloves, smashed

A large sprig of rosemary, leaves picked

2 tbsp olive or vegetable oil

500g tomatoes, ideally a mix of types and sizes, cut into chunks

400g tin beans (black, white or kidney beans), drained and rinsed

Sea salt and black pepper

For the miso dressing

2 tbsp white/shiro miso paste

2 tbsp virgin rapeseed or olive oil

1 tbsp raw cider vinegar

¼ garlic clove, crushed

A pinch of dried chilli flakes, or ¼ fresh red chilli, deseeded and finely chopped

To serve (optional)

Punchy salad leaves, such as rocket, mizuna, chicory or watercress

Preheat the oven to 190°C/Fan 170°C/Gas 5. Cut the aubergine and potatoes into roughly 2cm cubes and put into a large roasting tray with the garlic and rosemary. Season with a pinch of salt and a twist of pepper, trickle over the oil and toss well. Roast for 30 minutes.

Take the tray out and give everything a stir. Add the chunks of tomato, tucking them in, and return the tray to the oven. Turn the setting up to 200°C/Fan 180°C/Gas 6 and roast for a further 10–15 minutes until the tomatoes are juicy and bubbling and the potato is tender. Scatter over the beans and put back in the oven for 5 minutes.

Meanwhile, in a bowl, whisk together the ingredients for the miso dressing.

Spoon the dressing over the hot veg and beans, then serve up. Bitter or peppery leaves, like chicory, watercress, rocket or mizuna, are lovely on the side.

CHEESE VARIATION

Omit the miso and chilli from the dressing, combining the rest of the ingredients for a more conventional vinaigrette. After dressing the hot veg and beans, crumble 50–75g goat's cheese, feta or blue cheese (such as Dorset Blue Vinney, Shropshire Blue or my favourite, Harbourne Blue) over them. Give it a few minutes to melt and elevate the veg to a new level of savouriness.

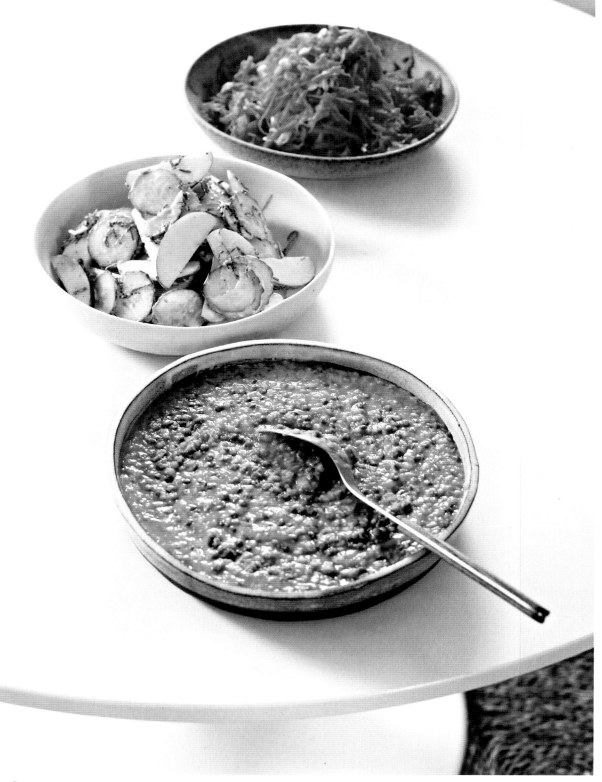

DOUBLE-DHAL
with carrot & raita salad

Nutty little Puy or beluga lentils are stirred into a freshly cooked dhal to give it extra body and texture, while crisp, raw carrot and a raita-style apple and cucumber salad lend plant-based goodness. Together, they make for a delicious, satisfying and healthy meal.

Serves 4

For the dhal

1 tbsp olive or vegetable oil

1–2 garlic cloves, sliced

1 tbsp curry powder

2 tsp cumin seeds

200g red lentils, rinsed

800ml veg stock (page 325) or water

400g tin Puy, beluga or green lentils, drained and rinsed, or 250g cooked lentils

1 tsp garam masala (optional)

Sea salt and black pepper

For the raita salad

2 medium crisp apples

½ cucumber (about 200g), sliced

A handful of mint leaves, shredded

3 tbsp natural yoghurt

A scrap of garlic (about ¼ clove), grated

For the carrots

About 400g carrots, coarsely grated

A couple of spring onions, trimmed and thinly sliced (optional)

Juice of 1 lemon

2 tbsp extra virgin olive oil

Set a large saucepan over a medium heat. Add the oil, sliced garlic, curry powder and cumin seeds. Cook gently for a couple of minutes, stirring often.

Before the garlic browns, add the rinsed red lentils, pour in the stock or water and bring to a gentle simmer. Cook, uncovered, for 20–25 minutes or until the lentils have broken down into a purée and the dhal is nice and thick. Stir the dhal regularly – ideally with a small whisk to help the lentils break down. If it gets too thick, add a splash of water.

While the dhal is cooking, prepare the raita salad. Quarter, core and thinly slice the apples. Place in a bowl with the cucumber, mint, yoghurt and garlic and turn gently together. In a second bowl, combine the grated carrots with the spring onions, if using, and the lemon juice and olive oil.

Once the dhal is cooked, stir in the tinned or pre-cooked lentils and cook for another minute or two, then season to taste with a pinch of salt and a twist of pepper. Stir in the garam masala, if you like. Transfer the dhal to a warm serving dish. Take it to the table with the grated carrot mix and the raita salad, and get everyone to help themselves.

VEG VARIATIONS
Grated raw beetroot makes a great alternative to the carrot here. Raw fennel, very thinly sliced or grated, is lovely instead of the apple in the raita salad.

ASIAN HOT POT

This is completely delicious and very filling! The mushrooms are fried 'hard' to start with, creating a lovely caramelised exterior that really adds to the flavour of the dish. I like to use black beans, but you can use kidney, cannellini or any other kind. The miso paste is optional but it does give the hot pot a boost of savoury, 'umami' character.

Serves 4

3–4 tbsp olive or vegetable oil

700g chestnut mushrooms, thickly sliced

½ large celeriac (about 500g) peeled and cut into 2cm cubes

A large thumb-sized piece of fresh ginger, grated

4 garlic cloves, sliced

2 x 400g tins beans (black, white or kidney), drained and rinsed

A bunch of spring onions, trimmed

A bunch of chard (200g), washed

About 2 tbsp white/shiro miso paste (optional)

2 tbsp soy sauce

Juice of 2 limes or 1 lemon, plus extra to taste

Sea salt and black pepper

3–4 tbsp chopped coriander, to finish (optional)

Set a large frying pan over a high heat. Add 2 tbsp of the oil, then half the mushrooms with a pinch of salt. Fry them 'hard' for 6–8 minutes, stirring only occasionally so they develop a rich golden-brown colour. If the mushrooms give out any liquid, cook until it's evaporated and keep going until they are nicely browned. Tip them into a very large saucepan or casserole. Repeat with the remaining oil and mushrooms.

Place the pan of mushrooms over a medium-high heat. Add the cubed celeriac with the ginger and garlic and fry for 2–3 minutes, stirring often. Tip in the beans and pour in enough water to just cover everything (about 700ml). Bring to a simmer and cook, uncovered, for 15 minutes or until the celeriac is just tender.

Meanwhile, cut the spring onions into 2cm slices and shred the chard into 1–2cm strips. Add them to the pan and stir well. Return to a simmer and cook for a further 5 minutes.

Take the pan off the heat. Scoop out a ladleful of the hot broth into a bowl and mix in 2 tbsp miso paste. Tip this thick liquid back into the hotpot, and add the soy and lime or lemon juice. Stir well. Taste and add more miso, lime/lemon, soy and/or pepper to taste. Ladle into bowls, finish with chopped coriander if you like, and serve.

VEG/PULSE VARIATIONS
In the summer, replace the celeriac with a mixture of waxy potatoes and carrots. Instead of chard, you can use spinach, spring greens or kale, removing the tough stalks. You can use any kind of tinned bean or pulse, including chickpeas or lentils.

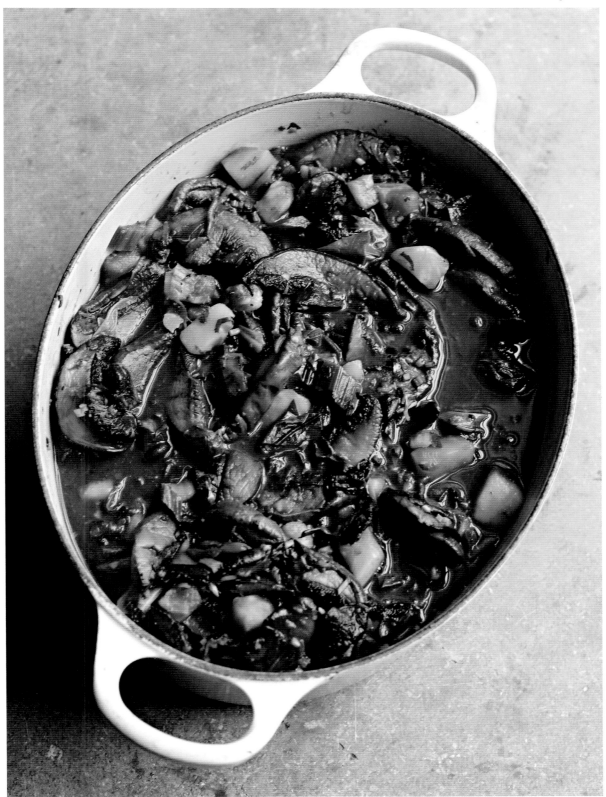

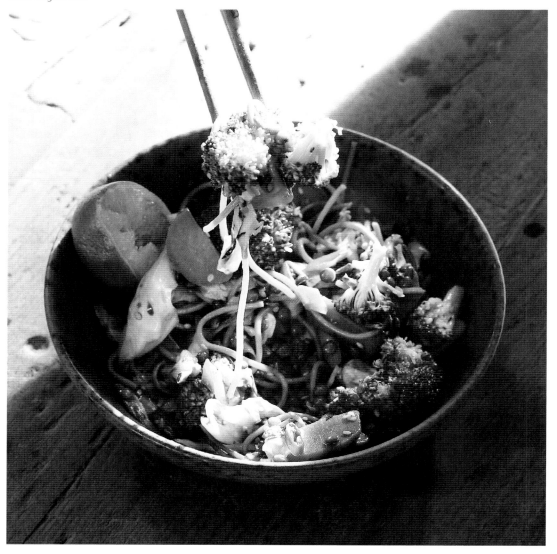

NOODLEY VEG STIR-FRY

There are a few simple rules to successful stir-frying: first, prepare all your veg before you begin, because stir-fries come together really quickly once you start cooking. Then, it's important not to crowd the pan, or the veg will soften but not colour – that's why I cook the veg here in two batches. And it's why I never attempt to cook a stir-fry for a crowd. You can double up this recipe and do each batch twice – to make it serve 4 or 5 – but I wouldn't go beyond that.

Caramelising the veg creates flavour, so don't be afraid to see a few golden-brown edges appearing on your veg – brassicas like cabbage are particularly delicious when lightly coloured.

And the final rule for me is to make this more about veg than noodles – so rather than stir-fried veg on top of a noodle mountain, a modest portion of the noodles is turned through the stir-fry at the end, for a pleasing tender texture amongst the crunchy veg.

I've gone for the most obvious mainstream veg – carrots, broccoli and cabbage – just to show how good they can be. But, of course, there's an endless variety of veg that are great in a stir-fry. You'll see a few suggestions below.

Serves 2

75–100g wholewheat, buckwheat or brown rice noodles (i.e. wholegrain)

Vegetable oil, for cooking

1 large or 2 medium carrots, sliced into thin half-moons

1 small head of broccoli, cut into small florets, stalk thinly sliced

½ small white or green cabbage, thinly sliced

2 garlic cloves, chopped

A bunch of spring onions, trimmed and sliced on the diagonal

½–1 fresh red or green chilli, sliced (and deseeded if you prefer less heat), or a pinch of dried chilli flakes

A handful of cooked lentils or cubed tofu (optional)

1–2 tbsp tamari or soy sauce

A trickle of toasted sesame oil (optional)

1 lime or lemon

Cook the noodles according the pack instructions, rinse thoroughly in cold water, toss with a few drops of oil and set aside.

Heat about ½ tbsp vegetable oil in a large wok or large frying pan over a high heat. When it is very hot, add the carrot(s) and broccoli and fry, tossing or stirring often but not constantly, for about 3–4 minutes, until starting to colour and become tender – but still with a bit of crunch. Transfer to a bowl.

Add a touch more oil to the pan then add the cabbage. Fry, tossing or stirring often, for a few minutes. Keep the heat high and allow the cabbage to colour in a few places. Throw the garlic, spring onions and chilli into the pan and fry for another minute.

Now add the carrot and broccoli back to the pan, along with the prepared noodles and lentils or tofu, if you choose to include some. Toss over the heat for a minute or two to thoroughly heat everything.

Turn off the heat and trickle over the tamari or soy sauce, sesame oil if using, and a good spritz of lime or lemon juice. Transfer to two large, warm bowls and eat straight away, squeezing over more lime or lemon if you like.

VEG VARIATIONS
Swap the carrot with parsnip or beetroot, and the broccoli with cauliflower. Try quartered Brussels sprouts in place of the cabbage. You can also use mangetout, French beans, courgette, sweet peppers, kohlrabi, celeriac… you name it.

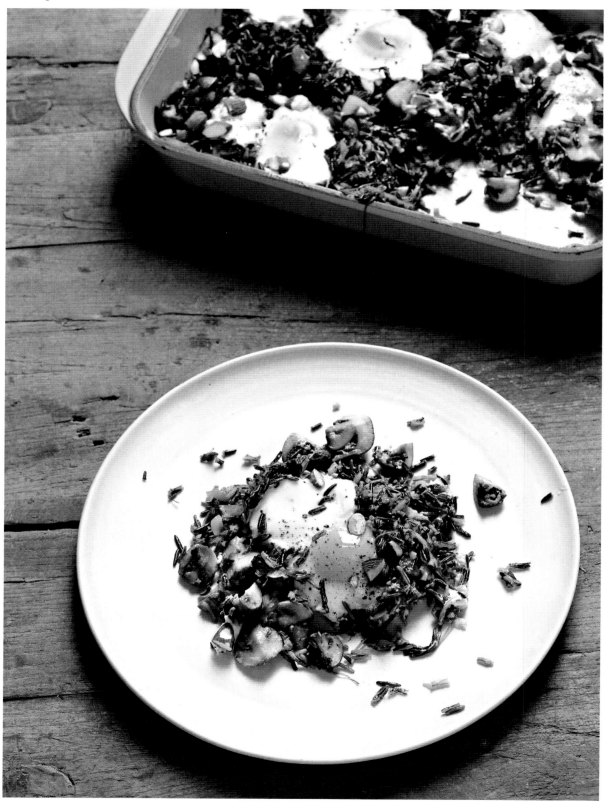

MUSHROOM & BLACK RICE 'CHACHOUKA'

A classic chachouka uses peppers and tomatoes, which are cooked together before being finished off with baked eggs (see below), but the concept is endlessly adaptable. Bake or roast almost any tasty combination of veg (plus grains and/or pulses if you like), then break in the eggs for the last 10 minutes of cooking, and you have a tasty, well-balanced supper. This is also a good way to use up leftover rice or other cooked grains.

Serves 4

150g black or red rice, or any other kind of wholegrain rice, pre-soaked if time

500g chestnut mushrooms, quartered

1 onion, roughly chopped

1–2 tbsp olive or vegetable oil

2 garlic cloves, chopped

2 small preserved lemons, finely diced, or finely grated zest of 1 lemon

250g spinach

2 tbsp crème fraîche

4 eggs

A handful of almonds, roughly chopped

Sea salt and black pepper

Cook the rice in plenty of gently simmering, lightly salted water for 20–35 minutes (the time will vary depending on the particular type of rice). Drain well. Meanwhile, preheat the oven to 190°C/Fan 170°C/Gas 5.

Put the mushrooms and onion into a large roasting dish, trickle with 1 tbsp oil and season with a pinch of salt and a twist of pepper. Roast for about 30 minutes, stirring once or twice, until the mushrooms are well coloured and the onion is tender. Stir in the garlic, diced lemons or lemon zest and the spinach. Return to the oven for 5–10 minutes, until the spinach is wilted.

Stir the cooked rice into the roasted veg. Dot over the crème fraîche and swirl it in a little. Make 4 shallow dips in the veg, to accommodate the eggs. Break the eggs into the dips. Pepper everything generously and scatter the chopped almonds over the veg, between the eggs. Return the dish to the oven for 8–10 minutes or until the egg whites are fully set but the yolks are still runny. Serve straight away.

CLASSIC CHACHOUKA

Fry 1 chopped onion and 2 sliced red peppers in an ovenproof wide pan with some cumin seeds and garlic until tender, about 20 minutes. Add 2 x 400g tins of tomatoes, roughly chopped, stir and simmer for 10–15 minutes to make a thick pulpy sauce. Stir in ½ tsp hot smoked paprika and check the seasoning. Then make 4 'hollows', break in 4 eggs and bake as above. Serve with wholegrain bread or cooked whole grains.

ROASTED PURPLE POWER

This is the roasted 'twin' of the lovely salad on page 254. The combination of sweet caramelised beetroot and onion, bitter radicchio, tomatoes and kidney beans is amazingly tasty – and colourful to boot.

Serves 2

1 large or 2 small–medium red onions, cut into wedges

2–3 medium beetroot (about 300g in total), scrubbed and cut into wedges

2 tbsp olive or vegetable oil

6–8 medium tomatoes, quartered, or 300g whole cherry tomatoes

1 head of radicchio, cut into thick wedges, or 2 red chicory bulbs, quartered lengthways

400g tin kidney beans, drained and rinsed

½ orange

Sea salt and black pepper

Preheat the oven to 190°C/Fan 170°C/Gas 5.

Put the onion and beetroot wedges into a large roasting tray. Add the oil, a pinch of salt and a twist of pepper and toss together lightly. Roast for about 45 minutes, taking the tray out and stirring a couple of times, until the beetroot is tender.

Add the tomatoes and the radicchio or chicory and toss lightly. Return to the oven for 15–20 minutes, until the radicchio is wilted and the tomatoes are soft and juicy. Throw in the kidney beans and return to the oven for 5 minutes, to heat them through. Squeeze over the juice of the orange and serve straight away.

VEG/PULSE VARIATIONS
You can replace the beetroot with other root veg, such as carrots, celeriac or parsnips, and the kidney beans with white beans or chickpeas.

FINISHING OPTIONS
Any of the above can be served with a spoonful of natural yoghurt or a crumbling of feta or goat's cheese, if you fancy – or a few dabs of my pestomega (page 278).

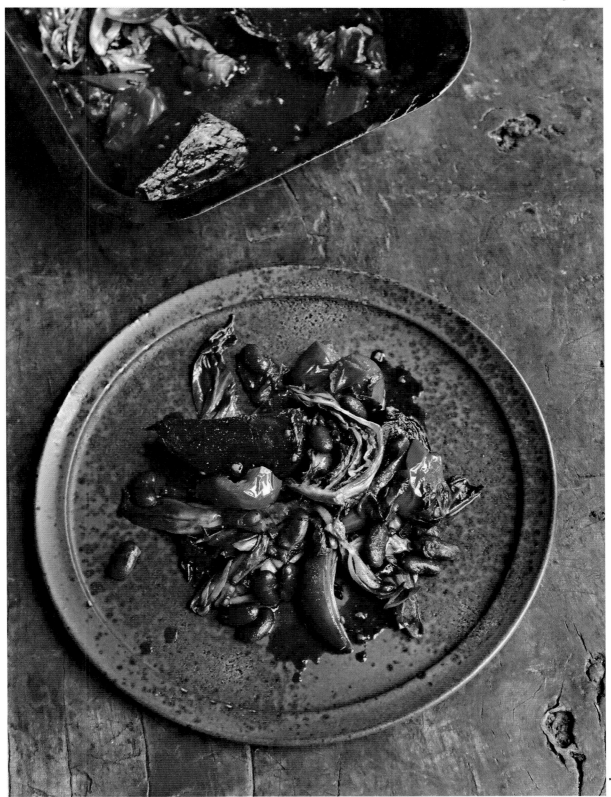

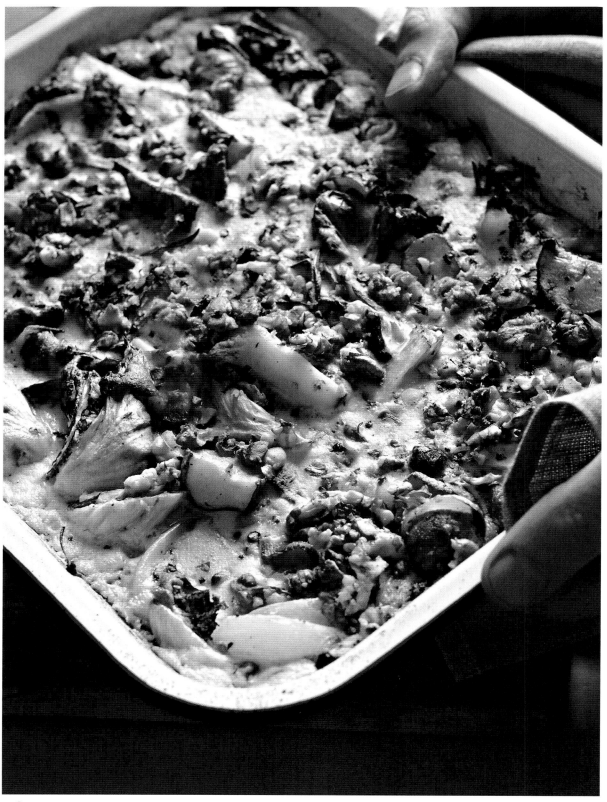

ARTICHOKE & RADICCHIO GRATIN

This is a dish full of creamy, bubbling comfort. It's also totally plant-based (so vegan), high in fibre, packed with pulses and nuts, and big on prebiotics (from the Jerusalem artichokes and onions) to nurture your gut.

Serves 4

400g Jerusalem artichokes, scrubbed and cut into chunks

2 large or 3 medium onions, cut into chunky wedges

1–2 tbsp olive or vegetable oil

A few bay leaves and/or sprigs of thyme or rosemary (optional)

1 head of radicchio, cut into 8 wedges, or 2 red or white chicory bulbs, quartered

½ x 400g tin white beans, such as cannellini, drained and rinsed (note, another ½ tin is used in the sauce)

A handful of buckwheat groats or smashed walnuts, or a mix

Sea salt and black pepper

For the creamy cashew sauce

350ml hot veg stock (page 325)

100g cashew nuts

½ x 400g tin white beans, such as cannellini, drained and rinsed

1 tsp English mustard

A scrap of garlic (about ¼ clove), finely grated

For the cashew sauce, pour the hot stock over the cashew nuts and leave them to soak for at least 10 minutes, or up to 30.

Preheat the oven to 190°C/Fan 170°C/Gas 5. Put the artichokes and onions into a large roasting dish. Trickle with 1 tbsp oil, tuck in any herbs you're using, and season lightly with salt and pepper. Toss well and roast for about 35 minutes, until the veg are tender.

Take out of the oven, stir well, then add the radicchio or chicory and a trickle more oil. Return to the oven for about 10 minutes, until the radicchio or chicory is wilted.

Meanwhile, make the sauce. Put the soaked cashews and veg stock, half tin of white beans, mustard, garlic and some black pepper into a blender and blitz until smooth.

When all the veg are cooked, add the other half tin of white beans and stir in. Trickle the cashew sauce over everything and give it all a stir. Scatter with the nuts or buckwheat groats and return to the oven for 10 minutes or until browned and bubbling, then serve.

VEG VARIATIONS
Parsnips or celeriac – or a combination – are the best replacements for Jerusalem artichokes if you can't get them (they are in season in the winter).

ALMOND VARIATION
You can use almonds instead of cashews, but they need longer soaking – at least 30 minutes but, better still, an hour.

SEARED HISPI CABBAGE & ORANGE
with citrus hummus & dukka

Searing cabbage in a hot pan gives it new layers of flavour and colour that are quite transformative. These charred wedges are delicious with juicy 'burnt' oranges, a creamy, tangy hummus and a scattering of dukka.

Serves 2

1 firm summer cabbage such as hispi/sweetheart (about 600g)

2–3 small oranges (or 4 clementines or 'easy-peelers')

About ½ tbsp rapeseed or olive oil

About 200g nutty citrus hummus (page 277), or good-quality shop-bought plain hummus

A little lemon or orange juice (or water)

A little extra virgin olive or rapeseed oil

A pinch of dried chilli flakes (optional)

Sea salt and black pepper

To finish

A handful of mint or parsley leaves, chopped (optional)

A good handful of dukka (page 281) or 30g toasted pumpkin seeds

Remove any dirty outer leaves from the cabbage and trim the stalk if necessary. Slice the cabbage in half, going down through the centre. Slice each half into four so you have 8 wedges, each still held together by a section of stalk at the centre. Don't worry if some of the leaves come free – they can all go into the pan.

To prepare the oranges, slice off the top and bottom ends then cut into thick, skin-on horizontal slices. You should get 3 or 4 slices from each orange. Set aside.

Put a large, non-stick frying pan over a medium-high heat (if you don't have a nice big pan, cook this in two batches). Brush the cabbage wedges sparingly with oil and season them lightly with salt and pepper. Add them to the hot pan and sear for 4–6 minutes, turning them a few times with tongs, and making sure you get lots of charring on all their surfaces. They shouldn't stick, but add a trickle more oil if you need to.

Meanwhile, get your hummus ready. It works best here thinned to a loose spoonable consistency, so add a dash of orange or lemon juice, or even water.

When the cabbage is nicely coloured and the stalk at the centre just yields to the tip of a knife (it should still be quite firm), transfer to a warm dish and keep warm. Brush the cut surfaces of the orange slices with a little more oil and add them to the pan. Sear for a few minutes, turning once, until they're nicely coloured and caramelised.

Arrange the seared oranges slices over the cabbage. Add the hummus in generous streaks or dollops, a trickle of extra virgin oil and a pinch of chilli flakes for a touch of heat if you wish. Add a sprinkle of chopped mint or parsley, if you like. Finish with a scattering of dukka or, more simply, toasted pumpkin seeds, and tuck in.

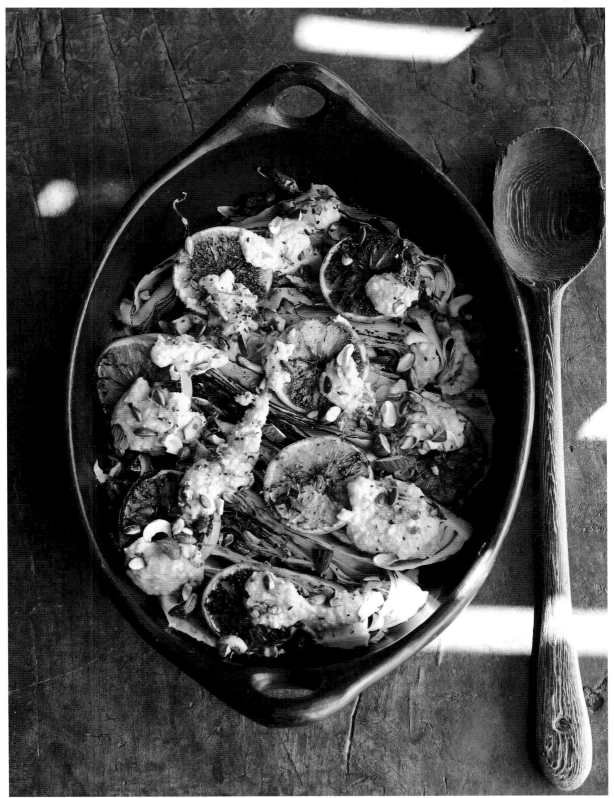

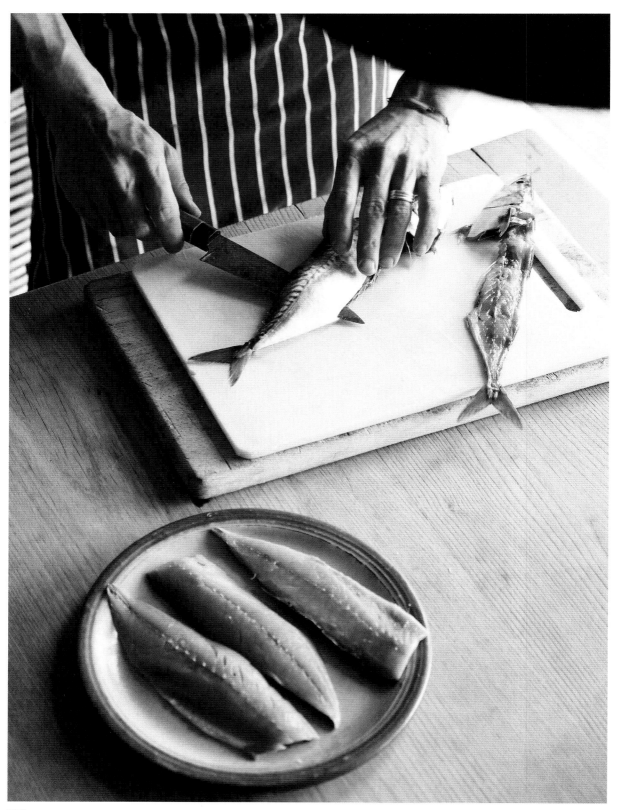

FEISTY FISH

I love eating fish, and I love feeding it to my family. It's one of the healthiest and most delicious protein-rich foods there is – full of nutrients and healthy fats, including those brain-boosting and body-bolstering omega 3s (see pages 43 and 125).

Fish and shellfish are so good for us, in fact, that many of us could probably do with eating more of them. But I know that some cooks lack confidence when it comes to cooking fish – and when it comes to buying it in the first place. I can understand that. It's not a cheap food; you don't want to shell out (sorry!) for something that might not be the freshest and finest; and you're understandably nervous of tricky cooking methods that might not give the results you hoped for.

The recipes here are so easy that there is no reason to be fish-shy. They are based on a forgiving approach to cooking fish – saucy and juicy – that includes a little margin for error. And all of them find the fish supported by – and agreeably flavoured with – some simple, rewarding veg, pulses and seasonings.

The species of fish you choose is flexible (that's an important principle in itself, to help keep fish stocks sustainable), so you don't need to feel pinned down. You can go for what's best and freshest on the day. You should always feel free to engage your fishmonger on that score; or if you're buying your fish in the supermarket, look for a margin of 2 or 3 days in the use-by date.

The truth is you don't need an extensive repertoire of fish recipes to enjoy a delicious and regular feed of fish. This little clutch will keep your piscine appetite piqued for many a meal.

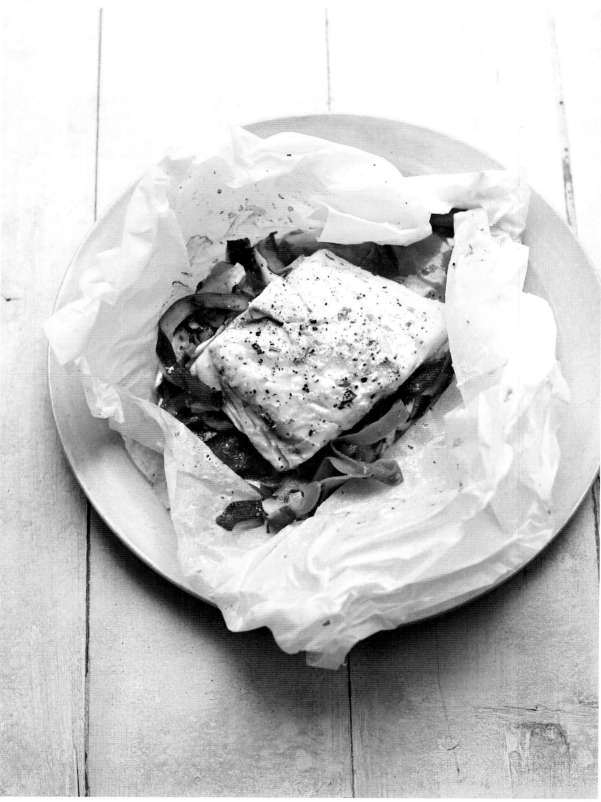

BAKED FISH & VEG PARCELS

This way of cooking fish is a real River Cottage favourite. You can use fillets of almost any fish, and vary the veg and seasoning according to what you have. It all cooks together to form a delicious pool of fragrant juice that will spill out of the parcel on to your plate.

Serves 4

500g courgettes (4 medium)

400g carrots

A bunch of spring onions, trimmed

2 garlic cloves, thinly sliced

A few sprigs of thyme, leaves picked and roughly chopped

A small bunch of parsley, leaves picked and chopped (optional)

3–4 tbsp olive oil

4 fish fillets (150–200g each), such as hake or coley, or sustainable (MSC-certified) haddock or cod

About 200ml white wine or cider, veg stock (page 325), or tomato passata

Sea salt and black pepper

Cooked whole grains (30–60g per serving), to serve

Preheat the oven to 200°C/Fan 180°C/Gas 6 and have ready a large baking tray with a rim (so no juices can escape). Tear off 4 large sheets of greaseproof paper or foil.

Cut the courgettes into thin ribbons or fine slices, using a mandolin, swivel veg peeler or a food processor fitted with a thin slicing blade. Put the courgettes into a large bowl. Ribbon or slice the carrots in the same way and add to the courgettes.

Finely slice the spring onions and add these too, along with the garlic, thyme, parsley if using, and 2 tbsp of the olive oil. Season with a pinch of salt and a twist of pepper. Toss together well with your hands.

Pile the veg in the middle of each sheet of paper or foil, dividing it equally. Place a fish fillet on top of each pile and season it with salt and pepper. Gather up the edges of the paper or foil and bring them up around the veg and fish. Pour a good splash of wine, cider, stock or passata into each parcel.

Crimp the top edges of the parcel together. With foil, you'll be able to seal the package completely; with paper, you can just scrunch it up so the fish is mostly covered. Place the parcels carefully on the baking tray. Bake in the oven for 15–20 minutes or until the fish is cooked through and the veg is just done (it will still be *al dente*).

Bring the parcels to the table and accompany with whole grains, to soak up the juices.

VEG VARIATIONS
Try swapping thinly sliced fennel, halved, slender asparagus spears, or some baby peas or petits pois for the courgettes. Halved cherry tomatoes can go in there too! And wafer-thin slices of young summer beetroot make a great swap for the carrot.

SPICY FISH FINGERS
with tomato & bean salad

I often coat my homemade fish fingers just with seasoned, beaten egg, rather than with flour and egg and breadcrumbs – to both simplify the process and cut back on the refined carbs. It works a treat. In this spicy version, I've used a bit of curry powder too. I serve these delicious fish bites with a well-seasoned tomato and bean salad, instead of the knee-jerk tomato ketchup – it's more filling and much better for you!

Serves 4

About 600g skinless white fish fillet, such as pollack, coley, sustainable (MSC-certified) cod or haddock

2 tbsp curry powder

2 eggs

Vegetable oil, for frying

For the tomato and bean salad

500g ripe sweet tomatoes (any size)

1 red onion, halved and thinly sliced

400g tin white beans, such as haricot or cannellini, drained and rinsed

½ cucumber (about 200g), diced into 1cm cubes (optional)

1 medium-hot fresh red chilli, deseeded and sliced

A small bunch of parsley, leaves picked and chopped (optional)

2 tbsp olive oil

1 tbsp red wine vinegar or raw cider vinegar

A scrap of garlic (about ¼ clove), finely grated

Sea salt and black pepper

Start with the salad. Roughly chop the tomatoes or, if you're using cherry tomatoes, just halve or quarter them. Put them into a large bowl and add the rest of the salad ingredients, seasoning with a pinch of salt and a twist of pepper. Tumble everything together gently then leave to sit while you make the fish fingers.

Cut the fish into large fingers, allowing 4 or 5 per person. Place the fish on a large plate and scatter over the curry powder, a pinch of salt and a twist of pepper. Turn the fish in the spices to coat it evenly.

Break the eggs into a bowl, season with salt and pepper and beat together. Put a large, non-stick frying pan over a medium heat and add enough oil to cover the base in a thin film. Have ready a plate lined with kitchen paper.

When the oil is hot, dip a piece of fish into the egg to coat, let the excess drain off, then lay in the hot frying pan. Repeat with the rest of the fish, cooking it in a couple of batches and adding an extra dash of oil to the pan if needed. Fry the fish fingers for 2–3 minutes on each side, until cooked through. Lift out onto the paper-lined plate.

As soon as all the fish fingers are done, bring them to the table, along with the tomato and bean salad, and tuck in.

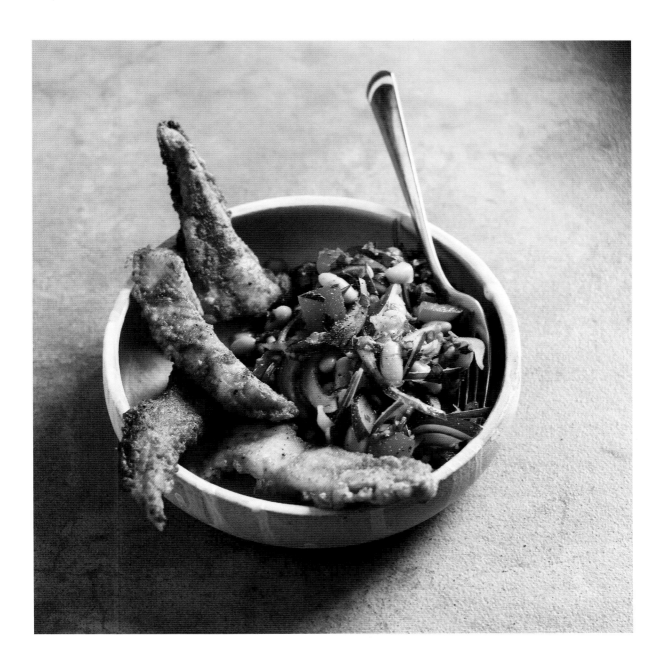

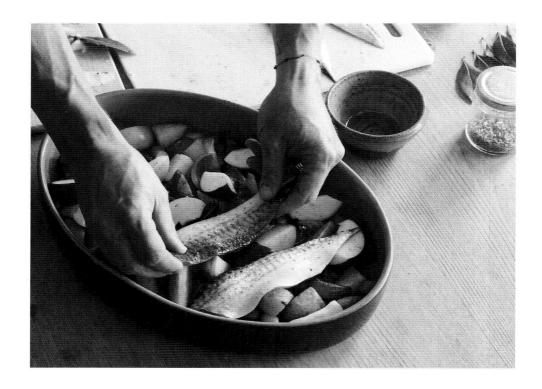

MACKEREL ON ROASTED VEG & FRUIT

This is a lovely variation of an old River Cottage favourite: baking mackerel over potatoes roasted with onions, bay leaves and lemon wedges. Here I've swapped around the veg and added some fruit – apples are lovely with mackerel – and a nice bit of spice.

Serves 4

300g new potatoes, peeled and cut into chunky cubes

4 large carrots, cut into chunky pieces

2 red onions, each cut into 8 wedges

1 garlic bulb, broken into cloves, peeled

2 tbsp olive oil

2 tart eating apples, cored and each cut into 8 wedges

1 tsp cumin, caraway or fennel seeds

2 very fresh large (or 4 medium) mackerel, filleted

8 bay leaves

Sea salt and black pepper

½ lemon, cut into 4 wedges, to serve (optional)

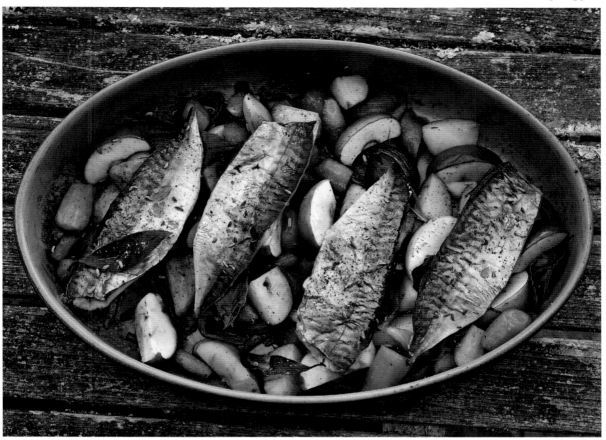

Preheat the oven to 200°C/Fan 180°C/Gas 6.

Put the potatoes, carrots, onions and garlic cloves into a large oven dish and trickle over most of the olive oil. Season with a pinch of salt and a twist of pepper and tumble everything together. Roast for 40–45 minutes, taking the dish out once or twice for a good stir, until the veg is looking golden and appetising.

Scatter the apple wedges into the dish and toss lightly with the roasted veg. Sprinkle over the spice seeds, saving a few for the fish. Lay the mackerel fillets, skin side up, on top. Brush or trickle the fish with a little more olive oil and tuck a bay leaf under and over each fillet. Sprinkle over the rest of the spice seeds and season with salt and pepper.

Return the dish to the top of the oven for 12–15 minutes or until the mackerel fillets are cooked and the skin is golden and blistered. Alternatively, you can finish it by placing the dish under a hot grill, to get a bit of crisp, golden blistering on the skin of the fish. The heat of the veg will cook the fish through from underneath as well. Serve at once, with lemon wedges for squeezing over, if you like.

FISH WITH FENNEL, TOMATOES & CHICKPEAS

Another nifty example of roasting fish fillets on top of fragrant, hearty veg, this easy, one-dish supper is full of delicious Mediterranean flavours. You can use any white fish.

Serves 4

2 large or 3 medium fennel bulbs, trimmed

1 large onion (red or brown), halved and sliced

4 garlic cloves, sliced

300g ripe tomatoes, cut into wedges, or whole cherry tomatoes

400g tin chickpeas, drained and rinsed

Finely grated zest and juice of ½ lemon

½ tsp hot smoked paprika or a good pinch of cayenne or dried chilli flakes

2 tbsp olive oil

2 sprigs of rosemary (optional)

About 600g white fish fillet, such as pollack, hake or coley, or sustainable (MSC-certified) haddock or cod, cut into 8 equal pieces

A small bunch of parsley, leaves picked and chopped, or a small bunch of chives, snipped (optional)

Sea salt and black pepper

Preheat the oven to 200°C/Fan 180°C/Gas 6.

Cut each of the fennel bulbs into 6–8 wedges and put them into a large roasting tray with the onion, garlic, tomatoes and chickpeas. Sprinkle with the lemon zest, smoked paprika, cayenne or chilli. Trickle over the olive oil and season with salt and pepper.

Tumble everything together so the oil and seasonings coat all the veg. Tuck in the rosemary sprigs, if using, then place in the oven. Bake for 35–40 minutes until the veg is golden and tender, taking it out and giving everything a good stir halfway through.

Take the tray from the oven. Season the pieces of fish with a pinch of salt and a twist of pepper, then nestle them, skin side up, amongst the veg. Return the tray to the oven for 10–12 minutes, or until the fish is just cooked through. If using parsley or chives, scatter over everything. Give the dish a good spritz of lemon juice and serve straight away.

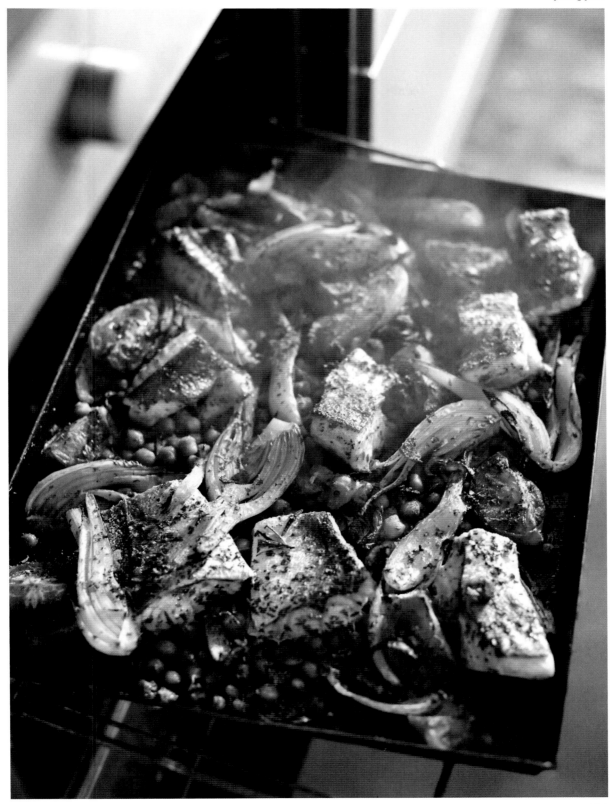

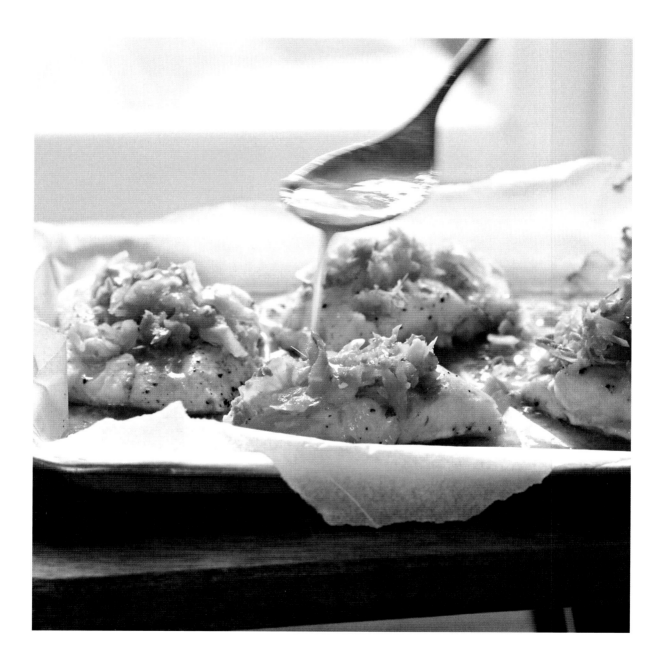

BAKED HAKE WITH KIMCHI BUTTER

Kimchi – Korean-style spicy fermented cabbage – is an amazing, all-in-one vegetable/ condiment/seasoning. It's also rich with friendly probiotic bacteria to nurture your gut. In this recipe, I cook the fish in a mix of kimchi 'juice' and butter for maximum flavour, but keep the kimchi itself uncooked, to preserve those wonderful friendly bacteria. It makes for an incredibly tasty fish dish. Serve it with broccoli, green beans or any other green veg and add a spoonful of brown rice or a few new potatoes if you're very hungry.

Serves 4

A little vegetable oil

4 pieces of hake, about 150g each (or use any chunky white fish)

125g live kimchi (ideally homemade, page 286)

30g unsalted butter, or 2 tbsp olive or rapeseed oil

Black pepper

Cooked whole grains or new potatoes, or wholegrain bread, to serve (optional)

Preheat the oven to 180°C/Fan 160°C/Gas 4. Line a roasting tray with greaseproof paper, oil very lightly and place the pieces of hake, skin side down on the paper.

Spoon the kimchi into a sieve over a smallish saucepan and press with a wooden spoon or spatula so that the tangy kimchi juice is squeezed out into the pan. Roughly chop the squeezed-out kimchi and set aside.

Add the butter or oil to the pan with the kimchi juice and heat gently, stirring, to melt the butter and combine the butter or oil with the juice.

Spoon the kimchi butter over the hake. Season with pepper and bake in the oven for 10–12 minutes until the fish is just cooked through.

Pile the squeezed-out kimchi on top of the fish, spoon over the juices from the tray and serve. For a more substantial meal, you can accompany the fish with whole grains or new potatoes, or simply offer a slice of wholegrain bread to mop up the lovely juices.

FRESH SARDINES WITH PANZANELLA SALSA

This is a delicious summery way to eat fresh sardines – and it's especially fine if the sardines are done on the barbecue. The side dish – a cross between a tomato salsa and a panzanella salad – cuts the richness of the sardines brilliantly. Fresh sardines vary a lot in size. By late summer, the lovely Cornish ones are quite chunky and three will make a hearty main, but you might need five smaller ones each.

Serves 2

6–10 fresh sardines (depending on size), gutted and descaled

Olive oil, for brushing

Sea salt and black pepper

For the panzanella salsa

A fairly large slice of wholegrain or rye sourdough or other wholemeal bread

½ garlic clove

About 2 tbsp olive oil

About 250g ripe cherry tomatoes, or larger tomatoes (or a mix)

A few chives, snipped, or 2–3 spring onions, thinly sliced

A small handful of basil or mint leaves (or both), torn

½ lemon

To serve (optional)

Lemon wedges

First prepare the panzanella salsa: toast (or barbecue) the sourdough slice, then lightly rub both sides with the cut surface of the garlic clove. Trickle over half the olive oil and leave for a minute so the oil is absorbed. Tear or cut into fairly small pieces.

Halve or quarter cherry tomatoes and/or roughly chop the bigger ones and place in a bowl with the sourdough pieces. Add the rest of the olive oil, the herbs and a little salt and pepper, and toss to combine. Leave to mingle while you cook the fish.

If you are cooking outdoors, heat up your barbecue ready for cooking. Or, if you're cooking indoors, get a ridged grill pan nice and hot. Brush the sardines with a little olive oil, season with salt and pepper and place on the hot grill/barbecue. Grill for about 3 minutes on one side, without moving (they are less likely to stick if they get nicely charred), then carefully turn them and grill for 2 or 3 minutes on the second side.

Transfer the sardines to serving plates. Give the salsa a re-mingle and spoon alongside. Grind over some pepper and serve with a lemon wedge if you like, to squeeze over.

VARIATIONS

Fresh sardines are a total joy but, if you can't get hold of them, this salsa works brilliantly with tinned sardines too. You can also serve it alongside all kinds of barbecued fish – it is especially good with mackerel and red mullet. It's lovely with barbecued chicken or pork chops, too. And if your barbecue plans don't pan out then you can simply roast your fish, or pan-fry the fillets.

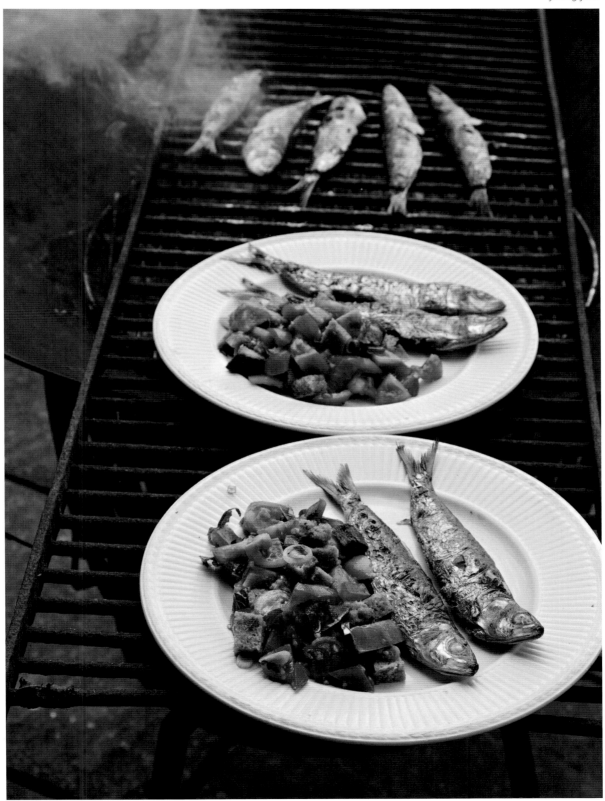

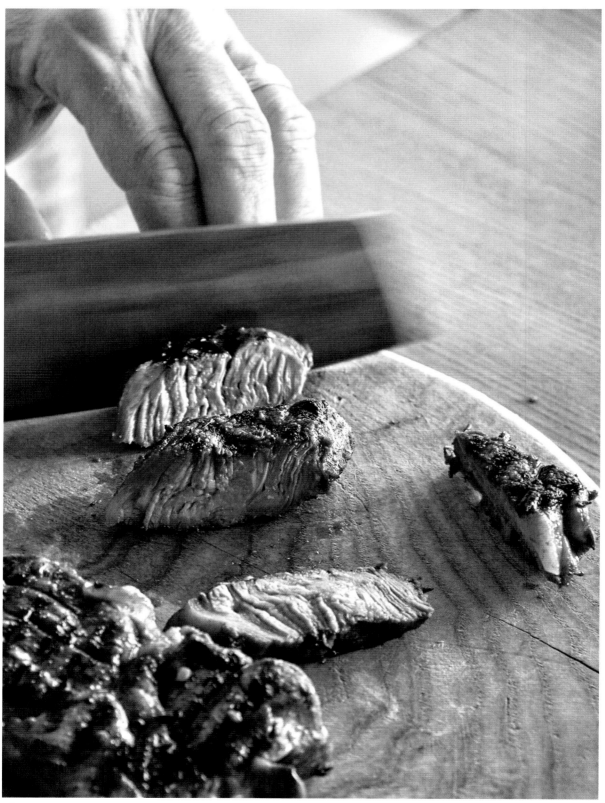

(LESS IS) MORE MEAT

This chapter pretty much sets out the way I like to eat meat these days. For a start, it contains less than 10% of the recipes in this book. That feels like a healthy proportion to me, and reflects the fact that I now have more days without meat than with. And when you look at the recipes themselves, you'll see that meat is always partnered with plenty of veg, whole grains or pulses. These other ingredients are not mere trimmings but equal partners in the feast; or even the main event, with the meat being the icing on the cake (metaphorically!)...

Let's not forget that good meat, for those who choose to eat it, is a good food – by which I mean that, in moderation, it's really good for you. Eating meat healthily certainly doesn't have to mean foregoing old favourites. But it's a good idea to take a fresh look at them, and make sure they are optimised for goodness as well as flavour. That's what I have done here with classics like chilli con carne, roast chicken and shepherd's pie – they've all got a whole veg boost without diminishing the pleasure of the meat. And they don't generally need an extra carb on the side.

I hope that eating less meat, less often, will also help you feel that you can afford to choose the best. If you're going to roast a chicken only once a month, say, you may be happy to spend the extra pounds that a good organic bird will cost. Similarly, with the other meats you'll find in these recipes, I'd urge you to choose organic, free-range, grass-fed or at the very least RSPCA Assured meat. You will enjoy better quality and flavour, just as the animals will have enjoyed more natural, contented lives.

ROAST CHICKEN WITH GARLIC & ROOTS

This is a brilliant way to roast a chicken: a load of lovely root veg is thrown in with it so the flavours mingle. You can happily swap or add in other root veg, such as celeriac, beetroot or sweet potato.

<u>Serves 4 (with some leftovers)</u>

1 free-range chicken (1.5–1.7kg)

2 medium leeks or onions, trimmed

1 whole garlic bulb, cloves separated and lightly bashed

A couple of bay leaves and/or sprigs of thyme or rosemary (optional)

4 tbsp olive or rapeseed oil

2 large or 3 medium carrots

1 large or 2 medium parsnips

2 large or 3 medium potatoes (about 250–300g)

Sea salt and black pepper

Take the chicken from the fridge an hour or two before cooking and leave it in a cool place to come to room temperature. Preheat the oven to 180°C/Fan 160°C/Gas 4.

Cut the leeks into chunks or the onions into wedges. Put into a large bowl with the garlic, and herbs if using. Add half the oil and some salt and pepper and toss together.

Place the chicken in a large roasting tin, untruss the legs and pull them gently away from the body, which will help to open up the cavity. Put the leeks or onions and garlic inside the chicken, but don't cram it full – air should still be able to circulate inside. If it doesn't all fit some can go in the tray with the rest of the veg.

Scrub or peel the carrots, parsnips and potatoes, cut into chunky pieces and put them into the bowl you dressed the leeks/onions in. Add the remaining oil, season and toss together. Arrange this veg around the bird in the roasting tin. Rub any seasoned oil left in the bowl over the chicken's skin, then give it another little dusting of salt and pepper. Turn the chicken upside down (it'll probably rest on one side of the breast, which is fine).

Roast the chicken for 20–25 minutes. Take it out of the oven, stir the veg in the roasting tin, turn the chicken breast side up and roast for another 20 minutes or so.

Remove from the oven again, spoon the garlic and leek/onion mix out of the chicken into the roasting tin and stir to mingle with the veg already there. Roast for another 15–25 minutes, until the chicken is cooked through. This skin should be golden and crispy, and the juices that run from the bird when you pierce the flesh between the thigh and the body should be completely clear. If you like using a probe thermometer, the thickest part of the meat should register at least 72°C.

Leave the whole thing to rest, covered in foil, for 10–15 minutes. Carve your chicken and serve with the veg from the roasting tin. A leafy green veg, or simple green salad, is a pleasing accompaniment.

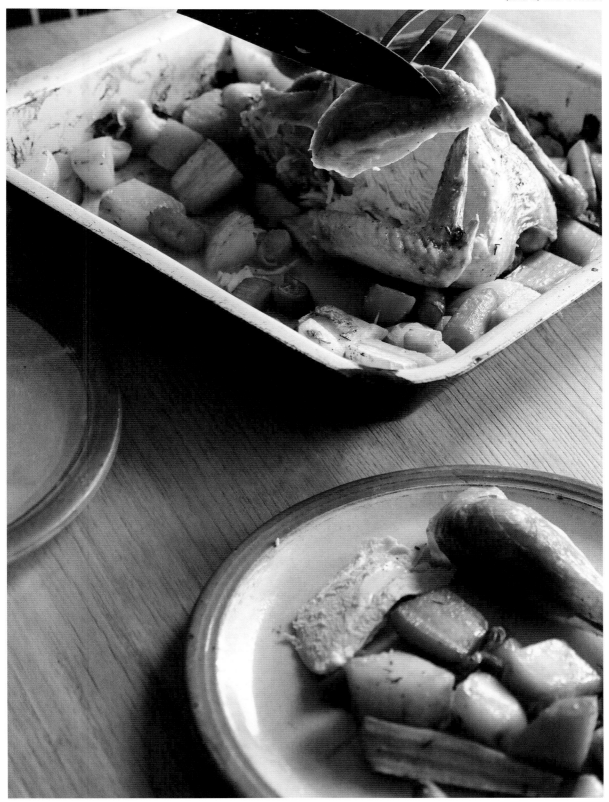

MOROCCAN-SPICED LAMB STEAKS
with herby barley tabbouleh

This is a lovely way to eat lamb steak: a modest but flavour-packed serving of meat on a zesty, herby tabbouleh. The meat is rubbed with dry spices – if I've got time, I roast whole spices briefly in a dry frying and grind them myself using a pestle and mortar, but if I'm on the fly, I'll use ready-ground spices.

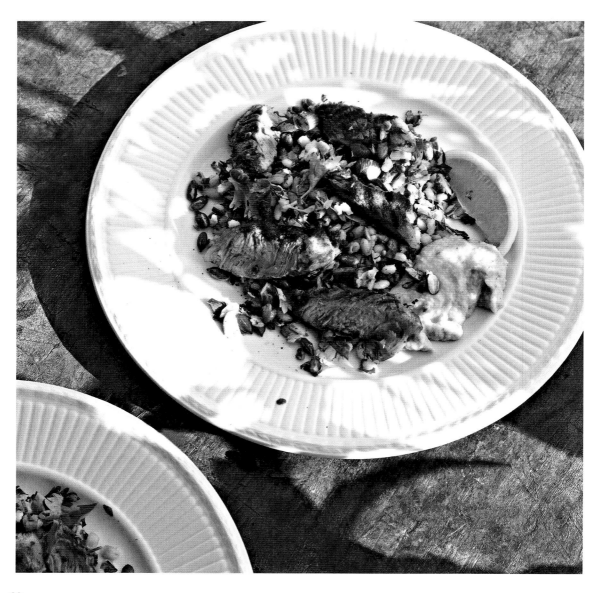

Serves 4

1 large or 2 medium lamb leg steaks
(about 300–350g in total)

A little olive or vegetable oil

For the spice rub

½ tsp ground cumin

½ tsp ground coriander

½ tsp ground mixed spice

A good pinch of hot paprika or cayenne

A good pinch of salt

For the herby tabbouleh

150g pearl barley, pre-soaked if time
(see page 249)

A large bunch of flat-leaf parsley, tougher
stalks removed

A bunch of coriander, leaves picked

A small bunch of mint, leaves picked

A small bunch of chives

Grated zest and juice of 1 lemon

Grated zest and juice of ½ orange

2 tbsp extra virgin olive oil

Sea salt and black pepper

To serve

Nutty citrus hummus (page 277), warmed

Dukka (page 281), optional

Lemon wedges

For the tabbouleh, cook the pearl barley in simmering water, according to the pack instructions until just tender (probably 25–30 minutes, quicker if pre-soaked), then drain and leave to cool. Roughly chop the parsley, coriander and mint, and finely snip the chives. Toss the herbs, citrus zest and juice, olive oil and some salt and pepper through the cooled pearl barley. Set aside to allow the flavours to mingle.

Meanwhile, combine the ingredients for the spice rub. Very lightly oil the lamb steak, then rub the spice mix all over it. Leave for about 30 minutes to come up to room temperature and absorb some of the flavour of the spices. Then gently scrape off excess spice mix so it doesn't burn in the pan.

Heat a heavy-based pan or griddle over a high heat. Add the seasoned lamb and 'dry-fry' for about 3 minutes on each side, for nicely pink meat (cook it a little longer if you prefer your lamb medium). Transfer to a wooden board to rest for a few minutes.

Divide the herby tabbouleh between serving plates. Slice the lamb steaks into roughly 2cm thick slices and arrange on the tabbouleh. Add a generous spoonful of warm hummus and finish with dukka if you like. Serve with lemon wedges, for squeezing over.

MEAT VARIATIONS
Instead of lamb steaks, use beef rump steak or try spicy lamb sausages such as merguez, or strips of leftover roast lamb – fried and seasoned with the spice mix.

TABBOULEH VARIATIONS
For a more classic tabbouleh, use cracked bulgar wheat instead of pearl barley. Or you can replace the barley with another cooked whole grain, such as spelt, pearl barley, farro (aka emmer), brown rice or even quinoa.

DUCK & BRAISED RED CABBAGE
with raisins & orange

Duck legs are roasted over red cabbage and onion until crisp-skinned, then shredded and tossed through the veg in this easy one-pot dish. Chunks of juicy orange go in at the end for a shot of fruity freshness. The sweet-and-sour fruity cabbage combination also makes a lovely, vibrant salad (see page 295).

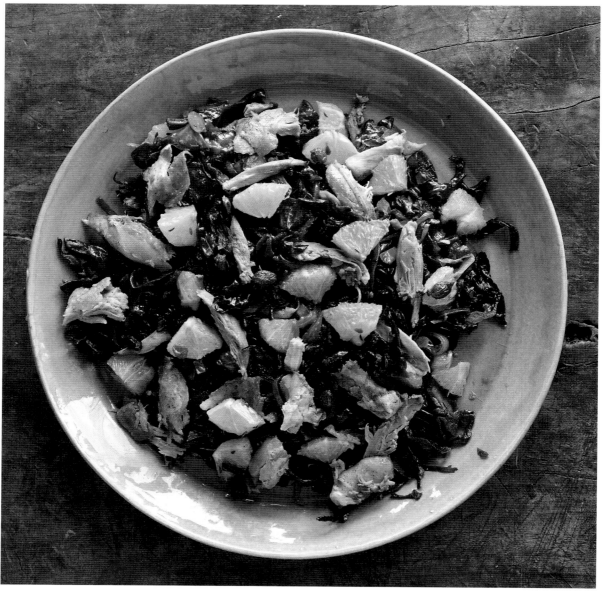

Serves 4

2 free-range duck legs

A trickle of olive or vegetable oil

1 medium red cabbage (about 700g), core trimmed out, very thinly sliced

2 garlic cloves, thinly sliced

1 red onion, thinly sliced

50g raisins

2 tsp caraway seeds (or use fennel, cumin or celery seeds)

½–1 medium-hot fresh red chilli, deseeded and sliced (or a pinch of dried chilli flakes)

2 oranges

Juice of ½ lemon

Sea salt and black pepper

Preheat the oven to 220°C/Fan 200°C/Gas 7. Put the duck legs, skin side up, into a large, deep roasting tray. Trickle over a little oil and season with salt and pepper. Rub or brush the oil and seasoning into the duck legs. Place in the hot oven and cook for 30 minutes.

Meanwhile, mix the cabbage, garlic, onion, raisins, caraway or other seeds and chilli together in a large bowl with a good pinch each of salt and pepper.

Take the tray from the oven and transfer the duck to a dish. Duck legs can be very fatty; if they are, you can tip out any excess fat from the tray at this point, but leave a little (the flavour's great), along with any juices and crispy bits, in the tray. Tip the cabbage mixture into the hot roasting tray, add a splash of water (½ small glass) and mix thoroughly.

Spread the cabbage mix out evenly, put the duck legs back on top, skin side up, and cover the tray with foil. Return the tray to the oven, lower the setting to 180°C/Fan 160°C/Gas 4 and cook for 45 minutes.

Take out the tray and give the cabbage a stir, working around the duck as you go. Return the uncovered tray to the oven for another 30 minutes or so – until the duck skin is golden and crisp and the meat is completely tender.

Meanwhile, use a sharp knife to slice the peel and pith away from the oranges. Quarter each orange and cut each quarter into small chunks, removing any pips as you go. Put the orange pieces in a fairly large bowl with any juice you can save while preparing the oranges, plus the lemon juice.

When the duck legs are done, transfer them to a warm plate to rest for a few minutes. Add half the orange pieces to the cabbage in the tray and gently toss them through. Keep the fruity veg covered in a warm place (for example, in the turned-off oven) while you prepare the duck. Using a couple of forks (and a knife if you need it), tear the duck into chunky shreds.

Take the tray from the oven, add the shredded duck and toss gently to combine with the cabbage and orange. Transfer to a warm platter or divide between warmed plates and spoon over any juices from the tray. Scatter over the rest of the orange pieces and serve. This dish doesn't cry out for a carb, but a spoonful or two of simply cooked brown rice goes well, and picks up the juices nicely.

SPICY CHICKEN LIVERS WITH LENTILS
& a herby yoghurt dressing

This is one of my favourite ways to eat chicken livers, and it works really well with lamb's or pig's liver too. It's very quick and easy. Simply cooked Puy lentils and some fresh spinach leaves, plus a herby yoghurt dressing, make a lovely meal of it.

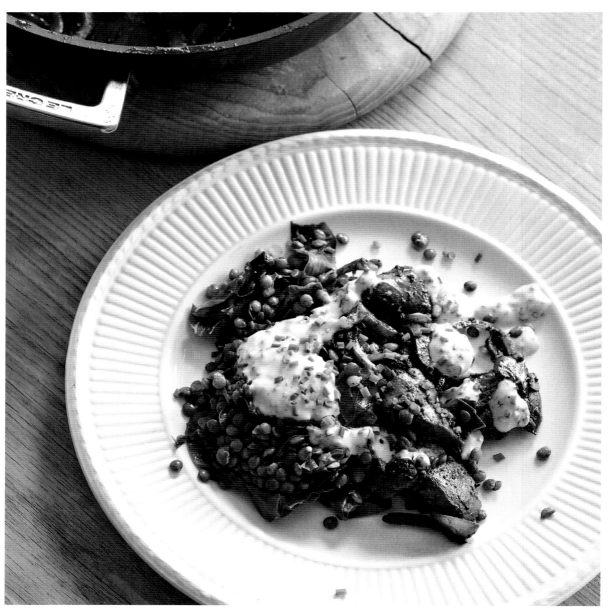

Serves 4

250g organic or free-range chicken livers (defrosted if frozen), or a 250g piece of very fresh lamb's or pig's liver

1 small red onion, very thinly sliced

1 tsp coriander seeds, lightly bashed (or use ground coriander)

1 tsp cumin seeds, lightly bashed (or use ground cumin)

A pinch of hot smoked paprika, cayenne or dried chilli flakes

1 garlic clove, thinly sliced

2 tbsp olive or vegetable oil

100g Puy lentils, soaked in cold water for 1–2 hours, if time

A good handful (50g) of whole baby spinach leaves, washed (or regular spinach, well washed, destalked and roughly chopped)

½ lemon

A small knob of butter or a dash of extra virgin olive oil

Sea salt and black pepper

For the dressing

About 150ml natural yoghurt

A small bunch of chives, parsley or mint (or a mix), chopped

A pinch of smoked paprika or cayenne

Trim the chicken livers of obvious sinews and cut any larger ones into 2 or 3 pieces. (If using lamb's or pig's liver, cut into thin slices (no more than 1cm) and then into thumb-wide strips). Put them into a large bowl with the onion, spices, garlic and 1 tbsp olive oil. Toss together, then cover and leave to marinate in a cool spot for at least 20 minutes, and up to an hour.

Drain and rinse the lentils if you've soaked them (or just rinse them if you haven't). Tip into a saucepan, cover with cold water and bring to the boil. Lower the heat a little and simmer for 12–15 minutes, until tender but still with a bit of bite. Drain thoroughly.

Rinse the pan, tip the still-warm lentils back in and return to the heat. Stir in another 1 tbsp oil and the spinach. Wilt the spinach with the lentils for 3–4 minutes, then remove from the heat. Add a good squeeze of lemon and a little salt and pepper; keep warm.

For the dressing, in a small bowl, mix the yoghurt with half of the chopped herbs and season with pepper and a pinch of smoked paprika, cayenne or chilli flakes; set aside.

Heat a large, non-stick frying pan over a high heat (no need for oil as the oil in the marinade will do the job). When it's hot, add the liver and onion mixture, spreading it out evenly. Cook for 4–5 minutes, keeping the pan really hot and turning or tossing the livers from time to time.

Check one liver in the thickest part: it should be still a bit pink inside but not raw-looking. Cook for a minute longer if necessary. Add the butter or olive oil to the pan and give the livers a final toss to bring everything together.

Divide the lentils and spinach between warm plates and add the livers and onion, along with any juices from the pan. Spoon on the yoghurt dressing, scatter over the rest of the chopped herbs and serve.

BAKED CHICKEN & VEG CURRY

This Thai-inspired aromatic trayful of chicken has oodles of sauce and plenty of veg and nuts. With two chicken pieces each, it makes a filling dinner for four without rice or bread. Or you can up the veg by 50%, accompany with brown rice and it will serve six.

Serves 4

1 tbsp coconut, olive or vegetable oil

1 chicken, jointed into 8 pieces (or 8 bone-in chicken portions, such as thighs)

2 medium or 1 large aubergine (about 400g in total), cut into chunky cubes

12 large shallots or 6 banana shallots, peeled and halved or quartered

200ml coconut milk

400ml chicken or veg stock (page 325)

A thumb-sized piece of fresh ginger, grated

4 garlic cloves, grated

1–2 medium-hot green chillies, sliced (and deseeded if you prefer less heat)

Grated zest and juice of 1 lime

2 lemongrass stems, halved lengthways

300g green beans, trimmed

About 50g cashew nuts

Sea salt and black pepper

A handful each of coriander and/or basil leaves, chopped, to finish

Preheat the oven to 200°C/Fan 180°C/Gas 6. When it is hot, add the oil to your largest roasting tray and put it into the oven for a couple of minutes to heat up. Take the tray from the oven and carefully add the chicken pieces. Use tongs to turn them over in the hot oil so they are coated, then place skin side up and season with salt and pepper. Return the tray to the oven and bake for 20 minutes.

Take out the tray and add the aubergine cubes and shallots, turning them in the chicken juices with a spoon and nestling them among the pieces of chicken. Return the tray to the oven for 20 minutes.

Meanwhile, put the coconut milk and stock into a saucepan. Add the grated ginger and garlic, chilli(es), lime zest and lemongrass stems. Bring to a simmer, stirring to blend everything together, then turn off the heat and leave to infuse for a few minutes.

Take the chicken out of the oven. Scatter the beans in between the chicken pieces and add the cashews. Pour on the fragrant, coconut liquor (the lemongrass can go in too). Return to the oven for a final 20 minutes. To check that the chicken is done, insert a probe thermometer into the thickest part of the meat – it should register at least 72°C; or cut into one piece – it should be opaque and steaming hot right down to the bone. Scatter over the chopped herbs, squeeze over the lime juice and the curry is ready.

VEG VARIATIONS
Replace the aubergines with sweet potato, cut into 2–3cm cubes, adding them at the start with the chicken. You can also swap the green beans for another green veg (such as broccoli florets), or a 400g tin of chickpeas or beans, drained and rinsed.

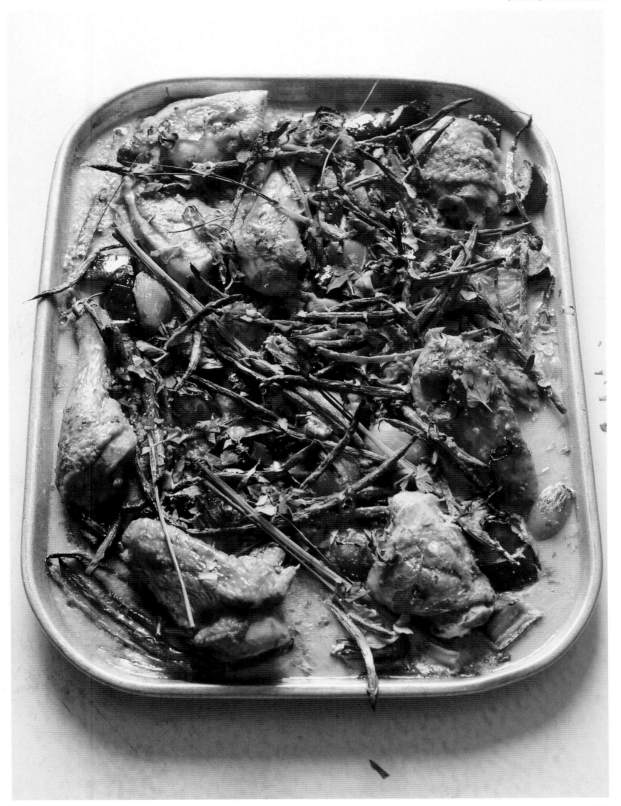

CHUNKY BEEF CHILLI

I've dialled down the meat for this big panful of warming chilli, and more than matched it with lots of veg. It tastes even better the day after it's made, so leftovers are a treat. Instead of serving it with a baked spud or white rice, I suggest a green salad. If you do serve it with brown rice (or another whole grain) the quantities will stretch to feed eight.

Serves 6–8

Olive or vegetable oil, for frying

About 200g free-range pork belly (rind on or off), cubed

800g chuck or stewing steak, cubed

150ml red wine (optional)

2 medium onions, halved and thinly sliced

4 medium carrots, halved and thickly sliced

4 garlic cloves, sliced

1 tsp dried chilli flakes

2 tsp each cumin and coriander seeds, crushed (or 1 tsp each ground)

1 tsp smoked paprika

1 star anise (optional)

½–1 fresh red chilli, sliced (optional)

A few strips of pared orange zest

3–4 sprigs of thyme (optional)

400g tin tomatoes

About 1 litre hot beef stock, or veg or chicken stock (page 325)

1 large sweet potato (300–400g), peeled and cubed (or you can use squash)

2 x 400g tins beans (cannellini, kidney or butter beans), drained and rinsed

Sea salt and black pepper

Set a large heavy frying pan over a high heat and add a dash of oil. When hot, add the pork with some salt and pepper. Cook briskly for several minutes, turning the meat from time to time, until browned all over. Transfer to a large flameproof casserole dish. Repeat the browning process with the beef, doing it in two batches so as not to crowd the pan, seasoning it as you go and adding a dash more oil to the pan if necessary.

When all the meat is browned and transferred to the casserole, reduce the heat under the pan to low and pour in the red wine (or 150ml of the hot stock). It will bubble and hiss. Stir the liquid, scraping the pan with a spatula, to release all the caramelised meaty bits from the base of the pan. Bring to a simmer and set aside.

Meanwhile, add the onions, carrots, garlic, spices, chilli if using, orange zest, a pinch of salt and a twist of pepper, plus the thyme if using, to the casserole with the browned meat. Cook over a medium heat, stirring often, for 8–10 minutes to soften the veg.

Tip the liquid from the frying pan over the meat. Add the tomatoes and hot stock; if the liquor isn't enough to cover everything, add a little more stock or boiling water. Bring to a low simmer and cook very gently for 1½ hours or until the meat is becoming tender.

Add the sweet potato and beans (with a little more hot stock or water if needed) and cook for a further 30–45 minutes. Check that all the meat and veg are nice and tender, tweak the seasoning and the chilli is ready to serve.

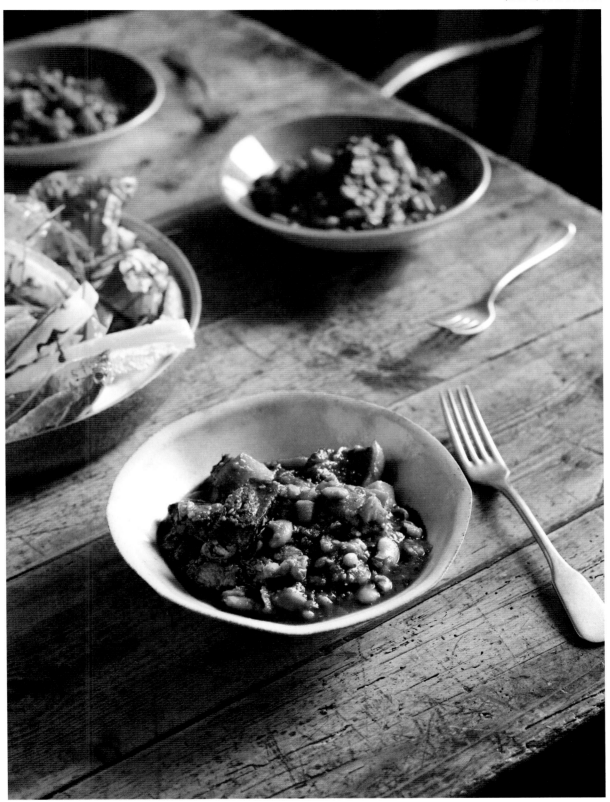

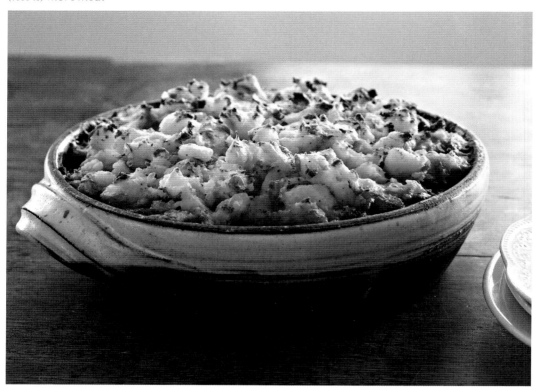

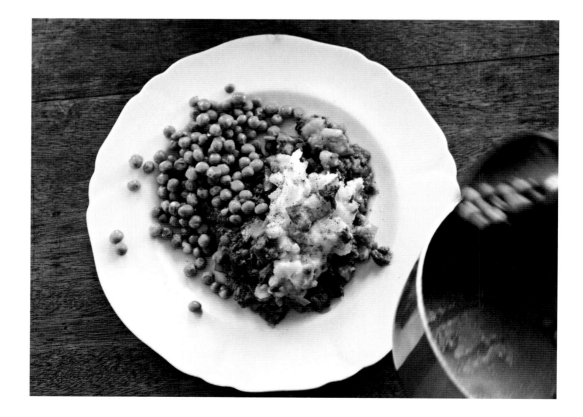

GARDENER'S PIE

This recipe takes the good old shepherd's pie and makes it much more veg-centric. The meat is still there, but it shares the limelight with lots of lovely plants...

Serves 5–6

About 4 tbsp olive or vegetable oil

300g chestnut mushrooms, roughly chopped

400g lamb or beef mince

2 large onions, chopped

3 medium carrots, chopped

1 celery stem, finely chopped

2 garlic cloves, chopped

300ml tomato passata

300ml hot veg or chicken stock (page 325) or hot water

About 800g potatoes, scrubbed but not peeled, cut into large bite-sized chunks

2 x 400g tins Puy, brown or green lentils, rinsed and drained, or 450g cooked lentils

1 rounded tbsp kimchi (page 286), roughly chopped, or a dash of Worcestershire sauce

3 tbsp extra virgin olive or rapeseed oil

Sea salt and black pepper

Heat 1 tbsp oil in a large saucepan. Add half the mushrooms and fry 'hard' until they release their juices. Keep going until these have evaporated, and the mushrooms are taking on a nice golden-brown colour (which adds flavour). Tip them into a large bowl and repeat with the second lot of mushrooms, adding a touch more oil.

Add a trickle more oil to the pan then add the mince and cook, again over a reasonably high heat, until any moisture it releases has evaporated and it is also getting some good brown colour (you may need to do this in two batches). Add to the mushrooms.

Heat another 1 tbsp oil in the pan and add the onions, carrots, celery and garlic. Sweat over a medium-low heat, stirring often, for 10 minutes, or until softening. Return the mushrooms, mince and any juices to the pan. Add the passata and stock or water. Bring to a simmer, lower the heat and simmer for 25–30 minutes, until the carrots are tender.

Meanwhile, preheat the oven to 190°C/Fan 170°C/Gas 5. Put the potatoes into a large pan, cover with water and bring to the boil, then simmer, covered, for about 15 minutes until completely tender. Drain and leave to steam in a colander for a few minutes.

Stir the lentils and chopped kimchi or Worcestershire sauce into the mushroom and mince mix. Taste and adjust the seasonings if needed, then transfer to an oven dish.

Tip the cooked potatoes back into their hot pan. Trickle in the oil and add a little salt and pepper, then use a potato masher to crush them into a rough mash. Spoon this on top of the mince and mushroom mix in the dish. Put the pie into the oven and bake for 15–20 minutes until the topping is golden brown. Alternatively, leave the pie to cool completely and refrigerate or freeze, to be cooked and served later on. Serve the pie with peas or petits pois, or a heap of wilted spinach or kale.

ROOTS, BANGERS & BEANS

Tasty and well-seasoned, a good sausage can go a long way. In this hearty winter stew, a few bangers partner up with lots of lovely root veg and some creamy white beans to create a filling, one-pot dinner that needs no accompaniment.

Serves 4

2 tbsp olive or vegetable oil

6 free-range 'butcher's banger' pork sausages, each cut into 4 pieces

A splash of dry cider or white wine (optional)

2 onions, chopped

2 medium carrots, quartered lengthways and thickly sliced

2 celery stems, chopped

½ head of celeriac or 2 medium parsnips, peeled and cut into chunky cubes

2 medium potatoes (about 250g in total), scrubbed or peeled and cut into chunky cubes

400g tin beans, such as cannellini or kidney, drained and rinsed

About 500ml hot veg or chicken stock (page 325) or hot water

Sea salt and black pepper

Chopped parsley, to finish (optional)

Heat 1 tbsp oil in a flameproof casserole or large saucepan. Add the chunks of sausage and cook over a medium heat, turning often, until they are well browned all over. Add the cider or wine (or just a splash of hot water from the kettle) and cook for a minute or two, stirring and scraping up any nice bits of browned sausage meat from the base of the pan. Transfer the sausages and the pan juices to a dish and set aside for a minute.

Heat another 1 tbsp oil in the casserole or pan. Add the onions, carrots and celery and cook for 10 minutes or so, until softened.

Return the sausages to the casserole with their juices and add the celeriac or parsnips, potatoes and beans. Add a pinch of salt and a grinding of black pepper and pour in enough stock or water to almost cover everything. Bring to a very gentle simmer. Cook, uncovered or partially covered, very gently over a low heat for about 40 minutes, until everything is tender. (Or cook with the lid on in the oven at 140°C/Fan 120°C/Gas 1.)

The potato should have broken down a little and thickened the sauce. If not, mash some of the veg and beans against the side of the dish with a fork and stir in. Check and adjust the seasonings if needed. Scatter over some chopped parsley if you like, and serve.

SUMMER VARIATION
After returning the sausages to the pan, add 4–5 thickly sliced new potatoes, the white beans and stock and simmer for 15 minutes. Add a couple of good handfuls of fresh peas, broad beans or green beans (or any combo) and 2 shredded little gem lettuces. Cook for a few minutes more, until all the veg are tender. Serve topped with a dollop of pesto or pestomega (page 278).

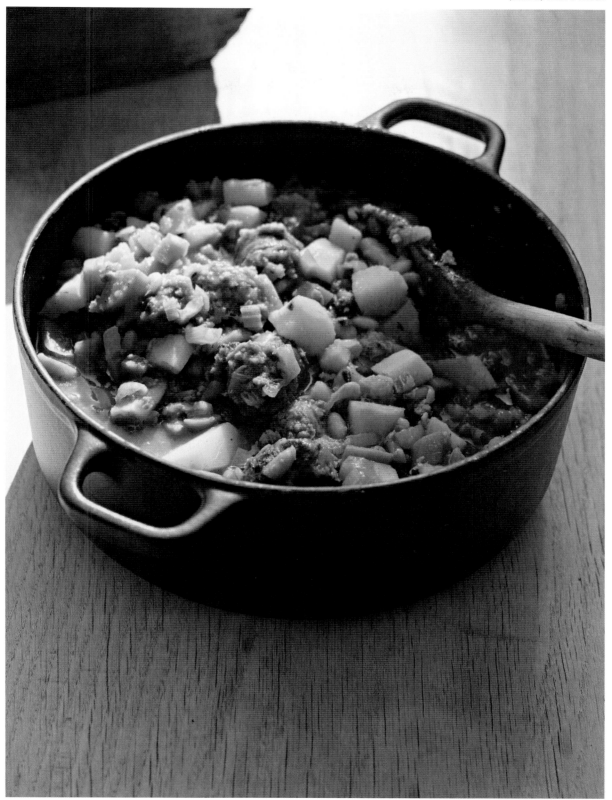

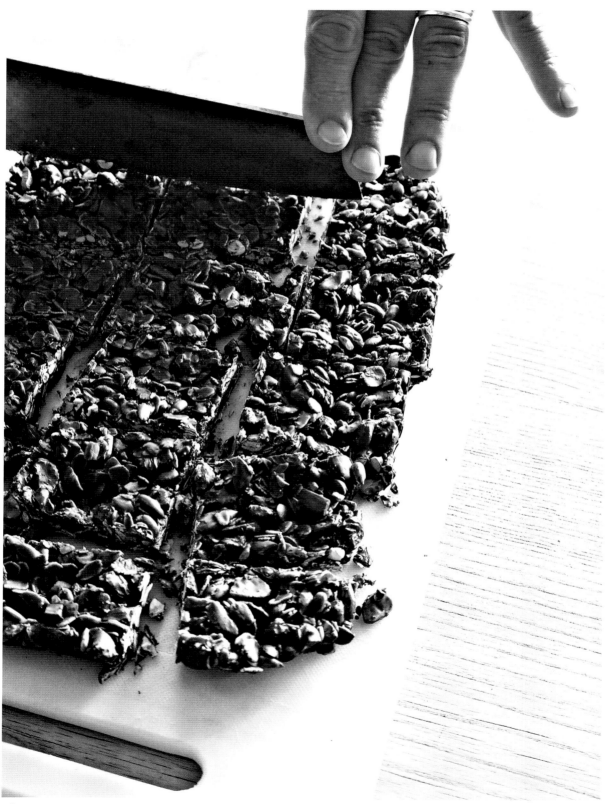

TREATS AND DRINKS

You may be familiar with the concept of the 'dessert tummy' – that extra bit of space we often seem to be able to find for something sweet at the end of a meal, even though we've just told ourselves we are full to bursting. And, as it turns out, this is not just an excuse to indulge. This is real physiological phenomenon. As my friend Dr Giles Yeo of Cambridge University explained to me (see page 31), the ancient, animal part of our brain is programmed to stock up with as much energy as possible, in case it's a long time before we eat again. So, even when our bellies don't have much room left, our brain tells us we still shouldn't miss an opportunity to squeeze in the most calorie-dense food we can. If something fatty, or sugary, or bliss-pointedly both (see page 100) is wafted in front of us, even when we are full, it's very likely to get a green light from our brain. It's an efficient evolutionary characteristic, but not very helpful these days.

For me the takeaway here is that no one should feel ashamed about having a sweet tooth – it's only natural. And although skipping puds and cutting back on sweet treats between meals is clearly a good idea, it isn't always easy or, in absolute terms, realistic. And I think, when it comes to food, 'never' is not a very helpful or healthy word.

The best way to satisfy these natural inclinations, however, is not to head for the sugar-laden, fat-heavy, highly-processed biscuits and chocolate bars we are so familiar with. As I've explained on page 100, those foods will mess with your mind as well as your body. Instead, it's entirely possible, and sensible, to take a much 'wholer' approach to making and baking treats and puds, which puts you in control of the ingredients.

Central to this endeavour are naturally sweet dried fruits and nuts (both whole and ground), and flours made with whole grains. They are the staples of the recipes that follow. You'll find that sugar and honey do appear in moderation – much reduced from conventional recipes. Yet I'm confident you won't feel in the least deprived: everything here is an unambiguous treat.

As you consciously go to work on reducing the sugar needed to keep that sweet tooth happy (as suggested on pages 104–5), these recipes can be particularly helpful. I'm not suggesting you tuck into them every day – it's best not to make a same time, same place habit of any sweet treats (see page 106). So just enjoy them occasionally. And as you build confidence and get more pleasure from less sweetness, you may want to reduce the sugar/honey quantities even further.

To round off this run of virtuous treats, I've addressed the drinks dilemma with some lovely alcohol-free tipples, to enjoy after a long day.

SEEDY ALMOND CAKE

To create this recipe, I started with a basic Victoria sponge and swapped out the white flour for a blend of wholemeal and ground almonds, reduced the sugar substantially and added extra nuts and seeds. The result is delicious – and you really do not miss all that sugar. I love to eat the cake still just warm from the oven, but it keeps well too. It's great with a cup of tea or, for a high-fibre, probiotic pud, enjoy it with a spoonful of kefir (page 246) or natural yoghurt, and a little heap of fresh berries or roasted fruit compote (pages 224–5). The poppy seeds aren't essential, but I love them for their look and their texture and, like any seed, they are rich in minerals.

Makes 8 slices

125g unsalted butter, softened

70g soft light brown sugar or light muscovado

Finely grated zest of 1 orange or lemon (optional)

100g wholemeal cake flour/fine plain wholemeal flour

2 tsp baking powder

100g ground almonds

25g sunflower seeds

25g poppy seeds (optional)

3 medium eggs

3 tbsp milk or water

About 20g flaked almonds or pumpkin seeds (or a mix)

Preheat the oven to 180°C/Fan 160°C/Gas 4. Line a 20cm round springform cake tin with baking paper.

Put the butter and sugar, and the orange or lemon zest if using, into a large bowl or a free-standing electric mixer. Use an electric hand whisk or the mixer to beat for a couple of minutes, until light and fluffy.

In a second bowl, thoroughly combine the flour, baking powder, ground almonds, sunflower seeds and poppy seeds, if using.

Add an egg and a spoonful of the dry ingredients to the butter and sugar mix and beat until evenly blended. Repeat to incorporate the remaining eggs. Tip in the remaining dry ingredients and fold together gently but thoroughly, finishing by folding in the milk or water to loosen the batter a little.

Spoon the mixture into the prepared tin and spread it gently and evenly. Scatter with the flaked almonds and/or pumpkin seeds. Bake in the oven for 35 minutes, or until risen and golden, and a skewer inserted into the centre comes out clean. Leave to cool, at least a little, on a wire rack.

Remove the cake from the tin and cut into slices to serve. It will keep in an airtight tin for up to 5 days, but you'll most likely finish it well before then.

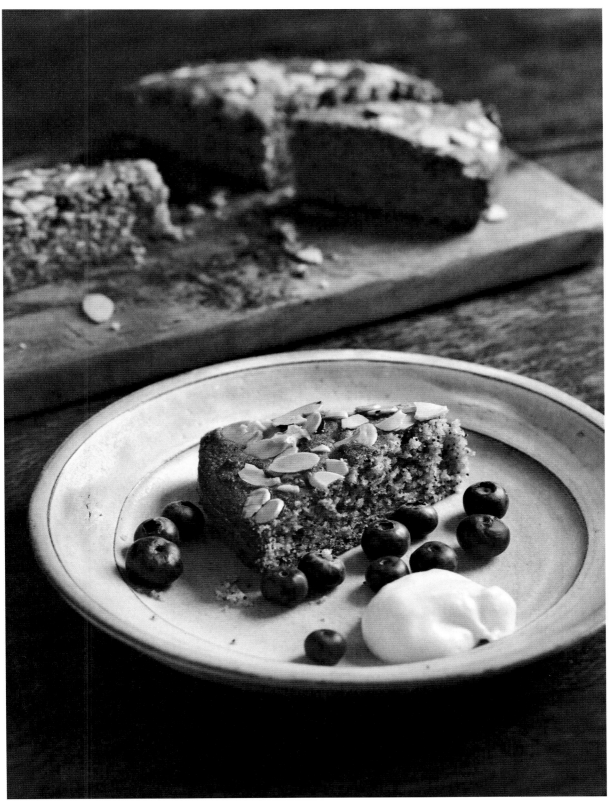

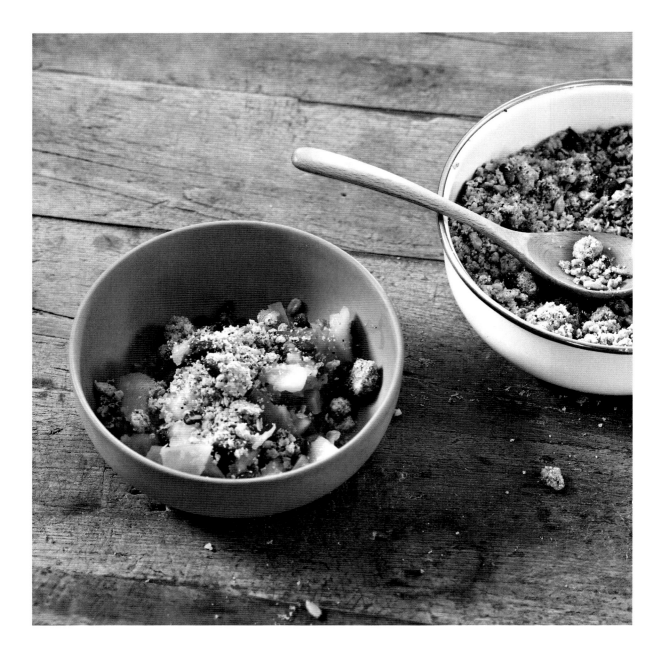

OATY SEEDY APPLE CRUMBLE

This uses sweet eating apples and raisins, so there's no need for added sugar, and the topping – made with whole grains, nuts and seeds – is baked separately. It's a treaty but healthy pud that you can repeat through the year with seasonal fruits. The crumble quantities are doubled here, to give you enough for a second outing. It keeps well.

Serves 4

4 large eating apples, cored and roughly chopped (no need to peel)

4 tbsp (about 60g) raisins or sultanas

Finely grated zest of 1 lemon, plus a good squeeze of the juice

Finely grated zest and juice of 1 large or 2 small oranges (about 100ml juice)

For the 'independent crumble'

50g fine plain wholemeal flour

50g ground almonds

50g porridge oats

50g mixed seeds, such as poppy, flax, sunflower and pumpkin

30g light muscovado or soft brown sugar

A pinch of salt (optional)

75g butter, chilled, or 75ml vegetable oil

Start with the independent crumble. Preheat the oven to 180°C/Fan 160°C/Gas 4. Put the flour, ground almonds, oats, seeds, sugar, and salt if using, into a large bowl and mix thoroughly. Use a coarse grater to grate the butter directly into the bowl – or chop into small pieces if that's easier. If using oil, trickle it in while stirring the dry mix. Now get your hands in there and squeeze and rub all the ingredients together. Don't worry about being light and delicate, the idea is to create a clumpy, nuggety mixture, with few or no dry crumbs left.

Transfer the clumpy mixture to a baking tray (with a rim) and spread it out evenly. Bake for 15–20 minutes until golden brown, removing once halfway through to stir well. Leave to cool completely.

For the apple compote, put the apples, raisins or sultanas, citrus zest and juice into a pan. Bring to a simmer and simmer gently for about 5 minutes, stirring occasionally and using the spoon to help crush the apple and break it down a bit (but not to a purée).

Serve the apple warm, each portion sprinkled with a couple of tablespoonfuls of the independent crumble. The remaining crumble (approximately half) can be stored in an airtight container in a cool place for up to 2 weeks.

FRUITY VARIATIONS

Scatter the crumble over a mix of lightly crushed raspberries, sliced strawberries and a few blueberries tossed with lemon juice and a trickle of honey. Or serve the crumble on top of any fruit compote – try the roasted plum or rhubarb on pages 224–5. Swirl the fruit with yoghurt for a 'fumble'.

RYE & BANANA COOKIES

These soft, cakey cookies are based on a recipe from my friend Rachel de Thample, who creates amazing gut-healthy ferments and whole food goodies. I love these particular treats, not only because they are delicious, satisfying, easy and full of good things, but because they are a brilliant way to use over-ripe bananas, as well as any end-of-the-packet bits and bobs from my nut, seed and dried fruit stash. The cookies also freeze well and can be popped into lunchboxes straight from the freezer.

<u>Makes 15 or 24 'bite-sized' cookies</u>

125g dark rye flour

150g porridge oats

½ tsp baking powder

1 tsp ground mixed spice

75g brown sugar

2 tsp ground flaxseed

120g raisins or chopped dried apricots

100g roughly chopped nuts or mixed seeds

2 ripe medium bananas, mashed

100g extra virgin olive oil, or coconut oil (melted)

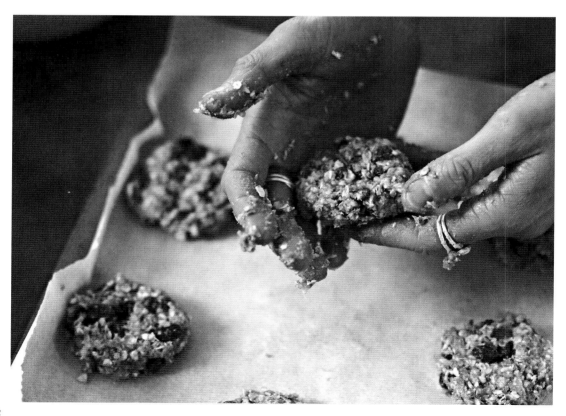

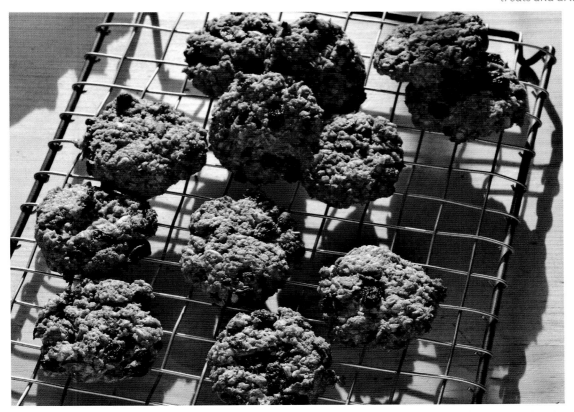

Preheat the oven to 180°C/Fan 160°C/Gas 4. Line 2 baking sheets with baking paper.

Put the flour, oats, baking powder, spice, sugar and ground flaxseed into a large bowl and mix thoroughly. Add the dried fruit and nuts or seeds and mix well again, separating any of the fruit if it's sticking together. Add the mashed bananas and the oil and mix again, really well.

Put tablespoonfuls of the mixture (dessertspoonfuls for bite-sized cookies) onto the prepared baking sheets, shaping them roughly into thick, round cookies. Bake for 12–15 minutes, until golden and starting to brown on the bases.

Leave to cool a little and then transfer to a rack to cool completely. Store in an airtight tin for up to 5 days, or for a few months in the freezer.

VARIATIONS

This flexible recipe is a great way to clear out the storecupboard! You can replace all or some of the rye flour with plain wholewheat flour or wholegrain spelt flour. The oats can be regular or jumbo, or you can use medium oatmeal. Any seeds or chopped nuts work well, and likewise any dried fruit. And if you fancy a touch of luxury, add chopped dark chocolate, or cacao nibs to the mix.

OATY NUTTY CHOCOLATE 'TIFFIN'

A virtuous way to enjoy chocolate (or a chocolate-y way to enjoy virtue).

<u>Makes 15–18</u>

75g jumbo oats

50g skinned whole almonds, roughly bashed or chopped

50g pumpkin seeds

25g sunflower seeds

150g dark chocolate (at least 70% cocoa solids), broken into chunks

50g coconut oil

100g raisins or chopped dried apricots

2 (half-thumb-sized) pieces of preserved ginger, excess syrup drained off, finely chopped

Preheat the oven to 200°C/Fan 180°C/Gas 6. Line a baking tin or dish, about 20 x 15cm, with baking paper or foil.

Spread the oats, almonds and seeds on a large baking sheet and toast in the oven for about 8 minutes, checking often, until the oats are crispy and the nuts are lightly browned. Tip onto a plate and leave to cool a little.

Put the chocolate chunks and coconut oil into a bowl over a pan of simmering water, or in a small saucepan over a very low heat, to melt very gently. Just before the chocolate is fully melted, remove from the heat and stir in the toasted oats, nuts and seeds (it's okay if they're still a bit warm, but they shouldn't be oven-hot). Add the raisins or chopped apricots and the ginger.

Spread the mixture evenly in the prepared tin and leave to set in the fridge. Cut into squares when completely cold.

TRAIL MIX VARIATION

The lovely tiffin squares are quite 'melty' on a warm day. For a more portable version, omit the coconut oil and ginger. Once the toasted oats, nuts and seeds are cold, mix them with 100g each chopped chocolate and raisins. You can carry a tablespoonful or two in a small snack box or tiffin tin.

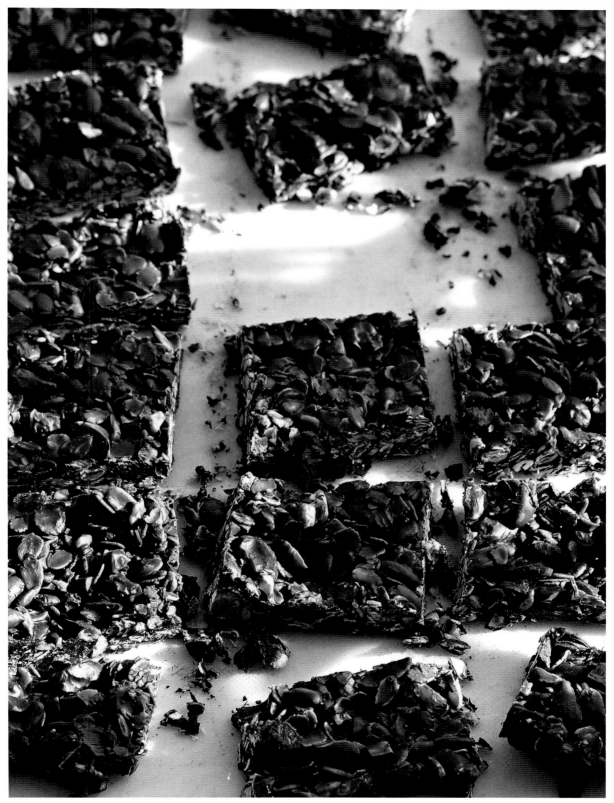

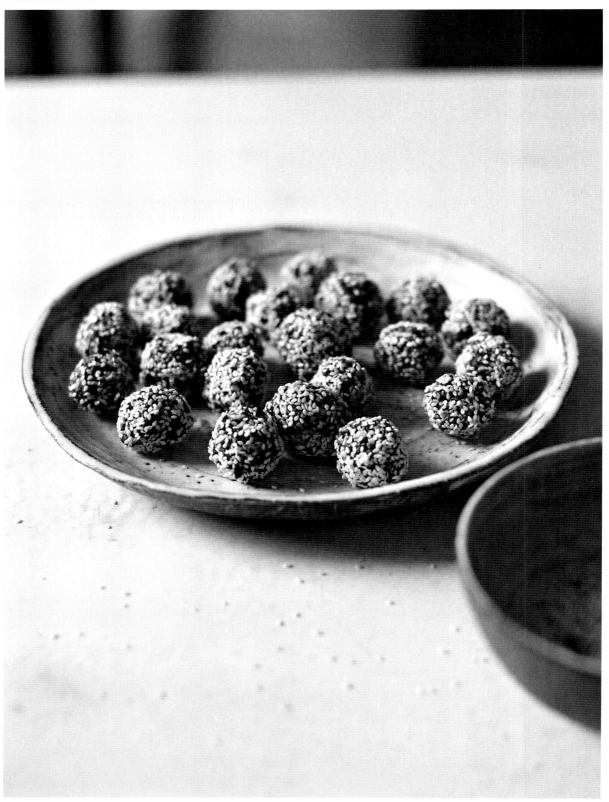

SEEDY, NUTTY, DATE & LIME BITES

These tempting little treats are sweet and sticky, but also fresh and zesty with lime. With a satisfying, slightly chunky texture from the raw almonds and seeds, they make a perfect, pick-me-up snack.

Makes 20

250g pitted dates

50g pumpkin seeds

50g skinned whole almonds

Finely grated zest and juice of 1 lime

1 tbsp cocoa powder or cacao powder

About 50g sesame seeds

Put all the ingredients except the sesame seeds into a food processor and blitz to a chunky, sticky paste. You will need to stop and scrape down the sides a few times to help everything get well amalgamated – but don't worry if there are some chunky bits of seed and nut remaining. It's all to the good.

Tip the sesame seeds onto a plate. Take heaped teaspoonfuls of the date mix and roll them into balls between your hands, then roll each one in sesame seeds to coat. Store in the fridge, or a cool place, and eat within a week.

NUTTY VARIATIONS

You can use walnuts or cashews instead of almonds.

COCOA-COATED BITES

You can roll the bites in extra cocoa powder instead of sesame seeds for a smooth finish if you prefer.

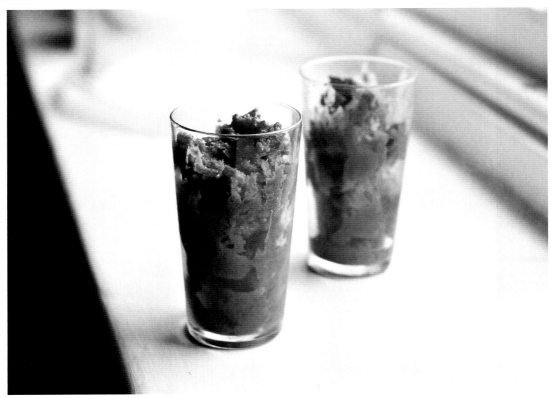

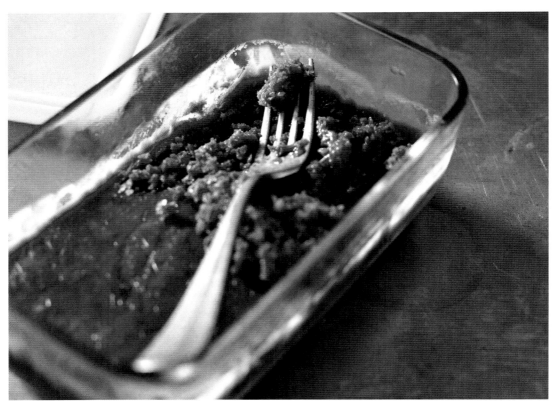

FRUITY GRANITAS (& LOLLIES)

Deliciously tangy and refreshing, a granita is a lovely way to enjoy an ice-cold treat of tart fruit with very little added sugar. My versions are essentially frozen compotes of cooked whole fruits, very lightly sweetened and frozen, then scratched up into fruity, icy shards when semi-defrosted. Or they can be frozen into lickable lollies. The vanilla and orange are optional, but both help to enhance the sweetness, so you can get away with less added sugar. The idea is to keep the 'added' sweetness to below 15% of the weight of fruit (typical recipes for ices have up to 50%). Honey, although it is a form of sugar (see page 98), somehow seems to deliver more sweetness to these chilly confections, spoon for spoon, than sugar. Of course, for the fruit, the riper and sweeter the better.

Serves 4

500g plums, gooseberries, blackcurrants, or rhubarb

2 tbsp water or the juice of 1 orange

¼ vanilla pod, split open, or ½ tsp vanilla extract (optional)

40–80g (2–4 tbsp) honey or soft brown sugar

Prepare the fruit: halve the plums and remove the stones (or do so after cooking). Cut rhubarb into 3–4cm lengths. Leave currants and berries whole, but remove any stalks.

Put the fruit into a saucepan with the water or orange juice, vanilla and 2 tbsp honey or sugar. Slowly bring to a simmer, stirring as the juices start to run, then simmer for a few minutes, until the fruit is collapsed, soft and juicy. Remove the vanilla pod, if used. Leave to cool for at least 15 minutes. (Remove plum stones if you haven't already.)

Purée the fruit using a stick blender or a jug blender. (You can do this when the fruit is still warm.) Taste for sweetness, and add a bit more honey or sugar only if you think it really needs it, stirring or blitzing again to dissolve it. Leave the purée to cool completely.

For a granita, freeze the mixture in a shallow tub or freezerproof dish until solid (at least 2 hours). Take out of the freezer 30–60 minutes before serving, scratch into shards with a fork then spoon into glasses. Alternatively, freeze the mixture in reusable lolly moulds.

FRUIT VARIATIONS

You don't need to cook fruit compotes for these granitas. You can make them (or the lollies) with crushed ripe, fresh berries, such as raspberries, strawberries, blackberries and blueberries, or a mixture. Blitz in the blender, adding as little honey or sugar as you can get away with, a dash of vanilla if you have it, and a tiny splash of cold water, if needed, to help them blend. Freeze and serve as above.

YOGHURT VARIATION

To give your granita (or lollies) a slightly creamier texture, stir about 250ml natural yoghurt into the cooled fruit purée before freezing.

Dry drinks

These are my favourite 'dry' drinks – i.e. non-alcoholic but nonetheless rather grown-up beverages. They are perfect for getting you past the 7 o'clock itch on alcohol-free days and very useful for weaning you off those SSBs too.

KOMBUCHA SUNRISE

I improvised this drink recently when we had somehow accumulated a slight glut of oranges, and everybody loved it. The berries not only add a burst of extra fruitiness, they give the classic 'sunset' effect as the drink blends from red to orange in the top of the glass.

Per person

About 100ml chilled freshly squeezed orange juice (about 1 large or 2 small oranges)

A few fine gratings of fresh ginger, or a pinch of ground ginger (optional, but adds a nice little kick)

A few ice cubes

200ml cold kombucha (page 244)

A small handful of strawberries or raspberries, crushed to a rough purée

A slice of orange, to finish (optional)

Pour the orange juice into a tall tumbler and stir in the ginger, if using. Add a couple of ice cubes and pour over the kombucha. Finally, spoon over the crushed berries. Stir the top of the drink (with a reusable metal straw) to mix in the berries a bit, but not right into the drink. You're after that sunset! Serve with a slice of orange, if you like.

APPLE AND BLACKBERRY 'MOONRISE' VARIATION
Use a good cloudy apple juice instead of the orange juice, or better still, blitz a cored and roughly chopped tart eating apple with about 100ml cold water. Use crushed ripe blackberries (ideally freshly picked) instead of the strawberries/raspberries. Proceed as above.

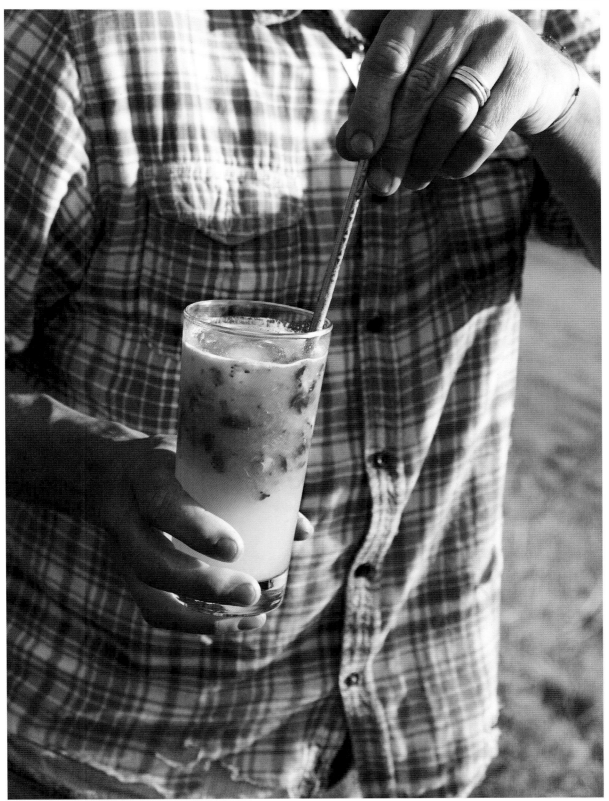

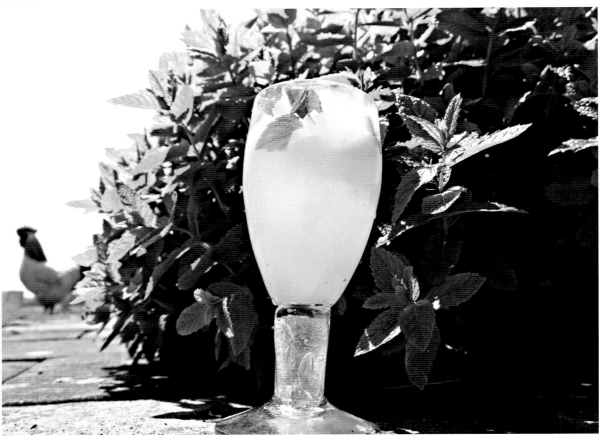

NO-JITO

A really refreshing glassful, made nicely tart by the cider vinegar (or citrus juice), which means you won't glug it too fast.

<u>Per person</u>

8–12 mint and/or lemon verbena leaves, plus an optional extra sprig to serve

25ml raw cider vinegar or lemon or lime juice, or 50ml orange juice

A few ice cubes

150ml chilled cloudy apple juice

Sparkling water, plain tap water or kombucha (page 244)

Bash or twist the herb leaves, or roughly chop them, and put into a tall glass. Add the cider vinegar and, if you can, leave to macerate for 10–20 minutes, though this isn't essential. Add the ice cubes and mix, then add the apple juice and mix some more. Finish with a splash of water or kombucha and a whole bruised sprig of mint or lemon verbena if you like.

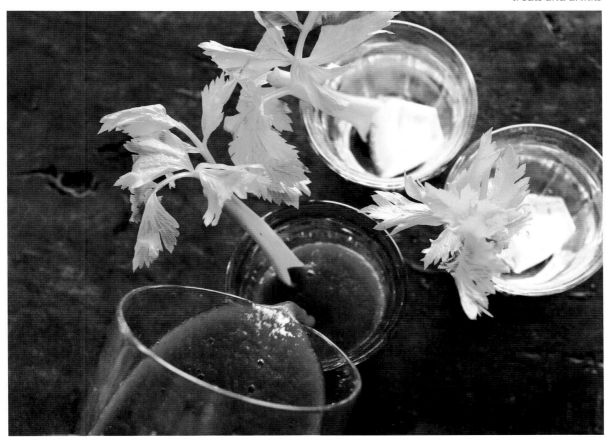

KIMCHI MARY

This is a brilliant version of a 'virgin' Mary cocktail, with the kimchi flavours giving a really complex aromatic dimension to the tomato juice.

Per person

200ml chilled tomato juice

2 generous tsp live kimchi (ideally homemade, page 286)

A good squeeze of lemon juice

½ large or 1 small celery stem, plus an optional extra stem to serve

Put all the ingredients into a blender and whiz for 40 seconds or so, until well blitzed. If you've got a punchy enough blender you won't need to strain it, but if there's a lot of celery fibres you might want to. Serve over ice, with a celery stem in each glass if you like.

INDEX

SOURCES

Katz, D L, Meller, S. Can we say what diet is best for health? www.annualreviews.org/doi/citedby/10.1146/annurev-publhealth-032013-182351 [page 16]

Jacka, F N, O'Neil, A, Opie, R *et al*. A randomised controlled trial of dietary improvement for adults with major depression (the 'SMILES' trial). *BMC Med* 15, 23 (2017). [page 18]

www.thelancet.com/journals/lancet/article/PIIS0140-6736(19)30500-8/fulltext. Global Burden of Disease study [page 18]

Coulthard H, Sealy A. Play with your food! Sensory play is associated with tasting of fruits and vegetables in preschool children. *Appetite*. 2017; Vol 113 pp.84–90. [page 25]

O'Keefe S, Li J, Lahti L *et al*. Fat, fibre and cancer risk in African Americans and rural Africans. *Nature Communications*, Art 6342 (2015). [page 26]

Cost of Constipation Report, Second Edition 2019, Bowel Interest Group/NHS. [page 28]

Kim S, de Souza R *et al*. Effects of dietary pulse consumption on body weight: a systematic review and meta-analysis of randomized controlled trials. *American Journal of Clinical Nutrition* (2016). [page 36]

EAT-Lancet Commission on Healthy Diets from Sustainable Food Systems, 2019. [page 44]

Clark M and Springman M. Multiple health and environmental impacts of foods, *PNAS* (2019); 116 (46) 23357–23362. [page 44]

Ann Gibbons www.nationalgeographic.com/foodfeatures/evolution-of-diet [page 56]

Eaton J, Iannotti L. Genome-nutrition Divergence: Evolving Understanding of the Malnutrition Spectrum. *Nutrition Reviews*, Issue 11 2017 pp934–950. [page 56]

Yang B, Wei J, Ju P, Chen J. Effects of regulating intestinal microbiota on anxiety symptoms: A systematic review. *General Psychiatry* (2019). [page 78]

Gardner C *et al*. Effect of Low-Fat v Low-Carbohydrate Diet on 12-Month Weight Loss in Overweight Adults and the Association with Genotype Pattern or Insulin Secretion. *JAMA* (2018); 319 (7): 667–679. [page 96]

www.hsph/Harvard.edu/news [page 97]

www.gov.uk/government/publications/saturated-fats-and-health-sacn-report [page 117]

de Souza R *et al*. Intake of saturated and trans unsaturated fatty acids and risk of all cause mortality, cardiovascular disease, and type 2 diabetes: systematic review and meta-analysis of observational studies. *BMJ* (2015); 351:h3978. [page 119]

www.gov.uk/government/collections/national-diet-and-nutrition-survey [page 120]

Estruch R *et al*. Primary Prevention of Cardiovascular Disease with a Mediterranean Diet. *New England Journal of Medicine* (2013); 368:1279–1290. [page 124]

www.imperial.ac.uk/news/176711/sugar-free-diet-drinks-better-healthy-weight [page 140]

www.ias.org.uk/Alcohol-knowledge-centre/Consumption.aspx [page 148]

Portion Distortion: How much are we really eating? British Heart Foundation report 2013, www.bhf.org.uk. [Page 172]

www.independent.co.uk/life-style/health-and-families/exercise-endorphin-high-time-how-long-motivation-study-10-minutes-wiggle-a8325661.html [page 201]

www.bsg.ox.ac.uk/news/wake-call-over-sleep-and-public-health-needed [page 204]

ACKNOWLEDGEMENTS

I have made *Eat Better Forever* with a fantastic team, many of whom I have now known and worked with for a decade or more. This book has presented a new set of challenges and my brilliant collaborators have risen to meet them all with exceptional energy and clear thinking (although for them, it isn't really exceptional – it's what they do). I owe them all a huge debt of thanks.

My key co-conspirator Nikki Duffy has been even more of a linchpin than usual. Her passion for the subject of this book (the power of good food to do us good), inspiring recipe ideas, exhaustive research and dogged flexibility (a concept which she has proved is not as oxymoronic as it sounds) have reached new heights – and throughout a very long period of inception, creation and production.

Gill Meller, with whom I've had the pleasure of working for almost two decades now, continues to craft and hone our recipes with his usual unflappable elan. I could wish for no finer fellow traveller on the path to making the good stuff even more delicious.

The wonderful photography of Simon Wheeler captures those recipes and the array of whole foods used to create them. It's been almost 20 years since we shot the *River Cottage Cookbook* together and his company and friendship, as much as his remarkable talent, have made every shoot day special.

At Bloomsbury, my new editor Rowan Yapp has taken over the reins of this careering culinary caravan with impressive calmness and control, brilliantly assisted by Kitty Stogdon. Thanks also to Ellen Williams (I think this is number 5!), Donough Shanahan, Maud Davies, Laura Brodie and Benjamin McConnell. And to Natalie Bellos and Lisa Pendreigh, who nurtured this book in its early stages.

Our project editor Janet Illsley has not only kept us all on task throughout a very intense production period but helped me to resolve many tricky editorial issues as we pulled the book together. And Sally Somers has once again given the book a thorough read and dotted my 'eyes' and crossed my 'teas'.

Lawrence Morton has brought his precise yet playful eye to our most difficult design conundrums yet. More than ever, this book looks and feels as good as it does because Lawrence is so great at what he does.

This book also stands on the shoulders of some giants of sensible food science and right-thing research into diet and health. They include Jacob Eaton, Giulia Enders, Professor Gary Frost, Professor Christopher Gardner, Dr Ifigenia Giannopoulou, Ann Gibbons, Professor Glenn Gibson, Professor Jason Gill, Professor Colin Greaves, Professor Martin Grootveld, Dr Kawther Hashem, Professor Corinna Hawkes, Professor Tony Howell, Professor Frank Hu, Dr Lora Iannotti, Professor Felice Jacka,

Professor Susan Jebb, Dr David Katz, Professor Russell Keast, Professor Clark Spencer Larsen, Professor Mark Mattson, Stephanie Meller, Dr Carlos Monteiro, Professor Kevin Morgan, Dr Michael Mosley, Professor Tim Spector, Mimi Spencer, Sasha Stephens, Professor Janice Thompson, Professor Anna Whittaker, Bee Wilson and Dr Giles Yeo.

And Dr Michelle Harvie has been a crucial part of team EBF from the outset, tirelessly reading copy, holding me to account rigorously on the science and the evidence, and helping me clarify my thinking on what sustainable healthy eating and weight loss really is, and how we can help as many people as possible to take it into their lives.

Sarah Turner has once again road-tested many of the recipes for me – her feedback is spot on, as ever. Hope Pointing and Alice Meller have assisted brilliantly on our photo shoots. Rachel de Thample has been a huge help with fermentation advice and recipe suggestions, and Naomi Devlin has generously shared her knowledge. And thank you to Patricia Smith and Katie Kelly, who tested the food variety audit.

Adam Croft, Helen Musgrave and Hannah Wright in the River Cottage garden, Harry Boglione at Haye Farm, Ash and Kate at Trill Farm, plus Millers Farm Shop, Colyton Stores, Ganesha and Washingpool, have all provided fantastic seasonal veg and whole foods. The Lyme Bay Fish Shack and Newlyn Fish Co. supplied super fresh fish.

The whole River Cottage team has helped us to make this book happen, even if they don't know it. Gelf Alderson continues to lead and inspire the kitchen team, and I've been subliminally absorbing his recipe ideas for years! Guy Baring has been a rock of support, personally and professionally, especially during the time I've been writing this book. And Stewart Dodd is a superb partner and leader for all our ideas and enterprises.

My brilliant Keo films colleagues on *Britain's Fat Fight* and *Easy Ways to Live Well* helped shape this book too, among them Alice Henley, Jackie Houdret, Helen Simpson, Callum Webster, Nick Angel, Will Anderson, Kari Lia and Andrew Palmer. Jo Murphy provided superb research (and emojis). And my fab co-presenters Steph McGovern and Dr Zoe Williams bravely lent their brains and bodies to the science of healthier living.

Antony Topping, ostensibly my agent, continues to be a collaborator, adviser and sounding-board without whom... let's not even go there.

And all of the above owe a huge debt of thanks (though nowhere near as big as mine) to the person who brings it all together, every day, Jess Upton. While I am dreaming of new plates, she is spinning others I can't even see.

Finally, none of this works without my family: Mum, Dad and Soph who have provided and shared the whole and the home-grown since year dot; Chloe, Oscar, Freddie and Louisa who give me love and support and life lessons, and are now cooking right back at me; and Marie, whom I love so much, and who grows and nurtures everything, and all of us, every day.

BLOOMSBURY PUBLISHING

Bloomsbury Publishing Plc

50 Bedford Square, London, WC1B 3DP, UK

29 Earlsfort Terrace, Dublin 2, Ireland

BLOOMSBURY, BLOOMSBURY PUBLISHING and the Diana logo are trademarks of Bloomsbury Publishing Plc

First published in Great Britain 2020

Text © Hugh Fearnley-Whittingstall, 2020
Photographs © Simon Wheeler, 2020
Except those on pages 27, 33, 42, 67 and 111 © Hugh Fearnley-Derome; page 190 © Marie Derome;
pages 24 and 64–5 © Freddie Fearnley-Derome

Illustrations © Andy Smith, 2020

Hugh Fearnley-Whittingstall, Simon Wheeler and Andy Smith have asserted their right under the Copyright, Designs and Patents Act, 1988, to be identified as author, photographer and illustrator, respectively, of this work.

For legal purposes the Acknowledgements on p.414 constitute an extension of this copyright page.

All rights reserved. No part of this publication may be reproduced or transmitted in any form or by any means, electronic or mechanical, including photocopying, recording, or any information storage or retrieval system, without prior permission in writing from the publishers.

The information contained in this book is provided by way of general guidance in relation to the specific subject matters addressed herein, but it is not a substitute for specialist dietary advice. It should not be relied on for medical, healthcare, pharmaceutical or other professional advice on specific dietary or health needs. This book is sold with the understanding that the author and publisher are not engaged in rendering medical, health or any other kind of personal or professional services. The reader should consult a competent health or medical professional before adopting any of the suggestions in this book or drawing inferences from it.

If you are on medication of any description, please consult your doctor or health professional before embarking on any fast or diet.

A catalogue record for this book is available from the British Library

Library of Congress Cataloguing-in-Publication data has been applied for

ISBN: HB: 978-1-5266-0280-0 ; eBook: 978-1-5266-0279-4

10 9 8 7 6 5 4

Project Editor: Janet Illsley
Designer: Lawrence Morton
Photographer: Simon Wheeler
Food Stylist: Gill Meller
Prop Stylist: Cynthia Inions
Illustrator: Andy Smith
Indexer: Hilary Bird

Printed and bound in Germany by Mohn Media.

[Insert FSC logo here]

To find out more about our authors and books visit www.bloomsbury.com and sign up for our newsletters.